Food and Health: Nutrition Science and Technology

Food and Health: Nutrition Science and Technology

Edited by Logan Bowman

SYRAWOOD
PUBLISHING HOUSE
New York

Published by Syrawood Publishing House,
750 Third Avenue, 9th Floor,
New York, NY 10017, USA
www.syrawoodpublishinghouse.com

Food and Health: Nutrition Science and Technology
Edited by Logan Bowman

International Standard Book Number: 978-1-68286-709-9 (Hardback)

Cataloging-in-Publication Data

Food and health : nutrition science and technology / edited by Logan Bowman.
p. cm.
Includes bibliographical references and index.
ISBN 978-1-68286-709-9
1. Nutrition. 2. Food. 3. Health. 4. Food industry and trade--Appropriate technology.
5. Nutrition--Technological innovations. I. Bowman, Logan.
TX353 .F66 2019
641.3--dc23

Printed in China.

TABLE OF CONTENTS

Preface IX

Chapter 1 **Alteration of starch hydrolyzing enzyme inhibitory properties, antioxidant activities, and phenolic profile of clove buds (*Syzygium aromaticum* L.) by cooking duration** 1
Stephen A. Adefegha, Ganiyu Oboh, Sunday I. Oyeleye and Kolawole Osunmo

Chapter 2 **Authenticity of raspberry flavor in food products using SPME-chiral- GC- MS** 12
Anne-Mette S. Hansen, Henrik L. Frandsen and Arvid Fromberg

Chapter 3 **Antioxidant activity and phenolic profiles of the wild currant *Ribes magellanicum* from Chilean and Argentinean Patagonia** 19
Felipe Jiménez-Aspee, Samanta Thomas-Valdés, Ayla Schulz, Ana Ladio, Cristina Theoduloz and Guillermo Schmeda-Hirschmann

Chapter 4 **Multivariate modeling of settling depth of apple fruit (Red Delicious variety) in water** 35
Kamran Kheiralipour and Farshid Marzbani

Chapter 5 **Maillard reaction products and potatoes: have the benefits been clearly assessed?** 40
DeAnn J. Liska, Chad M. Cook, Ding Ding Wang and John Szpylka

Chapter 6 **Rapid methods for extracting and quantifying phenolic compounds in citrus rinds** 56
Lembe Samukelo Magwaza, Umezuruike Linus Opara, Paul J. R. Cronje, Sandra Landahl, Jose Ordaz Ortiz and Leon A. Terry

Chapter 7 **Change in carbohydrate and enzymes from harvest to sprouting in garlic** 63
Kambiz Mashayekhi, Siamak Mohammadi Chiane, Manizheh Mianabadi, Farshid Ghaderifar and Seyyed Javad Mousavizadeh

Chapter 8 **Mathematical modeling of drying of potato slices in a forced convective dryer based on important parameters** 70
Samira Naderinezhad, Nasrin Etesami, Arefe Poormalek Najafabady and Majid Ghasemi Falavarjani

Chapter 9 **Effect of tamarind (*Tamarindus indica* L.) seed on antioxidant activity, phytocompounds, physicochemical characteristics, and sensory acceptability of enriched cookies and mango juice** 79
Sheilla Natukunda, John H. Muyonga and Ivan M. Mukisa

Chapter 10 **Development and quality characteristics of shelf-stable soy-agushie: a residual by-product of soymilk production** 93
Christina A. Nti, Wisdom A. Plahar and Nana T. Annan

Chapter 11 **Phytochemical, antimicrobial, and antioxidant activities of different citrus juice concentrates**......100
Ehigbai I. Oikeh, Ehimwenma S. Omoregie, Faith E. Oviasogie and Kelly Oriakhi

Chapter 12 **Nutritional composition of raw fresh cashew (*Anacardium occidentale* L.) kernels from different origin**......107
Ricard Rico, Mònica Bulló and Jordi Salas-Salvadó

Chapter 13 **Effect of green Spanish-style Manzanilla packaging conditions on the prevalence of the putative probiotic bacteria *Lactobacillus pentosus* TOMC-LAB2**......117
Francisco Rodríguez-Gómez, Verónica Romero-Gil, Pedro García-García, Francisco Noé Arroyo-López and Antonio Garrido-Fernández

Chapter 14 **Effects of maturity on physicochemical properties of Gac fruit (*Momordica cochinchinensis* Spreng.)**......134
Xuan T. Tran, Sophie E. Parks, Paul D. Roach, John B. Golding and Minh H. Nguyen

Chapter 15 **Influence of extraction methods on antioxidant and antimicrobial properties of essential oil from *Thymua danesis* subsp. *Lancifolius***......144
Yousef Tavakolpour, Marzieh Moosavi-Nasab, Mehrdad Niakousari and Soroush Haghighi-Manesh

Chapter 16 **Phenolic compounds, antioxidant, and antibacterial properties of pomace extracts from four Virginia-grown grape varieties**......151
Yixiang Xu, Sheanell Burton, Chyer Kim and Edward Sismour

Chapter 17 **Sensory quality of soymilk and tofu from soybeans lacking lipoxygenases**......160
Aijun Yang, Heather Smyth, Mridusmita Chaliha and Andrew James

Chapter 18 **Proximate, mineral, and antinutrient compositions of indigenous Okra (*Abelmoschus esculentus*) pod accessions: implications for mineral bioavailability**......169
Habtamu Fekadu Gemede, Gulelat Desse Haki, Fekadu Beyene, Ashagrie Z. Woldegiorgis and Sudip Kumar Rakshit

Chapter 19 **Rheological, baking, and sensory properties of composite bread dough with breadfruit (*Artocarpus communis* Forst) and wheat flours**......180
Adegoke H. Bakare, Oluwatooyin F. Osundahunsi and Joseph O. Olusanya

Chapter 20 **Methyl jasmonate effectively enhanced some defense enzymes activity and Total Antioxidant content in harvested "Sabrosa" strawberry fruit**......195
Mohammadreza Asghari and Ali Rashid Hasanlooe

Chapter 21 **Impact of type of child growth intervention program on caregivers' child feeding knowledge and practices: a comparative study in Ga West Municipality, Ghana** 202
Faith Agbozo, Esi Colecraft and Basma Ellahi

Permissions

List of Contributors

Index

PREFACE

Nutrition is the science that studies the effect of nutrients on the growth, reproduction and maintenance of the body, including health and disease. A healthy diet is largely achieved by the preparation and storage of food in a manner conducive to the preservation of nutrients and quality. Various deficiency-related diseases arise because of an unbalanced diet that does not consist of the appropriate nutrients in the right proportions. These include scurvy, anemia, blindness, goiter, etc. Similarly, many health conditions like obesity, diabetes, osteoporosis, etc. occur when there is an excess of certain nutrients in a regular diet. Nutrients are of two types, macro and micronutrients. Macronutrients are carbohydrates, fats, proteins, fiber and water. Micronutrients include vitamins and minerals. This book is a comprehensive text that addresses the vital aspects of food and health science. It strives to provide a fair idea about this discipline and to help develop a better understanding of the latest advances within this field. Scientists and students actively engaged in food and nutrition science will find this book full of crucial and unexplored concepts.

This book is a comprehensive compilation of works of different researchers from varied parts of the world. It includes valuable experiences of the researchers with the sole objective of providing the readers (learners) with a proper knowledge of the concerned field. This book will be beneficial in evoking inspiration and enhancing the knowledge of the interested readers.

In the end, I would like to extend my heartiest thanks to the authors who worked with great determination on their chapters. I also appreciate the publisher's support in the course of the book. I would also like to deeply acknowledge my family who stood by me as a source of inspiration during the project.

Editor

1

Alteration of starch hydrolyzing enzyme inhibitory properties, antioxidant activities, and phenolic profile of clove buds (*Syzygium aromaticum* L.) by cooking duration

Stephen A. Adefegha, Ganiyu Oboh, Sunday I. Oyeleye & Kolawole Osunmo

Functional food and Nutraceutical Unit, Department of Biochemistry, Federal University of Technology, P.M.B. 704, Akure 340001, Nigeria

Keywords

Antioxidant, clove bud, cooking duration, diabetes mellitus, polyphenol, vitamin C

Correspondence

Stephen A. Adefegha, Functional food and Nutraceutical Unit, Department of Biochemistry, Federal University of Technology, P.M.B. 704, Akure 340001, Nigeria.

E-mail: saadefegha@futa.edu.ng

Funding Information

Personal funds from the authors were used for the study.

Abstract

This study assessed the effect of cooking duration on starch hydrolyzing enzyme (α-amylase and α-glucosidase) activities, antioxidant (1,1-diphenyl-2 picrylhydrazyl [DPPH*], hydroxyl [OH*] radicals scavenging abilities and reducing power) properties, and phenolic profile of clove buds. Clove buds (raw) were cooked for 10 (SC_{10}) and 20 min (SC_{20}) and subsequently, their effects were assessed on enzyme activities, antioxidant properties, and phenolic profile. Inhibition of α-amylase and α-glucosidase activities and radicals scavenging abilities were altered by cooking in the trend; raw < SC_{10} > SC_{20}, with IC_{50} values ranging from 0.25 to 0.52 mg/mL and 0.10 to 1.50 mg/mL respectively. HPLC phenolic profile of the clove buds revealed significant ($P < 0.05$) changes in the amount of chlorogenic acid, quercitrin, quercetin, and kaempferol at different cooking duration. Thus, cooking duration may alter the phenolic compositions and nutraceutical potentials of clove bud by activation and/or deactivation of redox-active metabolites.

Introduction

Phenolic compounds are plant secondary metabolites, which are synthesized by plant adaptation to several biotic and abiotic stress conditions such as cold, water, infections drought, temperature, and nutrient deficiencies (Dicko et al. 1995). They are widely present in vegetables, fruits, legumes, cereals, nuts, and beverages, which upon consumption have been reported to reduce the development of several human degenerative diseases such as coronary heart disease, cancer, hypertension, diabetes, osteoporosis, and neurodegenerative diseases (Pandey and Rizvi 2009; Adefegha et al. 2014). There are thousands of phenolic phytochemicals which can be divided into at least 10 different groups depending on their basic chemical structure. Flavonoids constitute a very important group because of their capacity to protect living organism against free radicals and oxygenated reactive species (ORS) produced during the metabolism of oxygen (Wach et al. 2007; Adefegha and Oboh 2013; Lima et al. 2014; Oboh et al. 2015).

Diabetes mellitus (DM) is a metabolic disorder that occurs as a result of inability of the body to secrete insulin, or to make use of the insulin produced, or both. Insulin deficiency can lead to chronic hyperglycemia with disturbances of carbohydrate, fat, and protein metabolism (Adefegha and Oboh 2012; Oboh et al. 2015). The two major forms of diabetes are insulin-dependent diabetes mellitus (type-1 diabetes) and noninsulin-dependent diabetes mellitus (type-2 diabetes). Both insulin-dependent diabetes mellitus (IDDM) and noninsulin-dependent diabetes mellitus (NIDDM) share one central feature which is elevation of blood sugar (glucose) levels. NIDDM is the most common form of diabetes, accounting for 90% of the cases. Based on the World Health Organization (WHO) report, the occurrence of NIDDM affects more than 170 million people worldwide and it is estimated that by the year 2030, the total number of people having diabetes will reach 366 million (Fonseca 2006).

Clove bud (*Syzygium aromaticum* L. Merr. & Perry) is an unopened flower bud growing on the tree belonging to the family of Myrtaceae. It is a commonly consumed spice that is used in the preparation of several delicacies in many homes, therefore makes it a precious and valuable spice of the world (Milind and Deepa 2011). Clove bud is deep brown in color and possess intense odor and slightly astringent. They are consumed as whole spices or ground into powder and mixed with diets containing cereals, legumes, nuts, fruits, vegetables, milk, and milk products (Adefegha and Oboh 2013). Aside from its use in culinary purposes, it is also used in folklore for the management and treatment of inflammation, liver damage, cancer, diabetes, and other oxidative stress–induced diseases for several centuries, probably due to the abundance of bioactive compounds such as volatile (e.g., eugenol) and nonvolatile (e.g., polyphenols, tannin, terpenes and triterpenes, and sterols) constituents (Atawodi et al. 2011; Milind and Deepa 2011).

Earlier studies in our laboratory have shown in part the rationale behind the use of clove bud in the management of some pathologies including diabetes and hypertension (Adefegha and Oboh 2012, 2013; Adefegha et al. 2014). However, cooking methods and duration were not put into consideration in these studies. In Nigeria, clove bud is consumed both in its raw and cooked forms. The duration of cooking may affect both the bioactive constituents and the biological activities of the plant foods. Thus, this work was designed to evaluate the effect cooking duration on the phenolic constituents, antioxidant properties, and interaction of clove bud extracts (raw and cooked) on key enzymes linked to type-2 diabetes (α-amylase and α-glucosidase) in order to ascertain the best form by which clove bud can be used as nutraceutical and functional food.

Material and Methods

Sample collection and identification

The dried spice of clove bud was purchased at Oja Oba market in Akure metropolis, Nigeria. Authentication of the samples was carried out in the Department of Crop Soil and Pest Management, Federal University of Technology, Akure, Nigeria.

Chemicals and reagents

Chemicals and reagents used such as thiobarbituric acid (TBA), 1,10-phenanthroline, deoxyribose, gallic acid, Folin–Ciocalteau reagent were procured from Sigma-Aldrich, Inc., (St. Louis, MO), trichloroacetic acid (TCA) was sourced from Sigma-Aldrich, Chemie GmbH (Steinheim, Germany), hydrogen peroxide, methanol, sodium nitroprusside, Griess reagent, acetic acid, hydrochloric acid, sodium carbonate, aluminum chloride, potassium acetate, sodium dodecyl sulfate, iron (II) sulfate, potassium ferricyanide, and ferric chloride were sourced from BDH Chemicals Ltd., (Poole, UK). Except stated otherwise, all other chemicals and reagents were of analytical grades and the water was glass distilled.

Sample preparation

Ten grams of clove buds powder was steam cooked in 200 mL of distilled water for 10 (SC_{10}) and 20 min (SC_{20}), respectively, while another 10 g was soaked raw (SR) in 200 mL of distilled water for 1 h and filtered alongside the cooked portion. The filtrate from SR, SC_{10}, and SC_{20} was kept in the refrigerator for subsequent analysis.

α-Amylase inhibition assay

Raw and cooked clove bud extracts (0–200 μL) and 500 μL of 0.02 mol/L sodium phosphate buffer (pH 6.9 with 6 mmol/L NaCl) containing porcine pancreatic α-amylase (EC 3.2.1.1) (0.5 mg/mL) were incubated at 25°C for 10 min. To each tube, 500 μL of 1% soluble potato starch solution in 0.02 mol/L sodium phosphate buffer (pH 6.9 with 6 mmol/L NaCl) was then added to each tube. The reaction mixture was incubated at 25°C for 10 min and stopped with 1.0 mL of dinitrosalicylic acid color reagent. Thereafter, the mixture was incubated in a boiling water bath for 5 min, and cooled to room temperature. The reaction mixture was then diluted with 10 mL of distilled water, and absorbance was measured at 540 nm. The α-amylase inhibitory activity was calculated and expressed as percentage inhibition (Worthington 1993) using the formula below:

$$(\%)\,\text{Inhibition} = \left(\frac{\text{Abs}_{\text{ref}} - \text{Abs}_{\text{sam}}}{\text{Abs}_{\text{ref}}}\right) \times 100$$

where Abs_{ref} is the absorbance without sample and Abs_{sam} is the absorbance of the extract.

α-Glucosidase inhibition assay

Raw and cooked clove bud extracts (0–200 μL) and 100 μL of α-glucosidase (EC 3.2.1.20) solution in 0.1 mol/L phosphate buffer (pH 6.9) were incubated at 25°C for 10 min. Fifty microliters of 5 mmol/L *p*-nitrophenyl-α-D-glucopyranoside solution in 0.1 mol/L phosphate buffer (pH 6.9) and 3 mmol/L glutathione was added. The mixtures were incubated at 25°C for 5 min, before reading the absorbance at 405 nm in the spectrophotometer. The α-glucosidase inhibitory activity was expressed as percentage inhibition (Apostolidis et al. 2007). The formula for α-glucosidase inhibition (%) is as follows:

$$(\%)\,\text{Inhibition} = \left(\frac{\text{Abs}_{\text{ref}} - \text{Abs}_{\text{sam}}}{\text{Abs}_{\text{ref}}}\right) \times 100$$

where Abs_{ref} is the absorbance without sample and Abs_{sam} is the absorbance of the extract.

Free radical scavenging ability

The free radical scavenging ability of the extracts against 1,1-diphenyl-2-picrylhydrazyl (DPPH) free radical was evaluated as described by Gyamfi et al. (1999). Briefly, appropriate dilutions of the extracts (1 mL) were mixed with 1 mL of 0.4 mmol/L DPPH radicals in methanolic solution. The mixture was left in the dark for 30 min, and the absorbance was taken at 516 nm. The control was carried out by using 2 mL DPPH solution without the test samples. The DPPH free radical scavenging ability was subsequently calculated as percentage of the control using the following formula:

$$\text{DPPH}^{*}\text{scavenging ability}\,(\%) = \left(\frac{\text{Abs}_{\text{ref}} - \text{Abs}_{\text{sam}}}{\text{Abs}_{\text{ref}}}\right) \times 100$$

where Abs_{ref} is the absorbance without samples extract and Abs_{sam} is the absorbance of extracts.

Fenton's reaction (OH radical scavenging ability)

The ability of the extracts to prevent Fe^{2+}/H_2O_2-induced decomposition of deoxyribose was carried out using the method of Halliwell and Gutteridge (1981). Briefly, varied dilutions of the extracts were added to a reaction mixture containing 120 μL of 20 mmol/L deoxyribose, 400 μL of 0.1 mol/L phosphate buffer, 40 μL of 20 mmol/L hydrogen peroxide, and 40 μL of 500 μmol/L $FeSO_4$, and the volume was made up to 800 μL with distilled water. The reaction mixture was incubated at 37°C for 30 min, and the reaction was then stopped by the addition of 0.5 mL of 2.8% TCA, this was followed by the addition of 0.4 mL of 0.6% TBA solution. The test tubes were subsequently incubated in boiling water for 20 min. The absorbance was measured at 532 nm in spectrophotometer. The percentage (%) hydroxyl radical scavenging ability was subsequently calculated as follows:

$$\text{OH}^{*}\text{scavenging ability}\,(\%) = \left(\frac{\text{Abs}_{\text{ref}} - \text{Abs}_{\text{sam}}}{\text{Abs}_{\text{ref}}}\right) \times 100$$

where Abs_{ref} is the absorbance without samples extract and Abs_{sam} is the absorbance of extract.

Determination of reducing power

The reducing property of the extracts was determined by assessing the ability of the extracts to reduce $FeCl_3$ solution as described by Oyaizu (1986). A 500-μL aliquot of the extract was mixed with 2.5 mL of 200 mmol/L sodium phosphate buffer (pH 6.6) and 2.5 mL of 1% potassium ferricyanide. The mixture was incubated at 50°C for 20 min and then 2.5 mL of 10% trichloroacetic acid was added. This mixture was centrifuged at 650 rpm for 10 min. Five milliliters of the supernatant was mixed with an equal volume of water and 1 mL of 0.1% ferric chloride. The absorbance was measured at 700 nm and ferric reducing power was subsequently calculated and expressed as ascorbic acid equivalent (AAE).

Quantification of compounds by high-performance liquid chromatography coupled with diode array detection (HPLC-DAD)

Reverse phase chromatographic analyses were carried out under gradient conditions using C_{18} column (4.6 mm × 150 mm) packed with 5-μm diameter of the particles; the mobile phase was (A) acetonitrile:water (95:5, v/v) and (B) water:phosphoric acid (98:2, v/v), and the composition gradient was 5% of A until 10 min and changed to obtain 20%, 40%, 60%, 70%, and 100% of A at 20, 30, 40, 50, and 60 min, respectively, following the method described by Kamdem et al. (2013) with slight modifications. *Syzygium aromaticum* extracts were analyzed at a concentration of 15 mg/mL. The presence of 10 antioxidant compounds were investigated, namely, gallic acid, catechin, chlorogenic acid, caffeic acid, ellagic acid, quercetin, quercitrin, luteolin, kaempferol, and rutin. Identification of these compounds was performed by comparing their retention time and UV absorption spectrum with those of the commercial standards. The flow rate was 0.6 mL/min, injection volume 50 μL, and the wavelengths were 271 nm for gallic acid, 280 nm for catechin, 327 nm for chlorogenic, ellagic, and caffeic acids, and 365 nm for rutin, luteolin, quercitrin, kaempferol, and quercetin. The samples and mobile phase were filtered through 0.45-μm membrane filter (Millipore) and then degassed by ultrasonic bath prior to use. Stock solutions of standards references were prepared in the HPLC mobile phase at a concentration range of 0.030–0.250 mg/mL for catechin, quercetin, quercitrin, luteolin, kaempferol, and rutin, and 0.020–0.300 mg/mL for gallic, chlorogenic, caffeic, and ellagic acids. The chromatography peaks were confirmed by comparing its retention time with those of reference standards and by DAD spectra (200–500 nm). Calibration curve was determined as follows: for gallic acid: $Y = 13{,}568x + 1275.9$ ($r = 0.9996$); catechin: $Y = 11{,}985x + 1178.3$ ($r = 0.9998$); epicatechin: $Y = 12{,}643x + 1263.7$ ($r = 0.9995$); chlorogenic acid: $Y = 13{,}064x + 1187.6$ ($r = 0.9993$); caffeic acid: $Y = 12{,}876x + 1297.4$ ($r = 0.9997$); ellagic acid: $Y = 12{,}631x + 1243.9$ ($r = 0.9998$); rutin: $Y = 13{,}267x + 1265.8$ ($r = 0.9999$); isoquercitrin: $Y = 13{,}496x + 1273.2$ ($r = 0.9996$); quercitrin: $Y = 12{,}730x + 1308.5$ ($r = 0.9996$); kaempferol: $Y = 12{,}745x + 1289.5$ ($r = 0.9998$); and quercetin: $Y = 12{,}895x + 1362.7$ ($r = 0.9994$). All chromatography operations were carried out at ambient temperature and in triplicate. The limit of detection (LOD) and limit of quantification (LOQ) were calculated based on the standard deviation of the responses and the slope using three independent analytical curves, as defined by Boligon et al. (2013). LOD and LOQ were calculated as 3.3 and 10 σ/S, respectively, where σ is the standard deviation of the response and S is the slope of the calibration curve.

Determination of total phenol content

The total phenol content was determined according to the method of Singleton et al. (1999). Briefly, appropriate dilution of the raw and processed clove bud extracts were oxidized with 2.5 mL of 10% Folin–Ciocalteau reagent (v/v) and neutralized by 2.0 mL of 7.5% sodium carbonate. The reaction mixture was incubated for 40 min at 45°C and the absorbance was measured at 765 nm in the spectrophotometer. The total phenol content was subsequently calculated and presented as gallic acid equivalent (GAE).

Determination of total flavonoid content

The total flavonoid content of the extracts was determined using a slightly modified method reported by Meda et al. (2005). Briefly, 0.5 mL of appropriately diluted extracts were mixed with 0.5 mL methanol, 50 μL of 10% $AlCl_3$, 50 μL of 1 mol/L potassium acetate, and 1.4 mL water, and allowed to incubate at room temperature for 30 min. The absorbance of the reaction mixture was subsequently measured at 415 nm and the total flavonoid content was calculated as quercetin equivalent (QE).

Determination of vitamin C content

Vitamin C content of the water extracts was determined using the method of Benderitter et al. (1998). Seventy-five microliters of DNPH (2 g dinitrophenyl hydrazine, 230 mg thiourea, and 270 mg $CuSO_4{\cdot}5H_2O$ in 100 mL of 5 mol/L H_2SO_4) was added to 500 μL of reaction mixture (300 μL of extract with 100 μL 13.3% TCA and water). The reaction mixtures were subsequently incubated for 3 h at 37°C, then 0.5 mL of 65% H_2SO_4 (v/v) was added to the medium, followed by absorbance measurement at 520 nm. The vitamin C content of the extracts was subsequently calculated as AAE.

Data analysis

The results of the three replicates were pooled and expressed as mean ± standard deviation (SD). Student's t-test, one-way analysis of variance (ANOVA), and least significance difference (LSD) were carried out (Zar 1984). A $P \leq 0.05$ was considered statistically significant. EC_{50} was determined using linear regression analysis.

Results

The result of the α-amylase inhibitory effect of the raw and processed clove bud extracts is presented in Figure 1. Clove bud (raw and cooked) extracts inhibited α-amylase activity in a dose-dependent manner and the EC_{50} values are reported in Table 1. The result revealed that the extract of clove bud cooked for 10 min (SC_{10}) had the highest α-amylase inhibitory activity (IC_{50} = 0.25 mg/mL). The effect of cooking duration on the α-amylase inhibitory activity clove bud follows the trend; raw < SC_{10} > SC_{20}

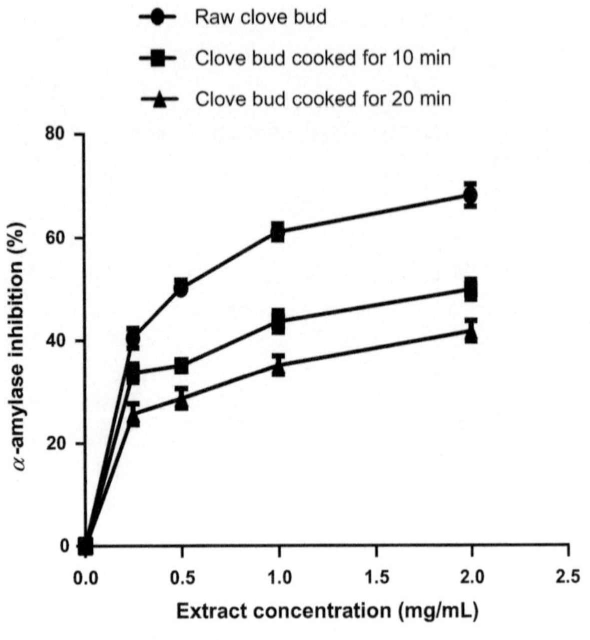

Figure 1. α-Amylase inhibition of clove bud extracts. Values represent mean ± standard deviation of triplicate readings (N = 3).

with IC_{50} values ranging from 0.25 to 0.50 mg/mL. Also, α-glucosidase inhibitory activity (Fig. 2) of the extract from the clove bud cooked for 10 min had the highest α-glucosidase inhibitory activity (IC_{50} = 0.25 mg/mL). The trend (raw < SC_{10} > SC_{20}) observed on the effect of cooking duration on the α-glucosidase inhibitory activity of clove buds is similar to that of the α-amylase inhibitory effect of the clove buds.

The DPPH* scavenging ability of raw and cooked (10 and 20 min cooked) clove bud extracts and the extract concentration that scavenged 50% (EC_{50}) are presented

Table 1. EC_{50} (mg/mL) values for the radicals (DPPH*, OH*) scavenging abilities, α-amylase and α-glucosidase inhibitory activities of raw and cooked (for 10 min and 20 min) clove buds.

Parameter	Raw	Cooked for 10 min	Cooked for 20 min
DPPH* scavenging ability	1.40 ± 0.05^a	1.10 ± 0.02^b	1.50 ± 0.04^c
OH* scavenging ability	0.15 ± 0.01^a	0.10 ± 0.00^b	0.13 ± 0.02^c
α-Amylase inhibition	0.48 ± 0.04^a	0.25 ± 0.06^b	0.50 ± 0.06^c
α-Glucosidase inhibition	0.50 ± 0.02^a	0.25 ± 0.04^b	0.52 ± 0.03^c

Values represent mean ± standard deviation of triplicate readings (n = 3).
Values with the same superscript letter on the same row are not significantly different (P > 0.05).

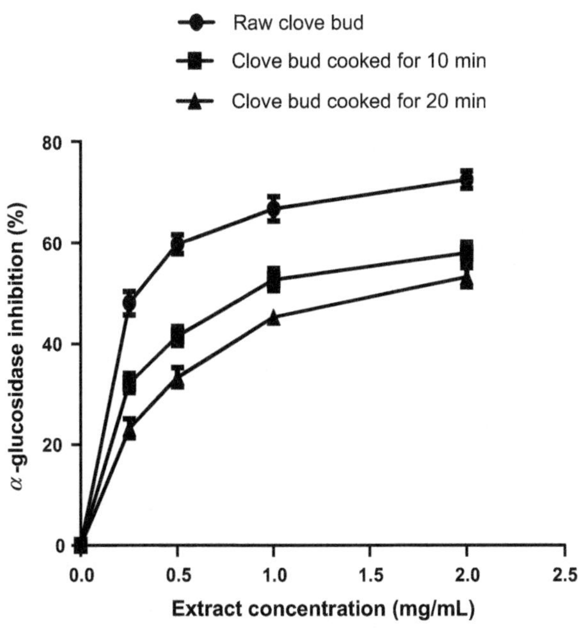

Figure 2. α-Glucosidase inhibition of clove bud extracts. Values represent mean ± standard deviation of triplicate readings (N = 3).

in Figure 3 and Table 1 respectively. The results revealed that SC_{10} (EC_{50} = 1.10 mg/mL) had the highest DPPH* scavenging ability, followed by raw (EC_{50} = 1.40 mg/mL) clove bud extract, while SC_{20} (EC_{50} = 1.50 mg/mL) had the least DPPH* scavenging ability. Furthermore, OH* scavenging ability of the clove bud extracts (Fig. 6) followed the similar trend in a concentration-dependent manner (0–0.30 mg/mL) with SC_{10} (EC_{50} = 0.15 mg/mL) having the highest OH* scavenging ability (Table 2). The ferric reducing antioxidant power (FRAP) of the extracts were assessed based on their ability to reduce Fe^{3+} to Fe^{2+}. The result of the reducing property of the clove buds extracts (raw, SC_{10}, and SC_{20}) is presented as AAE. SC_{10} had significantly (P < 0.05) higher ferric reducing antioxidant properties than the raw and SC_{20} (Fig. 4).

HPLC phenolic fingerprinting of raw, SC_{10}, and SC_{20} revealed the presence of gallic acid (t_R = 11.07 min; peak 1), catechin (t_R = 16.29 min, peak 2), chlorogenic acid (t_R = 21.83 min; peak 3), caffeic acid (t_R = 25.01 min; peak 4), ellagic acid (t_R = 29.76 min; peak 5), rutin (t_R = 37.54 min; peak 6), quercitrin (t_R = 44.98 min; peak 7), quercetin (t_R = 48.61 min; peak 8), kaempferol (t_R = 54.11 min; peak 9), and luteolin (t_R = 61.27 min; peak 10) (Fig. 5 and Table 2). The phenolic acids are gallic acid, chlorogenic acid, ellagic acid, caffeic acid, while the flavonoids present are (−) catechin, rutin, quercitrin, quercetin, kaempferol, and luteolin. Rutin, kaempferol, and luteolin values (Table 2) are in the trend: SC_{10} > SC_{20}, while quercitrin, quercetin, and catechin are in the trend: raw > SC_{10} > SC_{20} (Table 2). Furthermore, the phenolic acids

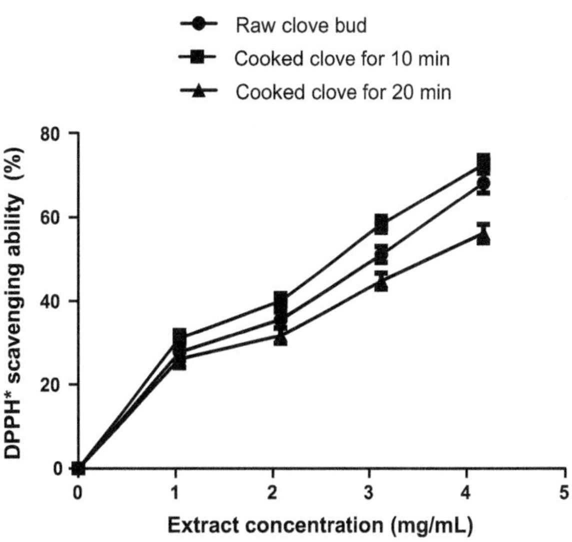

Figure 3. The effect of cooking time DPPH* scavenging ability of clove bud extracts. Values represent mean ± standard deviation of triplicate readings (N = 3).

Table 2. Phenolic composition of *Syzygium aromaticum* extracts.

	Syzygium aromaticum				
Compounds	Raw (mg/g)	10 min (mg/g)	20 min (mg/g)	LOD (μg/mL)	LOQ (μg/mL)
Gallic acid	14.07 ± 0.02^{a}	8.03 ± 0.01^{a}	8.19 ± 0.03^{a}	0.015	0.053
Catechin	1.85 ± 0.03^{b}	1.69 ± 0.01^{b}	1.16 ± 0.01^{b}	0.030	0.098
Chlorogenic acid	20.13 ± 0.01^{c}	15.02 ± 0.02^{c}	17.82 ± 0.02^{c}	0.009	0.031
Caffeic acid	13.98 ± 0.03^{a}	13.76 ± 0.03^{d}	13.27 ± 0.01^{d}	0.026	0.084
Ellagic acid	1.61 ± 0.02^{b}	1.57 ± 0.01^{b}	8.59 ± 0.01a	0.013	0.049
Rutin	9.11 ± 0.01^{d}	13.92 ± 0.01^{d}	3.41 ± 0.03^{e}	0.007	0.023
Quercitrin	30.26 ± 0.03^{e}	24.01 ± 0.03^{e}	20.47 ± 0.02^{f}	0.018	0.059
Quercetin	29.71 ± 0.02^{e}	21.86 ± 0.01^{f}	19.08 ± 0.01^{f}	0.010	0.034
Kaempferol	20.47 ± 0.01^{c}	21.73 ± 0.02^{f}	20.95 ± 0.03^{f}	0.036	0.119
Luteolin	9.28 ± 0.05^{d}	14.05 ± 0.01^{d}	8.57 ± 0.02^{a}	0.014	0.045

Results are expressed as mean ± standard error of mean (SEM) of three determinations. Averages followed by different superscript letters differ by Tukey test at $P < 0.05$.

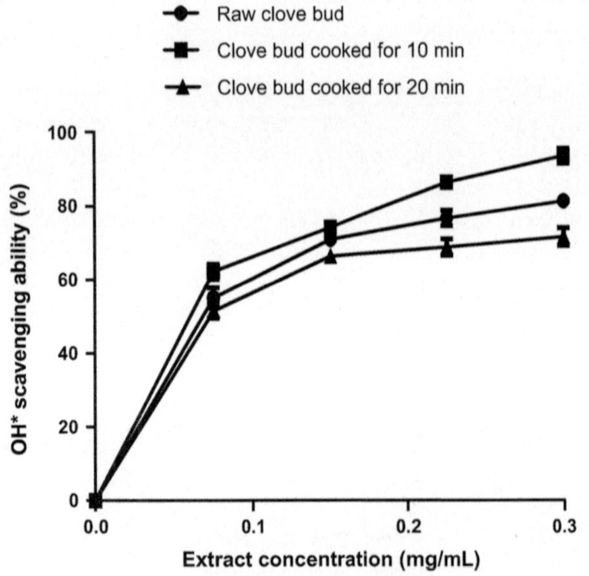

Figure 4. OH* scavenging ability of clove bud extracts. Values represent mean ± standard deviation of triplicate readings ($N = 3$).

(gallic and chlorogenic acids) are in the trend: raw > SC_{10} < SC_{20}. The result showed that there was no significant ($P > 0.05$) difference in ellagic acid content of the raw and SC_{10} but higher in SC_{20}. The result of the total phenol and flavonoid contents of the clove bud extracts (raw, SC_{10}, and SC_{20}) are presented in Figures 6 and 7 respectively. The results indicated that extract from SC_{10} had significantly ($P < 0.05$) higher total phenol and flavonoid contents than the raw clove bud extracts, while SC_{20} had the least. Conversely, the result of the vitamin C content revealed a significant ($P < 0.05$) decrease with increase in cooking duration. The trend (raw > SC_{10} > SC_{10}) is observed as shown in Figure 8.

Discussion

Cooking represents an indispensable prerequisite in obtaining safe and high-quality food products. It confers better hygienic quality, palatability, and makes food more digestible (Adefegha and Oboh 2011). In this study, the effect of cooking duration was assessed on the antidiabetic potentials of clove buds via its inhibition on amylase and glucosidase activities, antioxidant (radicals [DPPH* and OH*] scavenging and FRAP) effects, phenolic profiling, as well as total phenolics (phenol and flavonoid) and vitamin C contents.

Inhibition of enzymes related to carbohydrate hydrolysis (α-amylase and α-glucosidase) has been accepted as one of the therapeutic approach in the management of type-2 diabetes. The inhibition of α-amylase and α-glucosidase delay carbohydrate digestion thereby reduces rate of

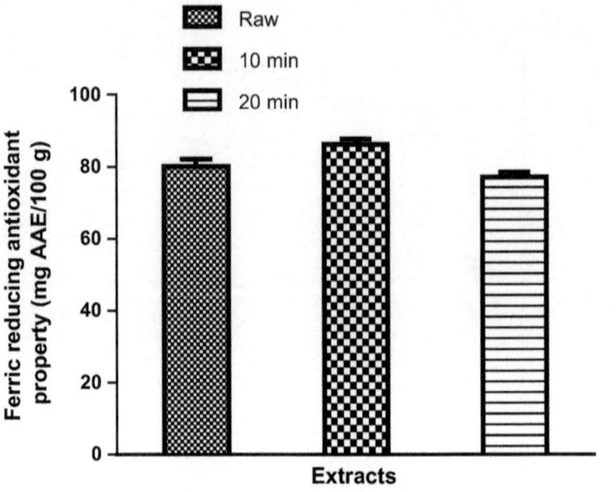

Figure 5. Ferric reducing antioxidant properties of clove bud extracts. Values represent mean ± standard deviation of triplicate readings ($N = 3$).

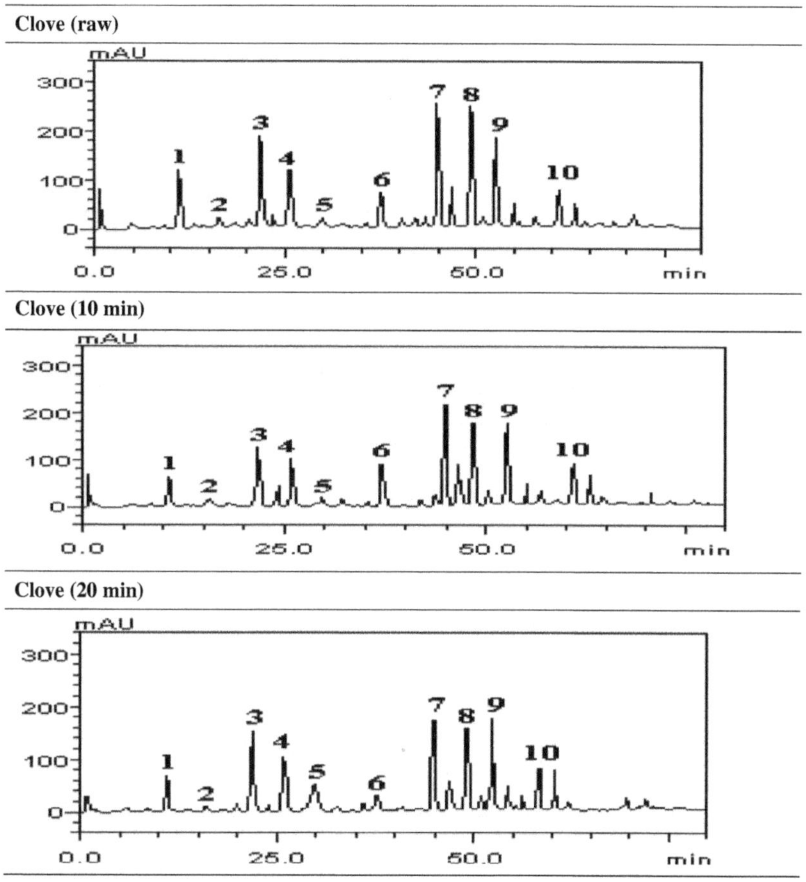

Figure 6. Representative high-performance liquid chromatography profile of *Syzygium aromaticum* extracts. Gallic acid (peak 1), catechin (peak 2), chlorogenic acid (peak 3), caffeic acid (peak 4), ellagic acid (PEAK 5), rutin (peak 6), quercitrin (peak 7), quercetin (peak 8), kaempferol (peak 9), and luteolin (peak 10).

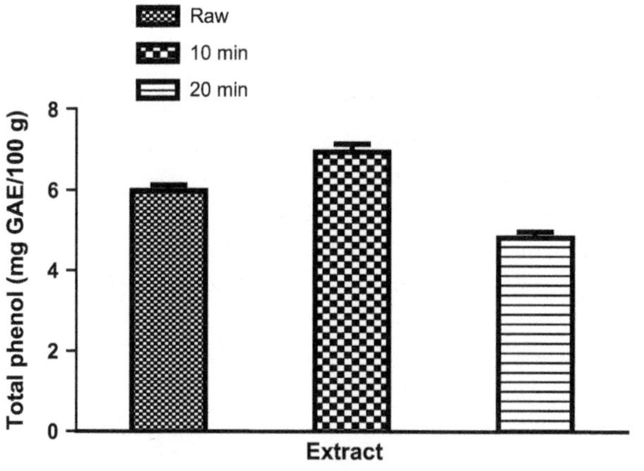

Figure 7. Total phenol content of the clove bud extracts. Values represent mean ± standard deviation of triplicate readings ($N = 3$).

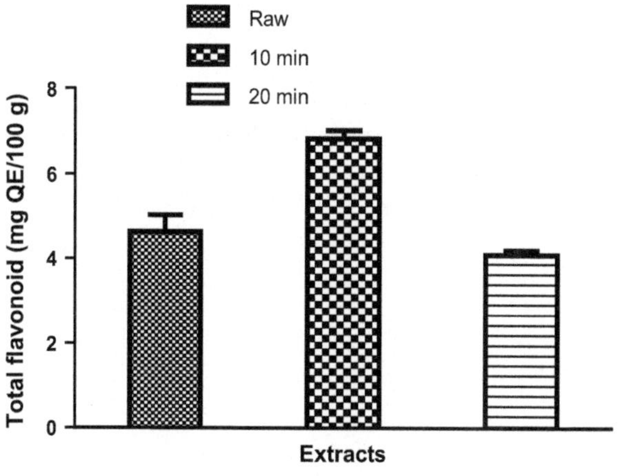

Figure 8. Total flavonoid content of the clove bud extracts. Values represent mean ± standard deviation of triplicate readings ($N = 3$).

glucose production and consequently causes reduction in postprandial hyperglycemia especially in patients with type-2 diabetes (Shim et al. 2003). From this study, all the extracts inhibited α-amylase and α-glucosidase activities in concentration-dependent manner (0–2 mg/mL) and these biological effects (Figs. 1, 2) may be attributed to

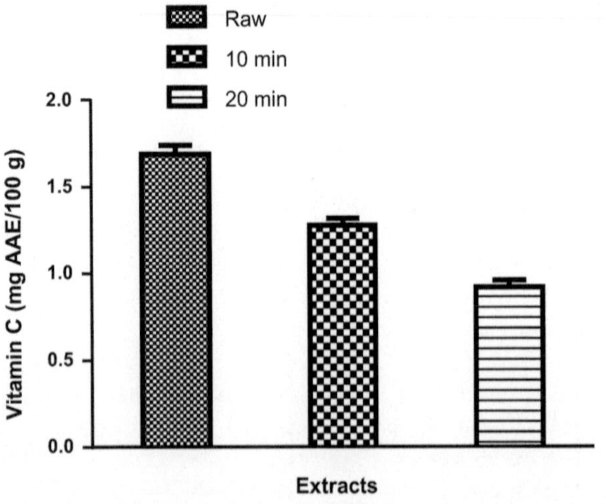

Figure 9. Vitamin C content of the clove bud extracts. Values represent mean ± standard deviation of triplicate readings ($N = 3$).

the presence of phenolic compounds such as phenolic acids and flavonoids (Table 2). Flavonoids such as kaempferol, rutin, and luteolin (which were found to be higher in SC_{10}) have been reported to reduce the risk of type-2 diabetes probably due to their stronger inhibition of α-amylase and α-glucosidase (Kim et al. 2000; Knekt et al. 2002; Oboh et al. 2015). It is worth noting that SC_{20} had the lowest α-amylase and α-glucosidase inhibitory effects and these may have resulted from the damage/loss of physiologically active phytochemicals through prolonged cooking duration as evidence in the phenolic contents (Figs. 7, 8) that have α-amylase and α-glucosidase inhibitory activities. Nevertheless, the determined α-amylase inhibitory activity of the clove buds agreed with earlier reports of plant phytochemicals from some spices such as *Allium* spp., red and white ginger inhibitory effects on α-amylase and α-glucosidase activity in vitro (Nickavar and Yousefian 2009; Oboh et al. 2010).

Free radicals have been reported to play a major role in diabetic complications (Mohamed et al. 1999). Hence, steady consumption of dietary antioxidants to boost the endogenous antioxidant defense system is one of the accepted practical approach by which free radical–mediated oxidative stress in DM may be curtailed. The antioxidative properties of plant secondary metabolites occur by diminishing the production of free radicals or by neutralizing and/or scavenging radicals produced during normal body metabolism or reducing/chelating the transition metals present in foods. More so, termination of chain initiation step via scavenging of reactive species has been considered to be one of the antioxidant mechanisms of action (Melo et al. 2006; Dastmalchi et al. 2007). The result of the DPPH free radical scavenging ability of raw and cooked clove bud extracts revealed that SC_{10} caused significant ($P < 0.05$) increase in the DPPH* scavenging ability compared to the raw clove buds, while prolonged SC_{20} led to the decline in the DPPH* scavenging ability. Similar trend of result was also observed in the OH* scavenging ability of raw and cooked clove buds, where SC_{10} significantly ($P < 0.05$) increased OH* scavenging ability than that of the raw extract, while the SC_{20} had the least OH* scavenging ability. The differences in the radicals scavenging abilities of the raw and cooked clove buds could be as a result of destruction and/or creation of redox-active phenolic compounds most especially flavonoid.

Reducing power is a novel antioxidation defense mechanism that involves electron and/or hydrogen atom transfers and reduces transition metals (Allhorn et al. 2005; Gocer and Gulcin 2011). This is because the ferric-to-ferrous ion reduction occurs rapidly in all reductants that have half-reaction reduction potentials above that of Fe^{3+}/Fe^{2+}, the values of the FRAP assay could express the corresponding concentration of electron-donating antioxidants. The trend of the result of the reducing power of the raw and cooked clove buds followed similar order as the total phenolic contents. Thus, this study agrees with previous studies where strong correlation were established between antioxidants properties of plant foods and their phenolic content (Adefegha and Oboh 2011, 2012; Carlonia et al. 2013). However, the antioxidant effects of the raw clove buds may be altered by cooking duration via the activation and/or deactivation of redox-active metabolites/phenolics during the heat processes.

The presence of phenolic compound has been reported to contribute immensely to the enhancement of protective potentials of plant and plant-based food against some degenerative diseases (Boyer and Liu 2004). Flavonoids have also been reported to possess antioxidative properties with the ability to lower cellular oxidative stress—a major culprit in the pathogenesis of various neurodegenerative diseases, such as Alzheimer's disease, Parkinson's disease, and amyotrophic lateral sclerosis (Adefegha et al. 2014)—via radicals scavenging and metals chelating effects, activation of antioxidant enzymes, and inhibition of oxidases (Altunkaya and Gökmen 2009; Muthiah et al. 2012).

The phenolic compound identified and quantified in the different clove bud extracts (raw, SC_{10}, and SC_{20}) may indicate that the spice under investigation is rich in phytochemicals with possible physiological importance. Furthermore, the extracts contained rutin, quercitrin, quercetin, and kaempferol as the major flavonoid composition, while chlorogenic acid was found to be present as the major phenolic acid. From the result, catechin, quercitrin, and quercetin contents decreased with increase in cooking duration. This trend agrees with earlier studies where thermal processing was reported to cause reduction in flavonoid content of foods based on the magnitude and extent of heat and duration (Viña and Chaves 2008; Zhang et al. 2010). The effects of cooking duration on the phenolic contents (total phenol and flavonoid) presented in Figs. 7, 8 revealed that SC_{10} increased the total phenol and flavonoid contents when compared to that of raw clove buds. This could be attributed to the release of stored total phenolics in cell wall bound pectins by thermal processing and breakage in the supramolecular structures or softened the plant matrix (Bunea et al. 2008; Ferracane et al. 2008). However, decreased contents of total phenol and flavonoid were observed in SC_{20} when compared to that of SC_{10}. This observation agreed with the assertion that prolonged cooking duration could lead to thermal destruction or heavy loss of polyphenols (El-Sohaimy 2013). From this study, the effect of the cooking duration on the phenolic contents of clove buds followed the trend: raw < SC_{10} > SC_{20} (Figs. 7, 8).

Plant foods including fruits, vegetables, and spices are good source of vitamin C (Babalola et al. 2010). Vitamin C is a prominent exogenous antioxidant that defends the body against free radicals, maintains blood vessel flexibility, improves blood circulation in the arteries, and protects against esophageal and stomach cancer (Block et al. 1992; Pandey and Rizvi 2009 Bashandy and Alwasel 2011). In this study, cooking significantly ($P < 0.05$) decreased the vitamin C content of clove buds. Hence, agreed with the report of Zhang and Hamauzu (2004) and Adefegha and Oboh (2011) that the loss in vitamin C contents with respect to cooking may be due to the thermal instability of vitamin C (ascorbic acid). Thus, the trend of the effect of cooking duration on the vitamin C content of clove buds observed in this study followed the order: raw > SC_{10} > SC_{20} as shown in Figure 9.

Conclusion

The higher phenolic content, antioxidant properties, and inhibition of key enzymes (α-amylase and α-glucosidase) linked with type-2 diabetes by SC_{10} compared to that of raw showed that consumption of moderate cooked clove bud with respect to time may indicate that potential antioxidant and antidiabetic agents are preserved and enhanced. However, prolonged cooking as in SC_{20} may lead to destruction of antioxidant and antidiabetic agents thereby reducing the nutritional quality and nutraceutical potentials of clove bud.

Conflict of Interest

None declared.

References

Adefegha, S. A., and G. Oboh. 2011. Enhancement of total phenolics and antioxidant properties of some tropical green leafy vegetables by steam cooking. J. Food Process. Preserv. 35:615–622.

Adefegha, S. A., and G. Oboh. 2012. Inhibition of key enzymes linked to type 2 diabetes and sodium nitroprusside-induced lipid peroxidation in rat pancreas by water extractable phytochemicals from some tropical spices. Pharm. Biol. 50:857–865.

Adefegha, S. A., and G. Oboh. 2013. Phytochemistry and mode of action of some tropical spices in the management of type-2 diabetes and hypertension. Afr. J. Pharm. Pharmacol. 7:332–346.

Adefegha, S. A., G. Oboh, O. M. Adefegha, A. A. Boligon, and M. L. Athayde. 2014. Antihyperglycemic, hypolipidemic, hepatoprotective and antioxidative effects of dietary clove (*Szyzgium aromaticum*) bud powder in a high-fat diet/streptozotocin induced diabetes rat model. J. Sci. Food Agric. 94:2726–2737.

Allhorn, M., A. Klapyta, and B. Åkerström. 2005. Redox properties of the lipocalinα1microglobulin: reduction of cytochrome C, hemoglobulin, and free iron. Free Rad. Biol. Med. 38:557–567.

Altunkaya, A., and V. Gökmen. 2009. Effect of various anti-browning agents on phenolic compounds profile of fresh lettuce (*L. sativa*). Food Chem. 117:122–126.

Apostolidis, E., Y. I. Kwon, and K. Shetty. 2007. Inhibitory potential of herb, fruit, and fungal enriched cheese against key enzymes linked to type 2 diabetes and hypertension. Innov Food Sci. Emerg. Technol. 8:46–54.

Atawodi, S. E., J. C. Atawodi, B. Pfundstein, B. Spiegelhalder, H. Bartsch, and R. Owen. 2011. Assessment of the polyphenol components and in vitro antioxidant properties of *Syzygium aromaticum* (L.) Merr. & Perry. EJEAChe. 10:1970–1978.

Babalola, O. O., O. S. Tugbobo, and A. S. Daramola. 2010. Effect of processing on the vitamin C content of seven Nigerian green leafy vegetables. Adv. J. Food Sci. Tech. 2:303–305.

Bashandy, S. A., and S. H. Alwasel. 2011. Carbon tetrachloride-induced hepatotoxicity and nephrotoxicity in rats: protective role of vitamin C. J. Pharmacol. Toxicol. 6:283–292.

Benderitter, M., V. Maupoil, C. Vergely, F. Dalloz, F. Briot, and L. Rochette. 1998. Studies by electron paramagnetic resonance of the importance of iron in the hydroxyl scavenging properties of ascorbic acid in plasma: effects of iron chelators. Fundam. Clin. Pharmacol. 12:510–516.

Block, G., B. Patterson, and A. Subar. 1992. Fruits, vegetables and cancer prevention. A review of epidemiological evidence. Nutraceuticals Cancer 18:1–29.

Boligon, A. A., T. F. Kubica, D. N. Mario, T. F. de Brum, M. Piana, R. Weiblen, et al. 2013. Antimicrobial and antiviral activity-guided fractionation from Scutia buxifolia Reissek extracts. Acta Physiol. Plant 35:2229–2239.

Boyer, J., and R. H. Liu. 2004. Apple phytochemicals and their health benefits. Nutr. J. 3:12.

Bunea, A., M. Andjeldkovic, C. Socaciu, O. Bobis, M. Neacsu, R. Verh'e, et al. 2008. Total and individual carotenoids and phenolic acids content in fresh, refrigerated and processed spinach (*Spinacia oleracea* L.). Food Chem. 108:649–656.

Carlonia, P., L. Tianob, L. Padellab, T. Bacchettic, C. Customud, A. Kayd, et al. 2013. Antioxidant activity of white, green and black tea obtained from the same tea cultivar. Food Res. Int. 53:900–908.

Dastmalchi, K., H. J. D. Dorman, M. Kosar, and R. Hiltunen. 2007. Chemical composition and in vitro antioxidant evaluation of a water soluble Moldavian balm (*Dracocephalum moldavica* L.) extract. Lebensm.-Wiss. Technol. 40:239–248.

Dicko, M. H., H. Gruppen, C. Barro, A. S. Traore, W. J. H. van-Berkel, and A. G. J. Voragen. 1995. Impact of phenolics and related enzymes in sorghum varieties for the resistance and susceptibility to biotic and abiotic stresses. J. Chem. Ecol. 31:2671–2688.

El-Sohaimy, S. A. 2013. The effect of cooking on the chemical Composition of Artichoke (*Cynara scolymus* L.). Afr. J. Food Sci. Technol. 3:182–187.

Ferracane, R., N. Pellegrini, A. Visconti, G. Graziani, E. Chiavaro, C. Miglio, et al. 2008. Effects of different cooking methods on antioxidant profile, antioxidant capacity, and physical characteristics of artichoke. J. Agric. Food Chem. 56:8601–8608.

Fonseca, V. A. 2006. Pp. 2–3Clinical diabetes: translating research into practice. Saunders Elsevier, Philadelphia.

Gocer, H., and I. Gulcin. 2011. Caffeic acid phenethyl ester (CAPE): correlation of structure and antioxidant properties. Inter. J. Food Sci. Nutr. 62:821–825.

Gyamfi, M. A., M. Yonamine, and Y. Aniya. 1999. Free-radical scavenging action of medicinal herbs from Ghana: *Thonningia sanguinea* on experimentally-induced liver injuries. Gen. Pharmacol. 32:661–667.

Halliwell, B., and J. M. C. Gutteridge. 1981. Formation of a thiobarbituric-acid-reactive substance from deoxyribose in the presence of iron salts: the role of superoxide and hydroxyl radicals. FEBS Lett. 28:347–352.

Kamdem, J. P., E. O. Olalekan, W. Hassan, I. J. Kade, O. Yetunde, A. A. Boligon, et al. 2013. *Trichilia catigua* (Catuaba) bark extract exerts neuroprotection against oxidative stress induced by different neurotoxic agents in rathippocampal slices. Ind. Crop Prod. 50:625–632.

Kim, J. S., C. S. Kwon, and K. H. Son. 2000. Inhibition of glucosidase and amylase by luteolin, a flavonoid. Biosci. Biotecnol. Biochem. 64:2458–2461.

Knekt, P., J. Kumpulainen, R. Järvinen, H. Rissanen, M. Heliövaara, A. Reunanen, et al. 2002. Flavonoid intake and risk of chronic diseases. Am. J. Clin. Nutr. 76:560–568.

Lima, G. P. P., F. Vianello, C. R. R. Corrêa, A. S. Campos, and M. G. Borguini. 2014. Polyphenols in fruits and vegetables and its effect on human health. Food Nutr. Sci. 5:1065–1082.

Meda, A., C. E. Lamien, M. Romito, J. Millogo, and O. G. Nacoulma. 2005. Determination of the total phenolic, flavonoid and proline contents in Burkina Faso honey, as well as their radical scavenging activity. Food Chem. 91:571–577.

Melo, E. A., V. L. A. Lima, M. I. S. Maciel, A. C. S. Caetano, and F. L. L. Leal. 2006. Polyphenol, ascorbic acid and total carotenoid contents in common fruits and vegetables. Braz. J. Food Technol. 9:89–94.

Milind, P., and K. Deepa. 2011. Clove: a champion spice. Int. J Res. Ayurveda Pharm. 2:47–54.

Mohamed, A. K., A. Bierhaus, S. Schiekofer, H. Tritschler, R. Ziegler, and P. P. Nawroth. 1999. The role of oxidative stress and NFKappa B activation in late diabetic complications. BioFactors 10:157–167.

Muthiah, P. L., M. Umamaheswari, and K. Asokkumar. 2012. In vitro antioxidant activities of leaves, fruits and peel extracts of citrus. Int. J Phytopharmacy 2:13–20.

Nickavar, B., and N. Yousefian. 2009. Inhibitory effects of six Allium species on α- amylase enzyme activity. Iran. J. Pharm. Res. 8:53–57.

Oboh, G., A. J. Akinyemi, A. O. Ademiluyi, and S. A. Adefegha. 2010. Inhibitory effects of aqueous extract of two varieties of ginger on some key enzymes linked to type-2 diabetes in vitro. J. Food Nutr. Res. 49:14–20.

Oboh, G., O. M. Agunloye, S. A. Adefegha, A. J. Akinyemi, and A. O. Ademiluyi. 2015. Caffeic and Chlorogenic Acids Inhibit Key Enzymes Linked to Type-2 diabetes (In vitro): A Comparative Study. J Basic and Clin Physiol Pharmacol 26:165–170.

Oyaizu, M. 1986. Studies on products of browning reaction: antioxidative activity of products of browning reaction prepared from glucosamine. Jpn. J. Nutr. 44:307–315.

Pandey, B. K., and I. S. Rizvi. 2009. Plant polyphenols as dietary antioxidants in human health and disease. Oxid. Med. Cell Longev. 2:270–278.

Shim, Y. J., H. K. Doo, S. Y. Ahn, Y. S. Kim, J. K. Seong, I. S. Park, et al. 2003. Inhibitory effect of aqueous extract from the gall of *Rhuz chinensis* on alpha-glucosidase activity and postprandial blood glucose. J. Ethnopharmacol. 85:283–287.

Singleton, V. L., R. Orthofor, and R. M. Lamuela-raventos 1999. Analysis of total phenols and other oxidation substrates and antioxidants by means of Folin–Ciocaltau reagent. Methods Enzymol. 299, 152–178.

Viña, S. Z., and A. R. Chaves. 2008. Effect of heat treatment and refrigerated storage on antioxidant properties of pre-cut celery (*Apium graveolens* L.). Int. J. Food Sci. Technol. 43:44–51.

Wach, A., K. Pyrzynska, and M. Biesaga. 2007. Quercetin content in some food and herbal samples. Food Chem. 100:699–704.

Worthington, V., ed. 1993. Alpha amylase. Pp. 36–41. Worthington enzyme manual. Worthington Biochemical Corp, Freehold, NJ.

Zar, J. H. 1984. Biostatistical analysis. Prentice-Hall Inc, Upper Saddle River, New Jersey, USA.

Zhang, D., and Y. Hamauzu. 2004. Phenolics, ascorbic acid, carotenoids and antioxidant activity of broccoli and their changes during conventional and microwave cooking. Food Chem. 88:503–509.

Zhang, M., H. Chen, J. Li, Y. Pei, and Y. Liang. 2010. Antioxidant properties of tartary buckwheat extracts as affected by different thermal processing methods. LWT- Food Sci. Technol. 43:181–185.

2

Authenticity of raspberry flavor in food products using SPME-chiral-GC-MS

Anne-Mette S. Hansen, Henrik L. Frandsen & Arvid Fromberg

National Food Institute, Technical University of Denmark Mørkhøj Bygade 19, Søborg DK-2860, Denmark

Keywords
Authenticity, chiral-GC-MS, enantioselective GC, raspberry flavor, SPME, α-ionone

Correspondence
Arvid Fromberg, National Food Institute, Technical University of Denmark, Mørkhøj Bygade 19, DK-2860 Søborg, Denmark.

E-mail: arfr@food.dtu.dk

Funding Information
No funding information provided.

Abstract

A fast and simple method for authenticating raspberry flavors from food products was developed. The two enantiomers of the compound (E)-α-ionone from raspberry flavor were separated on a chiral gas chromatographic column. Based on the ratio of these two enantiomers, the naturalness of a raspberry flavor can be evaluated due to the fact that a natural flavor will consist almost exclusively of the R enantiomer, while a chemical synthesis of the same compound will result in a racemic mixture. Twenty-seven food products containing raspberry flavors where investigated using SPME-chiral-GC-MS. We found raspberry jam, dried raspberries, and sodas declared to contain natural aroma all contained almost only R-(E)-α-ionone supporting the content of natural raspberry aroma. Six out of eight sweets tested did not indicate a content of natural aroma on the labeling which was in agreement with the almost equal distribution of the R and S isomer. Two products were labeled to contain natural raspberry flavors but were found to contain almost equal amounts of both enantiomers indicating a presence of synthetic raspberry flavors only. Additionally, two products that were labeled to contain both raspberry juice and flavor showed equal amounts of both enantiomers, indicating the presence of synthetic flavor.

Introduction

Authenticity of food products is often used as a parameter of quality in marketing. Food products containing only natural ingredients are preferred by many consumers who are willing to pay a higher price for such products. Natural aroma components are often more expensive than their synthetic equivalent making counterfeit an economical benefit. Counterfeit of aroma components is misleading to the consumers and is illegal according to European legislation (European Parliament 2008) where the term "Natural" can be used only for flavors containing exclusively natural flavoring substances. A natural flavor should be obtained by appropriate physical, enzymatic, or microbiological processes from the material of vegetable, animal, or microbiological origin (European Parliament 2008).

The flavor of raspberries consist of many different aroma compounds all contributing more or less to the characteristic perception of raspberries. Malowicki et al. investigated the volatile composition of raspberries following stir bar sorptive extraction and identified some 30 compounds, including (Z)-hexenol, hexanal, (E)-2-hexenal, 2-heptanone, δ-octalactone, δ-decalactone, geraniol, α-ionone, β-ionone, and terpinen-4-ol as the major constituents (Malowicki et al. 2008a,b). Some of the flavoring substances are chiral and the enantiomeric composition in raspberry extracts was characterized by chiral GC-MS, α-ionone occurs mainly in the R-form (97–100%), whereas δ-octalactone, δ-decalactone, and terpinen-4-ol occurs mainly in the S-form (80–100%) (Malowicki et al. 2008a,b). Also, Werkhoff et al. (1991) found an enantiomeric composition of α-ionone in raspberry extract sampled by a head space of 99.9% R-form and 0.1% S-form (Werkhoff et al. 1991). The enantiomeric composition of α-ionone and δ-decalactone in raspberry extract was by chiral GC determined to 98–100% R-form for ionone and to 98–100% S-form for decalactone (Casabianca and Graff 1994). The enantiomeric composition of a number of chiral 4-alkylated-γ-lactones from C_5 to C_{12} was determined in extracts from apricot, mango, passion fruit, peach, raspberry and strawberry (Bernreuther et al. 1989;. Guichard et al. 1990). For all fruits, there seemed to be a preponderance of the R-form of the longer chained γ-lactones > C_8 whereas for the shorter chained γ-lactones some fruits had preponderance of the R-form, some of the S-form and some hardly showed enantiomeric excess. In both orange flowers and unifloral orange honey, the enantiomeric composition of linalool was 87–91% of the (+) form and 9–13% of the (−) form indicating the usefulness of chiral analysis in the authenticity assessment of unifloral honey (Verzera et al. 2014).

Ravid et al. (2010) assessed the authenticity of natural fruit compounds in food and beverages, using head space SPME chiral GC-MS. The enantiomeric composition of linalool, linalyl acetate, and limonene were characterized in bergamot oil, γ-decalactone, and γ-undecalactone in peach and nectarine products, γ-lactones in passion fruit products and α-ionone in raspberry products. The study showed that (E)-α-ionone in raspberry is efficiently adsorbed on an SPME fiber and occur almost exclusively as the R enantiomer, whereas (E)-α-ionone originating from chemical synthesis is a racemic mixture containing almost equal amounts of both enantiomers. In raspberries, the biosynthesis of (E)-α-ionone is catalyzed by stereospecific enzymes leading to a preponderance of (R)-(E)-α-ionone of more than 99% (Ravid et al. 2010). Consequently, the presence of (S)-(E)-α-ionone could be an indicator of adulteration with artificial aroma components (Aprea et al. 2009; Taylor and Linforth 2010).

Head space SPME is an attractive method to isolate and concentrate volatile compounds from complex samples such as foods because only little sample pretreatment is required. In this study, we investigated three different fiber coatings: divinylbenzene/polydimethylsiloxane (DVB/PDMS), carboxen/polydimethylsiloxane (CAR/PDMS), and divinylbenzene/carboxen/polydimethylsiloxane (DVB/CAR/PDMS) for the capabilities to extract volatile compounds, from raspberry aroma and in particular (E)-α-ionone, as this compound is the major enantiomeric compound bound to the extraction fiber. Furthermore, addition of sodium chloride during head space SPME was investigated for potential improvement of extraction efficiency. Finally, 27 raspberry containing and/or flavored samples of foods, beverages and sweets from the Danish market were analyzed for enantiomer composition of (E)-α-ionone to investigate whether the labeling were in compliance with the EU regulation. The samples set included sodas and sweets, products which have not previously been investigated for authenticity.

Materials and Methods

Samples

Samples of jam, sodas, sweets, dried raspberries, fruit bars, and yoghurts from the Danish retail market were purchased at different retailers, all declared to contain raspberries, natural flavor and/or flavor, see Table 1. Samples of fresh raspberries were obtained from the local retail market. Chemicals: Pure standard of α-ionone was purchased from Sigma-Aldrich (Steinheim, Germany). Sodium chloride was purchased from Merck (Darmstadt, Germany).

SPME fibers

SPME fibers were purchased from Supelco, (Supelco, Bellefonte, Pennsylvania, USA), all coated on a fused silica fiber and with a length of 1 cm; divinylbenzene (DVB)/polydimethylsiloxane (PDMS) 65 μm coating, carboxen (CAR)/(PDMS) 75 μm coating, and DVB/CAR/PDMS 50 μm DVB and 30 μm CAR on PDMS coating.

SPME-chiral-GC-MS method

The SPME fibers were used for extracting aroma compounds from raspberries and subsequent analysis, using automated headspace solid phase micro extraction (HS-SPME), using a GC-Combi PAL (CTC Analytical, Zwingen, Switzerland) on an Agilent 6890 gas chromatograph (GC) (Agilent Technologies, Inc., Wilmington, Germany) equipped with an Agilent 5979 Mass Selective Detector.

Samples of fresh raspberries were macerated with a fork prior to transfer to the sample vials. No sample preparation, except homogenization was performed on jam, soda, yoghurt, and dried raspberry samples. Sweets and the fruit bar were cut into 5 mm pieces prior to transfer to the sample vials. Approximately, 4 g of all samples was placed in a 10 mL headspace vial. The vial was heated to 60°C before the SPME fiber was exposed to the headspace. Extraction was carried out at 60°C for 30 min using agitation. Optimized extraction conditions were adapted from Cagliero et al. (2012). Hereafter, the analytes were thermally desorbed into the GC inlet at 230°C for 5 min in splitless mode. The GC was used with the following temperature program: 50°C for 5 min and then raised at 30°C/min to 100°C and raised again at 2°C/min to 145°C and finally 30°C/min to 200°C for 4 min (GC runtime: 35 min). For the method optimizing part, the following temperature program was used: 50°C for 7 min and then raised at 1.5°C/min to 180°C and raised again at 6°C/min to a final temperature of 200°C/min for 5 min (GC runtime: 102 min). The column was a β-DEX 225 (Supelco, USA) consisting of nonbonded 25% 2,3-di-O-acetyl-6-O-TBDMS-β-cyclode xtrin in a SPB-20 phase 0.25 mm × 30 m, 0.25 μm film thickness. Carrier gas was helium at 0.8 mL/min, 33 cm/sec. The transfer line temperature was 250°C,

Table 1. Sample description and R-(E)-α-ionone and S-(E)-α-ionone analyses in food and sweet samples from the Danish market.

Sample	Fruit content declared	Natural aroma declared	Aroma declared	R-α-ionone %	S-α-ionone %	Compliance with EU legislation
Jam #1	Raspberry, 35%			97.1	3.0	Yes
Jam #2	Raspberry, 50%			97.4	2.6	Yes
Jam #3	Raspberry, 50%			96.8	3.2	Yes
Jam #4	Raspberry, 45%			96.3	3.7	Yes
Jam #5	Raspberry, 40%			98.5	1.5	Yes
Jam #6	Raspberry, 45%			97.3	2.7	Yes
Soda #1			x	49.9	50.1	Yes
Soda #2			x	49.8	50.2	Yes
Soda #3		x		100	0	Yes
Soda #4		x		100	0	Yes
Soda #5			x	50.6	49.4	Yes
Dried raspberries #1	Dried fruits			100	0	Yes
Sweet #1, fruit gum			x	49.9	50.1	Yes
Sweet #2, fruit gum			x	49.9	50.1	Yes
Sweet #3, fruit gum			x	49.7	50.3	Yes
Sweet #4, fruit gum	Raspberry juice		x	50.4	49.6	?
Sweet #5, fruit gum	Raspberry juice		x	51.0	49.0	?
Sweet #6, lollipops			x	50.4	49.6	Yes
Sweet #7, fruit gum			x	50.2	49.8	Yes
Sweet #8, fruit gum			x	50.4	49.6	Yes
Fruit bar #1	Raspberry 1.3%	x		49.2	50.8	No
Yoghurt #1	Raspberry 14%			100	0	Yes
Yoghurt #2	Raspberry 7.5%			100	0	Yes
Yoghurt #3	Raspberry 1.7%	x		49.5	50.5	No
Yoghurt #4	Raspberry 7%	x		100	0	Yes
Yoghurt #5	Raspberry 8%	x		100	0	Yes
Yoghurt #6	Raspberry 6%			100	0	yes

MS source 230°C, MS Quad 150°C. The mass spectrometer was used in Electron Ionization (EI) mode, using Scan mode (*m/z* 40–400) for the method optimizing part using Nist library for identification of compounds. The mass spectrometer was operated in Single Ion Monitoring (SIM) for food samples, using *m/z* 121 as quantifier ion and 192, 136, and 93 as qualifiers to ensure the identity and purity of the peaks. Quality ratio control of the qualifiers were ±20% and quality control of the retention time was ±0.2 min. Samples were analyzed as single determinations, which were deemed sufficient because percentages of R-α-ionone close to 100 in the samples would indicate natural flavor whereas values close to 50 would indicate a synthetic flavor.

Results and Discussion

Before analyzing the samples, the analytical method was optimized in order to obtain a fast and reliable method for the documentation of the authenticity of raspberry flavor in food products. The optimization was performed using macerated raspberries as samples and included SPME fiber-coating selection and the influence of addition of sodium chloride to the samples. A full scan SPME GC-MS chromatogram of macerated raspberries, using a DVB/CAR/PDMS fiber is shown in Figure 1, where it appears that α-ionone and β-ionone are the highest peaks.

To study the influence of fiber coating on the SPME the following fiber types were selected, all coated on a fused silica fiber and with a length of 1 cm; divinylbenzene (DVB)/polydimethylsiloxane (PDMS) 65 μm coating, carboxen (CAR)/(PDMS) 75 μm coating and DVB/CAR/PDMS with 50 μm DVB coating/30 μm CAR on PDMS coating. Macerated raspberries were used as a basis model for the experiments. For this method optimizing study, only the ability to extract analytes from raspberries was investigated and the levels were therefore not quantified but based on comparison of peak areas and presented in Figure 2.

The three SPME fibers showed approximately similar abilities to extract the seven major chemical constituents from raspberry headspace. With the exception that octanol was not extracted by DVB/CAR/PDMS and CAR/PDMS. In addition β-phellandrene and nonanal were not extracted by CAR/PDMS. The DVB/CAR/PDMS fiber showed slightly better extraction efficiency for ionone and was therefore selected for the further studies.

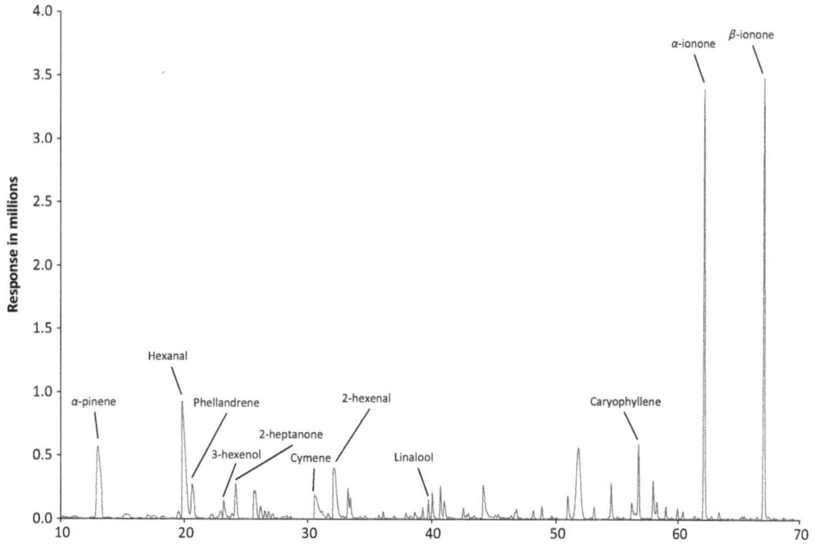

Figure 1. Full scan head space SPME GC-MS chromatogram of macerated raspberries, GC runtime 102 min.

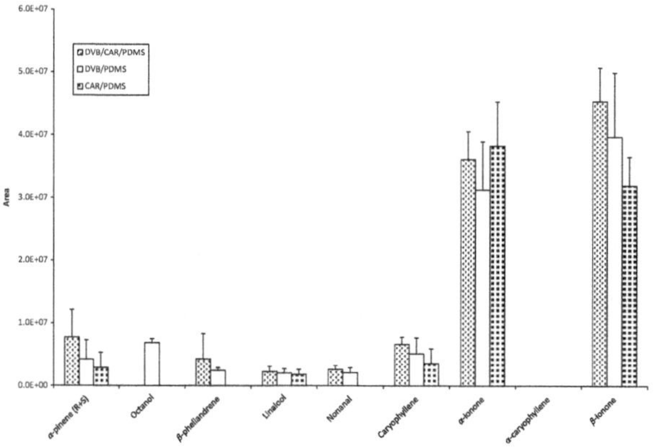

Figure 2. Peak areas for eight analytes extracted from raspberries with DVB/CAR/PDMS, DVB/PDMS, and CAR/PDMS SPME fibers.

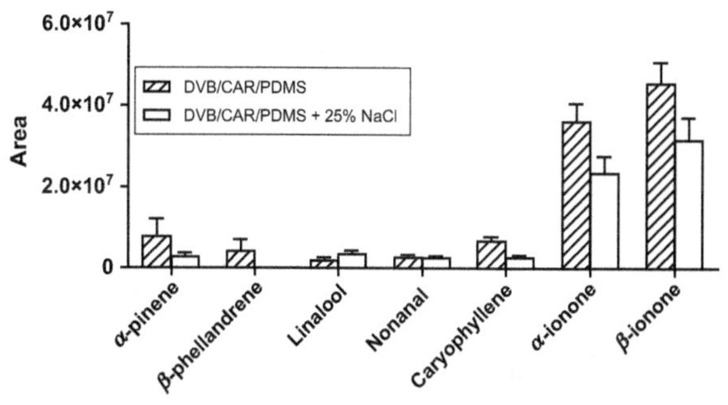

Figure 3. Peak area for seven analytes extracted from raspberries with DVB/CAR/PDMS SPME fiber with and without addition of NaCl.

Influence of addition of sodium chloride to samples

The effect of addition of sodium chloride to the matrix was investigated, as increased ionic strength usually improves the extraction efficiency of hydrophilic compounds (Kudlejova et al. 2012). Sodium chloride was added to the sample matrices to a concentration of 25 w/w % and analytes extracted with a SPME fiber coated with DVB/CAR/PDMS and presented in Figure 3.

From Figure 3 it is clear that addition of sodium chloride does not have a positive effect upon extraction of the majority of the analytes from raspberries. On the contrary it looks like the salt has a negative effect on the extraction especially for α-pinene, caryophyllene, α- and β-ionone. For the other compounds analyzed the effect was less pronounced. Only the extraction of linalool was a little higher when sodium chloride was added. Pawliszyn 2012 reported that the positive effect of salt increases with increased polarity of the analytes, which is in agreement with the results found in this study (Pawliszyn 2012).

The result for β-ionone is in agreement with the results of Yang and Peppard, who found that the extraction of β-ionone decreases with higher sodium chloride concentrations when extracted with a SPME fiber, coated with 100 μm PDMS (Yang and Peppard 1994).

Content of R-(E)-α-ionone and S-(E)-α-ionone in foods, beverages and sweets from the Danish market

For authenticity investigation of raspberry flavored foods, using head space SPME chiral GC-MS the most important compound is α-ionone. From the chromatogram in Figure 4, it can be seen that (S)-α-ionone is barely detectable in macerated raspberry (top) compared to the peak of

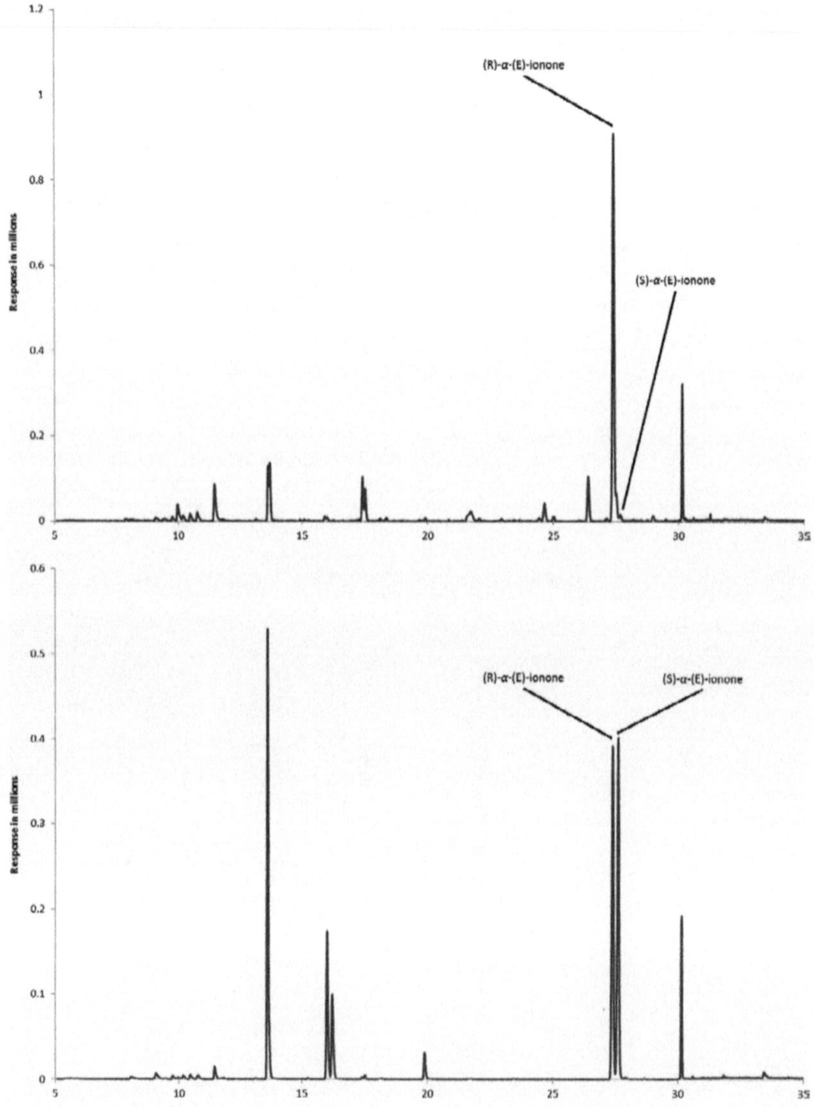

Figure 4. Chromatograms of raspberry jam containing primarily R-(E)-α-ionone (top) and of yoghurt containing synthetic raspberry aroma with both R-(E)-α-ionone and S-(E)-α-ionone (bottom).

(R)-α-ionone. This is in accordance with previously published results on the analyses of enantiomer ratios of α-ionone in raspberries showing that (R)-α-ionone constitutes more than 97% (Sewing et al., 2005; Ravid et al. 2010). On the contrary, synthetic raspberry aroma (Fig. 4 bottom) shows the presence of both enantiomers in almost equal amounts. Synthetic α-ionone can be added to natural raspberry flavor, that is, in order to fortify the flavor and/or reduce price. In that case, the enantiomer ratio will not be 50:50, but reflect the percentage of synthetic aroma added to the natural raspberry aroma and it would still be possible to detect (S)-α-ionone indicating a not purely natural flavor.

Twenty seven samples of food beverages and sweets from the Danish retail market were analyzed for enantiomer ratio of (E)-α-ionone using the described head space solid phase microextraction method, including chiral-gas chromatography combined with mass spectrometric detection, using the SIM mode. Table 1 present the results calculated as the percentage of R-(E)-α-ionone and S-(E)-α-ionone in all samples. Six samples of raspberry jam declared to contain between 35 and 50% fruit, all had a huge preponderance of the (R) enantiomer of α-ionone with the (S) enantiomer being barely detectable. These jams were all declared not to have any added aroma which the analyses confirmed.

Analyses of two out of five sodas declared to contain natural aroma only, showed that these contained only (R)-α-ionone which is in accordance with the declared content. The three sodas declared to contain aroma showed an enantiomer ratio of 50%, which is, also, in accordance with the declaration and confirmed that synthetic α-ionone had been added to the products.

The dried raspberries only contained the (R) enantiomer of α-ionone, so no synthetic α-ionone was added to this product. Six of the sweets samples had a 50:50 enantiomer ratio which is in accordance with the declared use of aroma in these samples. Two of the sweets were declared to contain raspberry juice concentrate, 5% as well as aroma. However, the content of ionone from this source must be very low as addition of raspberry juice containing exclusively the (R) enantiomer would have been expected to change the enantiomer ratio from the observed 50:50%. The fruit bar was declared to contain both 1.3% raspberry and natural aroma, however, the measured enantiomer ratio of 50:50% suggest that synthetic aroma was added to this product and accordingly the declaration is not compliant with legislation.

Finally, six yoghurt samples, declared to contain between 1.3% and 14% raspberries, were analyzed. Three of the samples were declared, in addition to raspberries, also to contain the natural aroma. For five of the raspberry yoghurt samples only the (R) enantiomer of α-ionone were found in the products indicating natural raspberries were used in the product. However, for yoghurt #3 declared to contain 1.7% raspberry and natural aroma, a 50:50 enantiomer ratio for R-α-ionone and S-α-ionone was observed indicating that synthetic α-ionone was added as aroma to this product contrary to the declared use of natural aroma.

Conclusions

A fast and simple headspace SPME-chiral-GC-MS method for analyses of authenticity of l raspberry flavor in foods has been developed and used to analyze samples of jams, sodas, sweets, fruits bars, dried raspberries and yoghurts. Raspberry jam, dried raspberries, and sodas declared to contain natural aroma all contained almost only R-α-ionone supporting the content of only naturally raspberry or naturally raspberry aroma used in the products. All sweets tested had an almost equal distribution between R-α-ionone and S-α-ionone indication that synthetic aroma was added to these products in agreement with the information from the declaration. For two out of the 27 products tested, the fruit bar and one of the raspberry yoghurts, both R-α-ionone and S-α-ionone was detected at an enantiomer ratio of 50% indicating the use of synthetic aroma in the products, which is in disagreement with the declared information on the products.

Acknowledgments

The authors thank Liljana Petrevska and Maud B. Andersen for skillful technical assistance.

Conflict of Interest

None declared.

References

Aprea, E., B. Franko, and C. Silvia. 2009. Investigation of volatile compounds in two raspberry cultivars by two headspace techniques: solid-phase microextraction/gas chromatography-mass spectrometry (SPME/GC-MS) and proton-transfer reaction-mass spectrometry (PTR-MS). J. Agric. Food Chem. 57:4011–4018.

Bernreuther, A., N. Christoph, and P. Schreier. 1989. Determination of the enantiomeric composition of γ-lactones in complex natural matrices using multidimentional capillary chromatography. J. Chromatogr. 481:363–367.

Cagliero, C., C. Bicchi, C. Cordero, P. Rubiolo, B. Sgorbini, and E. Liberto. 2012. Fast headspace-enantioselective GC–mass spectrometric-multivariate statistical method for routine authentication of flavoured fruit foods. Food Chem. 132:1071–1079.

Casabianca, H., and J. B. Graff. 1994. Enantiomeric and isotopic analysis of flavour compounds of some raspberry cultivars. J. Chromatogr. A 684:360–365.

European Parliament, C. of the E.U. 2008. Regulation (EC) No 1334/2008 of the European Parliament and of the Council of 16 December 2008 on flavourings and certain food ingredients with flavouring properties for use in and on foods and amending Council Regulation (EEC) No 1601/91, Regulations (EC, Available at http://eur-lex.europa.eu/LexUriServ/LexUriServ.do?uri=OJ:L:2008:354:0034:0050:en:PDF) (accessed 7 April 2013).

Guichard, E., A. Kustermann, and A. Mosandl. 1990. Chiral flavour compounds from apricots. Distribution of γ-lactone enantiomers and stereodifferentiation of di-hydroactinidiolide using multi-dimensional gas chromatography. J. Chromatogr. 498:396–401.

Kudlejova, L., S. Risticevic, and D. Vuckovic (2012). Sold-phase microextraction method development. Pp. 201–249 *in* J. Pawliszyn, ed., Handbook of solid phase microextraction. Elsevier, Waterloo, ON.

Malowicki, S. M. A., R. Martin, and M. C. Qian. 2008a. Volatile composition in raspberry cultivars grown in the Pacific northwest determined by stir bar sorptive extraction-gas chromatography-mass spectrometry. J. Agric. Food Chem. 56:4128–4133.

Malowicki, S. M. A., R. Martin, and M. C. Qian. 2008b. Comparison of sugar, acids and volatile composition in raspberry bushy dwarf virus-resistant transgenic raspberries and the wild type "meeker" (Rubus Idaeus L.). J. Agric. Food Chem. 56:6648–6655.

Pawliszyn, J. 2012. Theory of solid-phase microextraction. Pp. 13–59 *in* J. Pawliszyn, ed. Handbook of solid phase microextraction. Elsevier, London, UK. ISBN: 978-0-12-416017-0.

Ravid, U., M. Elkabetz, C. Zamir, K. Cohen, O. Larkov, and R. Aly. 2010. Authenticity assessment of natural fruit flavour compounds in foods and beverages by auto-HS-SPME stereoselective GC-MS. Flavour Fragr. J. 25:20–27.

Sewenig, S., D. Bullinger, U. Hener, and A. Hener. 2005. Comprehensive authentication of (E)-alpha(beta)-ionone from raspberries, using constant flow MDGC-C/P-IRMS and Enantio-MDGC-MS. J. Agric. Food Chem. 53:838–844.

Taylor, J. A., and S. T. Linforth. 2010. Food flavour technology. Blackwell Publishing Ltd., Oxford, United Kingdom. ISBN: 978-1-4051-8543-1.

Verzera, A., G. Tripodi, C. Condurso, G. Dima, and A. Marra. 2014. Chiral volatile compounds for the determination of orange honey authenticity. Food Control 39:237–243.

Werkhoff, P., W. Bretschneider, M. Guntert, R. Hopp, and H. Surbug. 1991. Chirospecific analysis in flavor and essential oil chemistry. Z. Lebensm. Unters. Forsch. 192:111–115.

Yang, X. G., and T. Peppard. 1994. Solid-phase microextraction for flavor analysis. J. Agric. Food Chem. 42:1925–1930.

3

Antioxidant activity and phenolic profiles of the wild currant *Ribes magellanicum* from Chilean and Argentinean Patagonia

Felipe Jiménez-Aspee[1], Samanta Thomas-Valdés[1], Ayla Schulz[1], Ana Ladio[2], Cristina Theoduloz[3] & Guillermo Schmeda-Hirschmann[1]*

[1]Laboratorio de Química de Productos Naturales, Instituto de Química de Recursos Naturales, Universidad de Talca, Talca, Chile
[2]Laboratorio Ecotono, INIBIOMA (CONICET)-Universidad Nacional del Comahue, Bariloche, Río Negro, Argentina
[3]Laboratorio de Cultivo Celular, Facultad de Ciencias de la Salud, Universidad de Talca, Talca, Región del Maule, Chile

Keywords
Antioxidant, comparative profiles, HPLC-DAD-MS, Patagonian currant, *Ribes magellanicum*

Correspondence
Guillermo Schmeda-Hirschmann, Laboratorio de Química de Productos Naturales, Instituto de Química de Recursos Naturales, Universidad de Talca, casilla 746, Talca, Chile.

E-mail: schmeda@utalca.cl

Funding Information
Financial support from FONDECYT Project N° 1120096 and CONICYT-PCHA/Doctorado Nacional/2013-21130048 (F. Jiménez-Aspee) and CONICYT-PCHA/Doctorado Nacional/2013-63130042 (S. Thomas- Valdés) are kindly acknowledged.

Abstract

The Patagonian currant *Ribes magellanicum* is highly valued due to its pleasant flavor and sweet taste. The aim of this study was to characterize its constituents and to assess their antioxidant and cytoprotective properties. For the fruit phenolic- enriched extract (PEE), total phenolics (TP), total flavonoids (TF), and antioxidant activity (DPPH, Ferric reducing antioxidant power (FRAP), and Trolox equivalent antioxidant activity (TEAC)) were determined. Argentinean samples presented better activity in the DPPH and FRAP assays. Best cytopro-tection against oxidative stress induced by H_2O_2 in AGS cells was found in one Argentinean sample at 500 μg mL^{-1} (65.7%). HPLC MS/MS analysis allowed the tentative identification of 59 constituents, including eight anthocyanins, 11 conjugates of caffeic- , ferulic- , and coumaric acid, and 38 flavonoids, most of them quercetin and kaempferol derivatives. Argentinean samples showed a more complex pattern of anthocyanins, hydroxycinnamic acids (HCA), and flavonoids. Cyanidin rhamnoside hexoside and cyanidin hexoside were the main anthocya-nins, accounting for 35 and 55% for the Argentinean and 60 and 27% for the ripe Chilean fruits. HCA content was about three times higher in Argentinean samples. The phenolic profiles of Chilean and Argentinean *Ribes magellanicum* show remarkable differences in chemical composition with higher HCA and flavonoid content in Argentinean samples.

Introduction

High intake of fruits and vegetables is inversely related to the incidence of several pathologies, including obesity (González-Castejón and Rodriguez-Casado 2011), age-related neurodegenerative diseases (Shukitt-Hale et al. 2008), cardiovascular diseases, diabetes, and certain types of cancer (Boeing et al. 2012). These health benefits have been attributed to the presence of polyphenols, especially flavonols, anthocyanins, proanthocyanidins, and phenolic acids (Liu 2003). Polyphenols possess a high antioxidant potential which may help to decrease or repair oxidative stress generated during physiological processes (Hollman 2001). Wild or cultivated berries are recognized as health-promoting fruits due to their high content of antioxidant phytochemicals (Zafra-Stone et al. 2007). Wild plants are often incorporated into traditional medicine or are used in a balanced diet, improving the state of well-being and reducing the risk of diseases. Nutraceuticals are generally defined as products that promote health in addition to their nutritional value. For this reason, it is relevant to identify, characterize and quantify the phytochemicals contained in these plants.

The fruits of the *Ribes* genus are gaining importance and are considered as promising crops with high economic value, especially since they are ranked second in consumer preferences after strawberries (Djordevic et al. 2010). The Patagonian region in South America provides a wide range of native plants due to the geographic and climatologic characteristics of its territory. The Patagonian wild currant (*Ribes magellanicum* Poir., Grossulariaceae) is a native species occurring in southern Chile and Argentina. This species has a long history of use among Amerindians of Patagonia and played a relevant role in their gathering for subsistence. It has a pleasant flavor and sweet taste with an intense purple color (Fig. 1). The fruits can be consumed fresh, in preserves and in syrups (Sparre 1984). In Chile and Argentina, these Patagonian currants are collected in the wild or cultivated in home gardens (Rapoport and Ladio 1999; Ladio et al. 2007; Eyssartier et al. 2011; Molares and Ladio 2012).

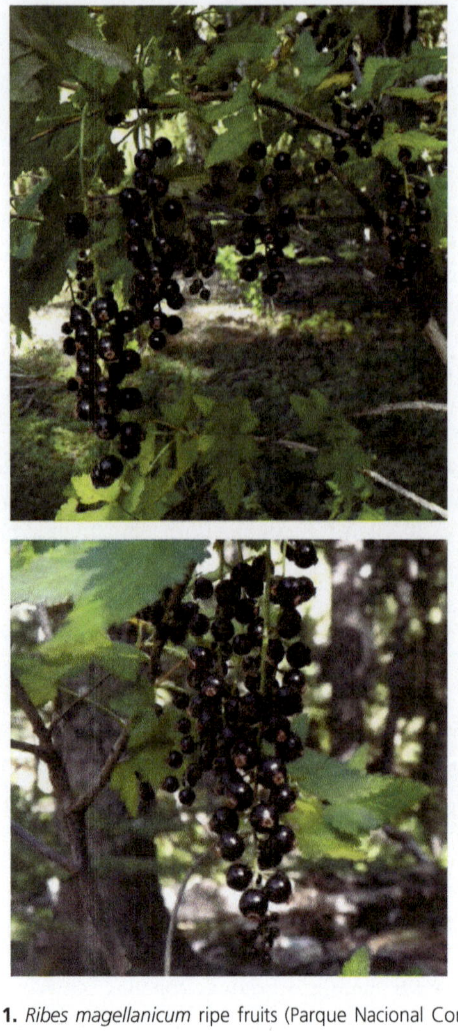

Figure 1. *Ribes magellanicum* ripe fruits (Parque Nacional Conguillio, Chile).

Scarce information has been published regarding the chemical composition and nutritional characteristics of Patagonian native berries. In *R. magellanicum* collected in southern Chile, the 3-glucoside, and 3-rutinoside derivatives of cyanidin are predominant among anthocyanins (Ruiz et al. 2013). Caffeoylquinic acid, feruloylquinic- and coumaroylquinic acids, quercetin hexoside, rutinoside and acetyl-derivatives, kaempferol-acetylhexoside and rutinoside derivatives, myricetin, and kaempferol were found in this berry in southern Chile (Ruiz et al. 2015). However, no information was found regarding phenolic profiling from Argentinean *R. magellanicum*.

While little is known about the wild Patagonian currant *R. magellanicum*, the chemical profiling of European currants has been extensively described, mainly for *Ribes nigrum* (black currants) and *Ribes rubrum* (red currants) (Määttä et al. 2003; Benvenuti et al. 2004; Anttonen and Karjalainen 2006; Kapasakalidis et al. 2009; Borges et al. 2010; Pinto et al. 2010; Gavrilova et al. 2011). *Ribes nigrum* contains *p*-coumaric, ferulic, and caffeic acid derivatives (Määttä et al. 2003; Gavrilova et al. 2011), as well as myricetin, quercetin, isorhamnetin, and kaempferol derivatives as the main flavonols (Zheng et al. 2012). *Ribes rubrum* presents caffeoyl and *p*-coumaroyl hexoside derivatives, rutin, (+)-catechin, and epigallocatechin (Gavrilova et al. 2011). Anthocyanins comprise up to 85% of the total phenolic content, whereas hydroxycinnamic acid derivatives just represent 1–6% of the total phenols in the currants (Gavrilova et al. 2011).

There is an increasing international interest in South American native berries, mainly due to their potential health benefits (Schreckinger et al. 2010). In this context, the aim of this work was to compare the chemical composition and antioxidant activity of *Ribes magellanicum* fruits from Chilean and Argentinean Patagonia. Following our studies on South American food plants, we now report the phenolic, flavonoid, and anthocyanin content and composition, antioxidant activity, and cytoprotection toward oxidative stress, as well as polyphenol profiling in *R. magellanicum*.

Materials and Methods

Chemicals

Folin-Ciocalteu phenol reagent, 2,4,6-tri(2-pyridyl)1,3,5-triazine (TPTZ), potassium chloride, sodium acetate, 1,1-diphenyl-2-picrylhydrazyl radical (DPPH), quercetin, gallic acid, L-glutamine, MTT, $AlCl_3$, and hydrogen peroxide were purchased from Sigma-Aldrich (St. Louis, MO). 2,2′-Azino-bis(3-ethylbenzothiazoline-6-sulfonic acid) diammonium salt

(ABTS), 6-hydroxy-2,5,7,8-tetramethylchroman-2-carboxylic acid (Trolox), potassium persulfate, sodium carbonate, sodium bicarbonate, acetic acid, $FeCl_3.6H_2O$, HPLC-grade methanol, and formic acid were purchased from Merck (Darmstadt, Germany). Quercetin-3-glucoside (99.14%), kaempferol-3-glucoside (99.37%), quercetin-3-glucuronide (95.91%), cyanidin-3-glucoside (99.21%), cyanidin-3-rutinoside (98.02%), delphinidin-3-glucoside (98.02%), *trans*-caffeic acid (99.81%), and 3-caffeoylquinic acid (98.95%) were from PhytoLab GmbH (Vestenbergsgreuth, Germany). Ultrapure water was obtained using a Barnsted EasyPure water filter (Thermo Scientific, Marietta, OH). Culture medium Ham F-12, penicillin, streptomycin, and fetal bovine serum (FBS) were obtained from Invitrogen Corp. Chemicals (Grand Island, NY).

Fruit material and sample preparation

Argentinean fruits were collected at the Provincia de Rio Negro, Arroyo Casa de Piedra (41°07′07″S; 71°27′56″W) (ripe fruits) (1) and Laguna Verde, Villa La Angostura (40°45′55″S; 71°38′41″W) (turning fruits) (2). Chilean fruits were collected at the Region de La Araucanía, Parque Nacional Conguillio (39°29′36″S; 71°41′53″W) (ripe fruits) (3) and Reserva Nacional Malalcahuello (38°25′13″S; 71°36′48″W) (turning fruits) (4). The collection places are shown in Figure 2. The samples from Chile were identified by Prof. Patricio Peñailillo (Universidad de Talca herbarium), whereas samples from Argentina by Prof. Ana Ladio, Universidad Nacional del Comahue.

Fruits were homogenized in a blender and extracted four times with MeOH:formic acid (99:1 v/v) in a 1:3 v/v homogenate:solvent ratio in the dark under sonication (15 min each). The combined extracts were dried under reduced pressure at 37°C. To obtain the phenolic-enriched extract (PEE), the samples were adsorbed into Amberlite XAD-7 resin. The Amberlite resin was preconditioned as follows: the resin was washed with 0.1N NaOH, rinsed with distilled water, washed with 0.1N HCl and rinsed with distilled water to remove acid, and stored with $MeOH:H_2O$ (1:9 v/v) until use. The concentrated MeOH extract was dissolved in water, filtrated and mixed with Amberlite XAD-7 in a 1:5 (extract:Amberlite) ratio and continuously stirred for 40 min. The resin was filtered, washed with water and phenolics were desorbed with MeOH. The MeOH solution was evaporated under reduced pressure at 40°C and freeze-dried for analysis, obtaining the phenolic enriched extract (PEE). The accuracy of the extraction method was evaluated by spiking a fruit sample with standard solutions of chlorogenic acid

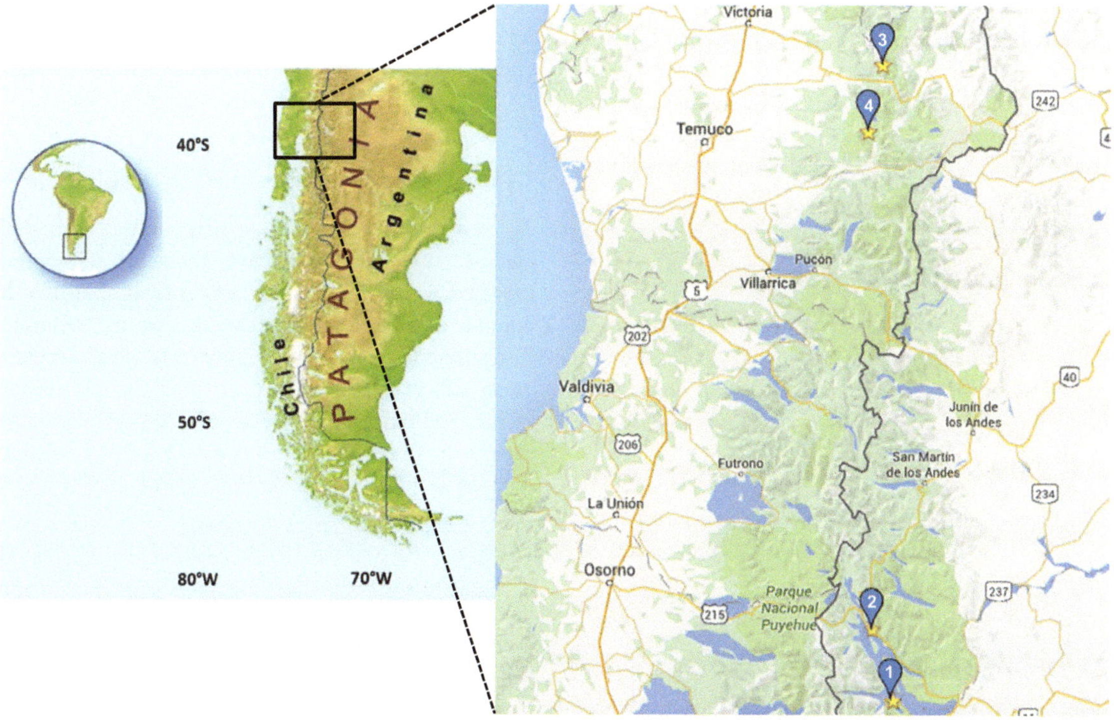

Figure 2. Map of Patagonia showing the geographic collection places of *Ribes magellanicum* fruits. Argentina: (1) Arroyo Casa de Piedra, (2) Laguna Verde, Villa La Angostura (Parque Nacional Nahuel Huapi). Chile: (3) Reserva Nacional Malalcahuello, (4) Parque Nacional Conguillio. Source: Google maps.

(78.9 mg Kg^{-1}), cyanidin-3-rutinoside (6.9 mg Kg^{-1}), and kaempferol-3-glucoside (6.9 mg Kg^{-1}). The recovery percentages of the standards were calculated by means of HPLC-DAD.

Total phenolic and total flavonoid content

The TP content was determined by the Folin–Ciocalteu method with slight modifications (Jiménez-Aspee et al. 2014). Stock solutions of 5 g L^{-1} were prepared in MeOH:H_2O 1:1. For TP, the results are expressed as grams of gallic acid equivalents per kilogram PEE (g GAE kg^{-1}). The TF content was determined as described by Simirgiotis et al. (2013). For TF, results are expressed as grams of catechin equivalents per kilogram PEE (g CatE kg^{-1}).

Scavenging of the 2,2-diphenyl-1-picryl hydrazyl

The free radical-scavenging activity of the samples was determined by the discoloration of the free radical DPPH (20 mg L^{-1}) as previously described (Jiménez-Aspee et al. 2014). Extracts were dissolved in MeOH: H_2O (1:1) to a final concentration of 300 mg L^{-1}. Serial dilutions of the stock solutions of each sample were prepared in 96-well plates. Methanol was used as the negative control and quercetin as the reference compound. Absorbance was measured at 517 nm in a universal microplate reader (Biotek Instruments Inc., ELx 800, Winooski, VT). The concentration of the extract that scavenges the DPPH radical by 50% (SC_{50}) is expressed as milligrams of PEE per liter of solution (mg L^{-1}) and was calculated using the OriginPro 8.0 software (OriginLab Corporation, Northampton, MA).

Ferric reducing antioxidant power

The FRAP assay was performed as previously described (Simirgiotis et al. 2013; Jiménez-Aspee et al. 2014). Samples were dissolved in MeOH:H_2O (1:1) to a final concentration of 300 mg L^{-1}. Absorbance was read at 593 nm using a Thermo Spectronic Helios Alfa spectrophotometer (Cambridge, U.K.). Quantification was performed using a standard curve of the antioxidant Trolox. Results are expressed as millimol Trolox equivalents per kilogram of PEE (mmol TE kg^{-1}).

Trolox equivalent antioxidant activity

ABTS radical-scavenging activity was determined according to Nenadis et al. (2004). The ABTS* was generated by mixing ABTS solution with potassium persulfate. The solution was stored in the dark for 16 h, and diluted with methanol to a final absorbance of 0.700 ± 0.050 at 734 nm. Determinations were carried out by mixing ABTS* with fresh standard (1 mmol L^{-1} Trolox) or PEE (100, 150, 200, 250, and 300 mg L^{-1}). Absorbance was read at 734 nm after 6 min. Results are expressed as μmol Trolox equivalents per gram of PEE (μmol L^{-1} TE g^{-1}).

AGS cell culture

Human epithelial gastric cells AGS (ATCC CRL-1739) were grown in Ham F-12 medium supplemented with 1 mmol L^{-1} L-glutamine, 1.5 g L^{-1} sodium bicarbonate, 100 g L^{-1} heat-inactivated fetal bovine serum (FBS), 100 IU mL^{-1} penicillin, and 100 mg L^{-1} streptomycin. Cells were grown as monolayers in a humidified incubator with 5% CO_2 in air at 37°C.

Cytotoxicity assay

Cytotoxicity values (IC_{50}, μg mL^{-1}) were required as a reference to determine the working concentrations of the PEEs in the cytoprotection experiment. Confluent cultures of AGS cells were treated during 24 h with the medium containing the lyophilized PEE samples at concentrations ranging from 0 up to 1000 mg L^{-1}. The samples were dissolved in the medium supplemented with 20 g L^{-1} FBS. Cells treated with the medium only were used as controls. Cell viability was determined at the end of the incubation by means of the MTT reduction assay (Cheli and Baldi 2011), and the concentration that inhibits 50% of cell viability was calculated (IC_{50}).

Cytoprotection against H_2O_2-induced stress

The cytoprotective activity of the extract was evaluated against H_2O_2-induced stress, following the previously reported methodology (Jimenez-Aspee et al. 2016). Briefly, confluent cultures of AGS cells were treated overnight with different concentrations of *Ribes magellanicum* PEEs (0, 62.5, 125, 250, and 500 mg L^{-1}). Extracts were dissolved in the medium supplemented with 20 g L^{-1} FBS and antibiotics. At the end of the incubation, culture medium was completely removed via vacuum aspiration. Then, oxidative stress was induced with 442 mg L^{-1} H_2O_2 for 2 h. The H_2O_2 solution was prepared using the medium without any supplements. Untreated cells were used as 100% viability controls. Cells treated with H_2O_2 only served as damage control. Quercetin was used as the reference compound (Heo et al. 2008). After the oxidative stress challenge, cell viability was determined by means of MTT reduction assay (Cheli and Baldi 2011). Each concentration was tested in quintuplicate and experiments were repeated twice. Results are expressed as a percentage of the viability control.

HPLC-DAD analysis

The PEEs were analyzed by HPLC coupled to a diode array detector to compare the samples and set the conditions for HPLC-DAD-MS/MS studies. The HPLC system used for DAD analysis was a Shimadzu equipment (Shimadzu Corporation, Kyoto, Japan) consisting of a LC-20AT pump, a SPD-M20A UV diode array detector, CTO-20AC column oven and a LabSolution software. A MultoHigh 100 RP 18-5 μ (250 × 4.6 mm) column (CS-Chromatographie Service GmbH, Langerwehe, Germany) maintained at 25 °C was used. The HPLC analyses were performed using a linear gradient solvent system consisting of 1% formic acid in water (A) and acetonitrile (B) as follows: 90% A to 75% A over 30 min, followed by 75% A to 90% A from 30 to 50 min, and finalizing with 90% A for 5 min. The flow rate was 1 mL min^{-1} and the volume injected was 20 μL. The compounds were monitored at 254, 320, 350, and 520 nm and spectra from 200 to 600 nm were recorded for peak characterization. The results of the HPLC-DAD chromatograms were compared with the HPLC-MS analysis. The compounds were identified based on the elution profile, retention time, UV, and mass spectra.

Quantification of main anthocyanins, hydroxycinnamic acids, and flavonols

Quantification of the main phenolics was carried out by HPLC-DAD using external calibration curves prepared with pure standards. For anthocyanins, two curves were prepared using the main anthocyanins occurring in the sample: cyanidin-3-glucoside (12.5–800 mg L^{-1}, $r = 0.9962$) and cyanidin-3-rutinoside (12.5–800 mg L^{-1}, $r = 0.9999$) and were measured at 520 nm. For hydroxycinnamic acids (HCA), a curve with 3-caffeoylquinic acid (10-800 mg L^{-1}, $r = 0.9990$) was carried out and measured at 320 nm. For flavonols, two curves were prepared using quercetin-3-glucoside (5–80 mg L^{-1}, $r = 0.9987$) and kaempferol-3-glucoside (5–80 mg L^{-1}, $r = 0.9997$), and measured at 350 nm. The samples were injected at 5 g L^{-1} twice and the peak areas at 320, 350, and 520 nm were determined. The peak areas were quantified through comparison with the corresponding calibration curve and results are expressed as mg equivalents of the corresponding standard per kg of PEE. For comparative purposes, an internal standard was added to samples in parallel before HPLC analysis. For HCA the internal standard was *trans*-caffeic acid (100 mg L^{-1}), for flavonols the internal standard was quercetin-3-glucuronide (40 mg L^{-1}), and for anthocyanins the internal standard was delphinidin-3-glucoside (100 mg L^{-1}). Previous HPLC analyses of the extracts were carried out to establish that these compounds were not detectable in the PEE.

Identification of phenolics by HPLC-ESI-MS/MS

Mass spectra were recorded using an HPLC HP1100 (Agilent Technologies Inc., Santa Clara, CA) liquid chromatography system connected through a split to an Esquire 4000 Ion Trap LC/MSystem (Bruker Daltoniks, Germany). Full-scan mass spectra were measured between *m/z* 150 and 2000 μ. Mass spectrometry data were acquired in the negative mode for all phenolic compounds except anthocyanins, which was acquired in the positive ion mode. Nitrogen was used as nebulizer gas at 27.5 psi, 350 °C and at a flow rate of 8 L min^{-1}. The mass spectrometric conditions were as follows: electrospray needle, 4000 V; end plate offset, −500 V; skimmer 1, 56.0 V; skimmer 2, 6.0 V; capillary exit offset, 84.6 V; and capillary exit, 140.6 V. Collision-induced dissociation (CID) spectra were obtained with a fragmentation amplitude of 1.00 V (MS/MS) using helium as the collision gas.

Statistical analysis

Determinations of TP, TF, DPPH, and FRAP were performed in triplicate and results are expressed as mean values ± SD. For the TEAC assay, a curve was plotted for each sample and a correlation coefficient with 95% confidence limit was established. Experiments with AGS cells were carried out twice using different cell preparations. Each concentration was tested in quintuplicate. Statistical differences between different treatments and their respective control were determined by one-way analysis of variance (ANOVA) and Dunnett's multiple comparison test. The level of significance was set at $P < 0.05$. The Spearman's correlation coefficient for nonparametric data with a significance level of $P \leq 0.05$ was used to determine the relationships among variables. Additionally, a multivariate statistical method was applied to the data set. The chemical descriptors for *Ribes* samples were: TP, TF, quantified phenolics, DPPH, and FRAP. Analyses were carried out using the software SPSS 14.0 (IBM, Armonk, NY) and the statistical package Statistica 12.7.207.0 (Dell Inc., Tulsa, OK).

Results and Discussion

Four *R. magellanicum* collections, including samples from Argentina and Chile, were assessed for TP and TF content, DPPH, FRAP, and TEAC antioxidant activity, cytoprotective effect against oxidative stress-induced toxicity, and phenolic composition. The PEE yield in terms of fresh fruit was as follows (in g kg^{-1}): Arroyo Casa de Piedra: 8.5; Laguna Verde, Villa La Angostura: 6.2; Parque Nacional Conguillio: 17.3; Reserva Nacional Malalcahuello: 3.0. The recovery of phenolic compounds was 117.21% for chlorogenic acid, 85.16% for cyanidin-3-rutinoside and 78.44% for kaempferol-3-glucoside. According to Burin et al. (2011) these ranges of recovery would indicate that the extraction method used was acceptable for the quantification of these compounds.

Total phenolic, total flavonoid content, and antioxidant activity

The TP and TF values were higher for ripe Argentinean fruits (320.0 g GAE kg^{-1} and 164.0 g CatE kg^{-1} compared with 117.0 g GAE kg^{-1} and 48.6 g CatE kg^{-1} for the ripe Chilean sample, respectively) (Table 1). When comparing Argentinean and Chilean *R. magellanicum*, samples showed large differences regarding antioxidant activity (Table 1). In the Argentinean collection of Arroyo Casa de Piedra, DPPH, FRAP, and TEAC values were of 6.2 mg L^{-1}, 4006.3 mmol TE kg^{-1} PEE, and 2856.9 μmol L^{-1} TE g^{-1} PEE, respectively. In the Chilean fruits, the best activity was found in the Parque Nacional Conguillio sample with a SC_{50} of 22.9 mg L^{-1} in the DPPH, 1182.4 mmol TE kg^{-1} PEE in the FRAP, and 1577.7 μmol L^{-1} TE g^{-1} PEE in the TEAC assay. According to Ruiz et al. (2013), the antioxidant effect from *R. magellanicum* was 64.1 μmol TE g^{-1} fresh fruit in the TEAC assay, whereas in the CUPRAC assay the value was 71.16 μmol TE g^{-1} fresh fruit (Ruiz et al. 2015). Among the Chilean Patagonian berries *R. magellanicum* showed the best CUPRAC activity and one of the best TEAC activities (Ruiz et al. 2013).

Cytoprotection against chemical oxidative damage

Under our assay conditions, PEEs were devoid of toxicity toward AGS cells, with IC_{50} values >1000 mg L^{-1}. In MRC-5 cells a 10,000 mg L^{-1} *Ribes nigrum* extract concentration induced 20% decrease in cell viability and was selected for further experiments (Jia et al. 2014). We selected 500 mg L^{-1} of PEE for the following studies as the highest concentration. *Ribes magellanicum* PEEs showed a significant cytoprotective dose-dependent effect against oxidative damage induced by H_2O_2 in AGS cells. Hydrogen peroxide (442 mg L^{-1}) caused a significant decrease in cell viability (57.3%) compared to untreated controls. Exogenous H_2O_2 can enter cells inducing cytotoxicity due to its high membrane permeability, and through Fenton reaction can form highly reactive ·OH species causing oxidative injury in cells (Halliwell et al. 1992; Halliwell 1994). The positive control quercetin (100 mg L^{-1}) did not protect cells from oxidative damage. From the Argentinean samples, Arroyo Casa de Piedra showed significant protective effect at 125 mg L^{-1} (20.0%), 250 mg L^{-1} (42.9%), and 500 mg L^{-1} (65.7%), compared with the H_2O_2 control (Fig. 3A). The sample from Villa La Angostura presented significant activity at 250 mg L^{-1} (22.9%) and 500 mg L^{-1} (42.9%) (Fig. 3A). From the Chilean samples, only the PEE from Conguillio presented significant activity at 250 mg L^{-1} (15.2%) and 500 mg L^{-1} (27.3%) (Fig. 3B).

Anthocyanins and other flavonoids may exert their protective antioxidant effects in humans before absorption into the systemic bloodstream by directly scavenging free radicals (Moskaug et al. 2005), thus protecting cells of the gastrointestinal tract (Halliwell et al. 2005). Black currant phenolics have previously demonstrated a protective effect against H_2O_2-induced oxidative stress in human fetal lung fibroblast MRC-5 cells (Jia et al. 2014), neuroblastoma SH-SY5Y human promyelocytic leukemia cells, and gastric cancer SGC-7901 cells (Ghosh et al. 2006). The authors attributed the improved viability of cells against H_2O_2 to the neutralization capabilities of black currant extracts against radical oxidants. Moreover, the extract was responsible for up-modulation of the antioxidant enzymes superoxide dismutase, catalase, and glutathione peroxidase (Jia et al. 2014). In a recent study

Table 1. Total phenolics (TP), total flavonoids (TF), and antioxidant activity of phenolic enriched extract (PEEs) from *Ribes magellanicum* from Argentina and Chile.

			Antioxidant activity		
Samples	TP (g GAE kg^{-1} PEE)	TF (g CatE kg^{-1} PEE)	DPPH (SC_{50} in mg PEE L^{-1})	FRAP (mmol TE kg^{-1} PEE)	TEAC (μmol L^{-1} TE g^{-1} PEE)
Argentina					
Arroyo Casa de Piedra	320.0 ± 0.0	164.0 ± 1.7	6.2 ± 0.3	4006.3 ± 106.5	2856.9
Laguna Verde, Villa La Angostura	59.0 ± 1.0	56.8 ± 0.3	10.6 ± 0.4	1616.3 ± 22.5	1414.3
Chile					
Parque Nacional Conguillio	117.0 ± 1.0	48.6 ± 0.3	22.9 ± 1.2	1182.4 ± 22.5	1577.7
Reserva Nacional Malalcahuello	48.0 ± 1.0	31.4 ± 0.6	24.2 ± 0.5	816.2 ± 15.0	1098.7

GAE, gallic acid equivalent; CatE, catechin equivalent; DPPH, diphenyl picryl hydrazyl radical; FRAP, ferric reducing antioxidant power; TEAC, Trolox equivalent antioxidant capacity; TE, Trolox equivalent. All determinations were carried out in triplicate and results are expressed as mean values ± SD.

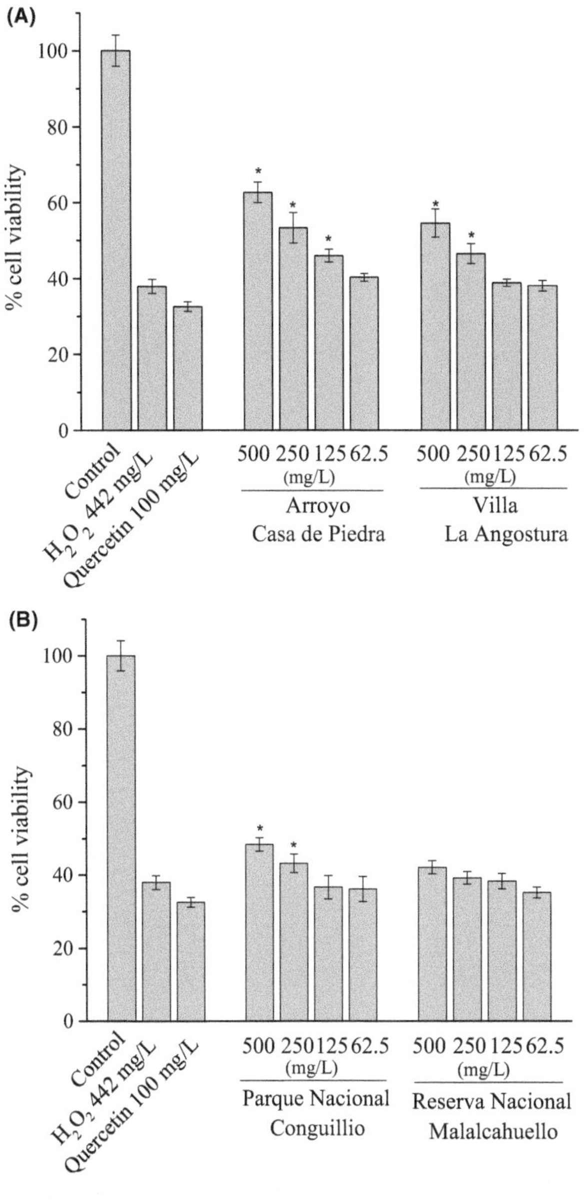

Figure 3. Cytoprotective effect of *Ribes magellanicum* PEEs against H_2O_2-induced oxidative stress on AGS cells. (A) Argentinean samples, (B) Chilean samples. The cell viability was determined by MTT reduction assay. Results are expressed as means ± SD ($n = 5$). $^*P < 0.05$ compared to H_2O_2 controls.

on another Patagonian berry, *Rubus geoides*, the fruit extract increased the intracellular GSH content and protected AGS cells against oxidative and dicarbonyl-induced stress (Jimenez-Aspee et al. 2016). In a study on the protective effect of *Rubus coreanus* on PC-12 cells against H_2O_2, the authors determined that cyanidin glycosides present in the fruit effectively diminished intracellular oxidative stress, whereas the nonanthocyanin fraction of the extract had no significant effect (Im et al. 2013). Our results show that the Argentinean samples were the most effective in preventing oxidative damage in human gastric epithelial AGS cells.

HPLC-DAD and HPLC-MS/MS analysis

All PEEs were compared by HPLC-DAD to get an insight into the chemical diversity of *R. magellanicum* fruits and to disclose similarities and differences in the composition according to the collection place and ripening stage. The HPLC chromatograms (at 254 nm) of ripe Argentinean and Chilean fruits are presented in Figure 4, whereas Figure 5 shows the HPLC trace of anthocyanins detected at 520 nm. HPLC MS/MS analysis allowed the tentative identification of 59 constituents, including anthocyanins, hydroxycinnamic acids, and flavonols. The tentative identification of the compounds is summarized in Table 2.

Anthocyanins

Two main anthocyanins were observed in the HPLC-DAD chromatograms of the ripe fruits (Fig. 5), showing UV maxima of 517 nm, in agreement with cyanidin derivatives. Positive ion MS allowed the identification of several minor constituents based on the selected ion chromatograms and MS/MS data. The main anthocyanins **17** and **18,** as well as compound **30** and **57,** showed in the MS/MS spectra a *m/z* ion at 287 amu, indicative of cyanidin. The compound **17** losses a deoxyhexose (146 amu) and a hexose (162 amu), whereas **18** showed the loss of 162 amu (hexose), in agreement with cyanidin rhamnosyl hexoside and cyanidin hexoside, respectively. The compound **57** showing the loss of hexose and additional fragments leading to cyanidin was tentatively identified as cyanidin hexoside derivative, whereas compound **30** losses 190 amu leading to cyanidin and was assigned as cyanidin derivative. Compounds **19** and **36** were minor constituents presenting in the MS/MS spectra a *m/z* ion at 303 amu, in agreement with delphinidin derivatives. The compound **19** shows the loss of 162 amu (hexose), whereas **36** losses a deoxyhexose (146 amu) and a hexose (162 amu). The compounds were assigned as delphinidin hexoside and delphinidin rhamnosyl hexoside, respectively. The MS^2 of compounds **32** and **33** shows a *m/z* ion at 317 and 331 amu, confirmed by selected ion chromatogram, in agreement with petunidin and malvidin derivatives, respectively. In *R. nigrum* four major anthocyanins distributed between cyanidin and delphinidin derivatives are responsible for more than 97% of total anthocyanin content (Slimestad and Solheim 2002) and are major contributors to the antioxidant activity (Borges et al. 2010). In *R. magellanicum* from southern Chile, Ruiz et al. (2013) reported the occurrence of delphinidin 3-glucoside and

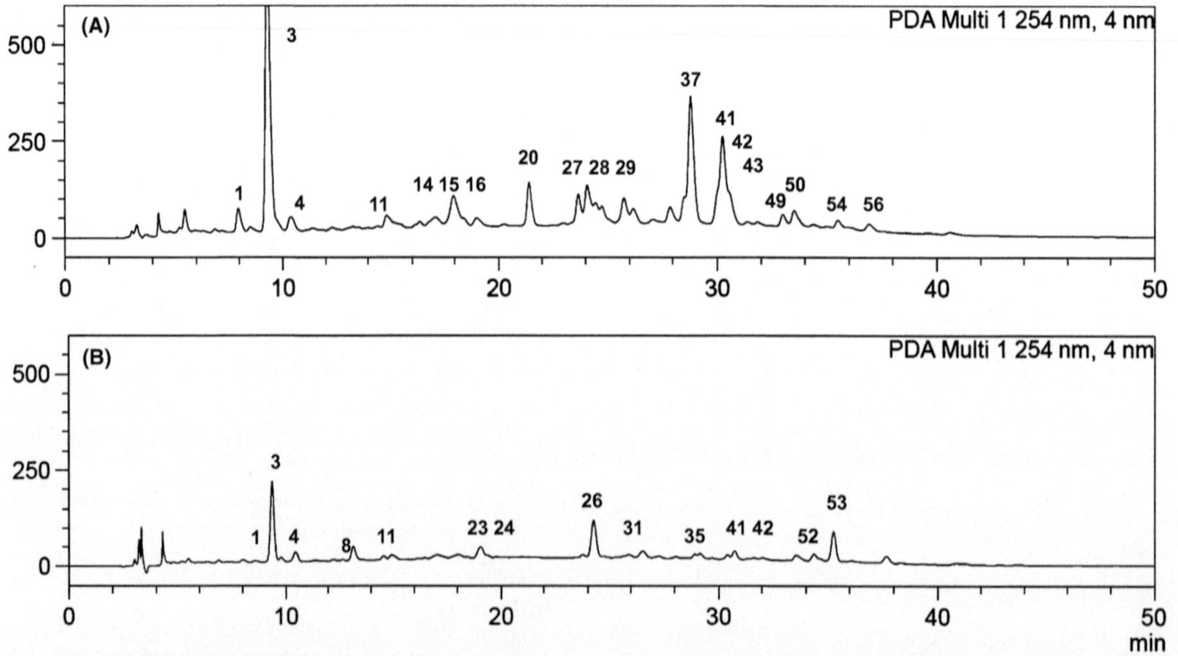

Figure 4. Representative HPLC-DAD chromatograms of *Ribes magellanicum* PEE at 254 nm. (A) Arroyo Casa de Piedra, Argentina; (B) Parque Nacional Conguillio, Chile. Peak numbers refer to Table 2.

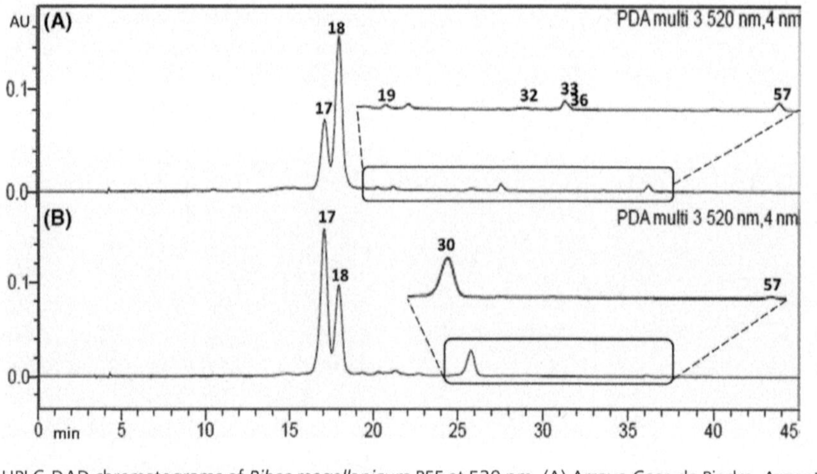

Figure 5. Representative HPLC-DAD chromatograms of *Ribes magellanicum* PEE at 520 nm. (A) Arroyo Casa de Piedra, Argentina; (B) Parque Nacional Conguillio, Chile. Peak numbers refer to Table 2.

3-rutinoside as minor anthocyanins and cyanidin 3-glucoside and 3-rutinoside as main compounds.

Hydroxycinnamic acids

Eleven hydroxycinnamic acid derivatives were detected in the *R. magellanicum* samples, including eight caffeic-, two ferulic-, and one coumaric acid conjugates. Selected ion chromatograms allowed clear identification of caffeoyl, coumaroyl, and feruloyl derivatives based on the *m/z* ions at 179, 163, and 193 amu, respectively. Compounds **1**, **3**, **6**, and **10** presented UV spectra compatible with caffeoylquinic acid/chlorogenic acid and a pseudomolecular ion of *m/z* 353 with product ions at 191 and 179 amu, respectively, and were characterized as caffeoylquinic acid isomers. Compound **3** was the main caffeoylquinic acid in all the samples, presenting MS^1 of 353, MS^2 191 and 135, and MS^3 of 172 and 127, compatible with 3-caffeoylquinic acid (Clifford et al. 2003). Compound **4** was identified as caffeic acid and compounds **5** and **8**,

Table 2. Tentative identification of phenolics in *Ribes magellanicum* fruits from Argentina and Chile by HPLC-DAD-ESI-MS.

Peak	Rt (min)	λ max (nm)	MW	$[M + H]^+$ or $[M - H]^-$	+/– ions	MS/MS	Tentative identification
1	8.4	324, 300, 238	354	353	–	191, 179	Caffeoyl quinic acid
2	8.5	324, 290 sh, 238	730	729	–	353, 179	Caffeoyl quinic acid derivative
3	8.8–8.9	325, 290 sh, 239	354	353	–	191, 179, 135	3-Caffeoyl quinic acid[1]
4	9.8	330, 215	180	179	–	134	Caffeic acid derivative
5	10.3		342	341	–	179	Caffeoyl hexoside
6	10.5	320 sh 281, 240	354	353	–	191, 179	Caffeoyl quinic acid isomer
7	10.9		290	289	–	245	Catechin/Epicatechin
8	12.6		342	341	–	179	Caffeoyl hexoside
9	13.7		464	463	–	417, 301	Q-hexoside
10	14.3	330 sh, 281, 240	354	353	–	191, 179, 173	Caffeoyl quinic acid isomer
11	14.6		368	367	–	193	Feruloyl quinic acid
12	16.0		368	367	–	193	Feruloyl quinic acid
13	15.9–16.1		448	447	–	285	K-hexoside
14	16.1		594	593	–	285	K-rhamnosidehexoside
15	16.4		466	465	–	285	K-derivative
16	16.8		594	593	–	447, 285	K-hexosiderhamnoside
17	16.4–17.3	517, 280	593	594	+	449, 287	Cyanidin rhamnosyl hexoside
18	18.7	517, 280	450	449	+	287	Cyanidin glucoside
19	20.1		466	465	+	303	Delphinidin hexoside isomer
20	20.6–20.8	352, 300 sh, 272	770	771	–	609, 591, 505, 301	Q-dihexosylrhamnoside
21	21.0		776	775	–	467, 313,163	Coumaroyl hexoside rhamnoside derivative
22	21.1		449	449	–	285	K derivative
23	21.3		626	625	–	463, 301	Q-dihexoside
24	21.5		610	609	–	463, 316	Myr dipentoside
25	21.9		742	741	–	609, 591, 475, 301	Q-pentoside derivative
26	22.3	353, 300 sh, 270	610	609	–	463, 301	Q-hexosiderhamnoside
27	23.1		626	625	–	463, 301	Q-dihexoside
28	24.1		656	625	–	316	Myr hexoside pentoside
29	24.6		480	479	–	316, 179	Myr hexoside
30	24.6		478	477	+	287	Cyanidin derivative
31	25.4–25.6		610	609	–	463, 343, 301	Q-rhamnoside hexoside
32	25.5		620	619	+	487, 317	Petunidin derivative
33	27.8		952	951	+	634, 557, 476, 331	Malvidin rhamnoside derivative
34	28.0–28.3	353, 300 sh, 270	610	609	–	463, 301	Q-hexoside rhamnoside
35	28.1–28.4		464	463	–	316, 179	Myr pentoside
36	28.1		612	611	+	465, 303	Delphinidin rhamnosyl hexoside
37	28.5		464	463	–	301	Q-hexoside
38	29.1–29.2	348, 300 sh, 296	566	565	–	433, 301	Q-dipentoside
39	29.3–29.4		610	609	–	301	Q-hexoside rhamnoside
40	29.5		915	914	–	895, 771, 447, 284	K-trihexoside conjugate
41	29.5–29.6	348, 297	448	447	–	285	K-hexoside
42	29.7		464	463	–	301	Q-hexoside
43	29.8–29.9		580	579	–	447, 429, 285	K-pentoside hexoside
44	30.4		594	593	–	447, 285	K-rhamnoside hexoside
45	30.4–30.5		610	609	–	447, 285	K-dihexoside
46	30.5		652	651	–	593, 301	Q-conjugate
47	30.8		506	505	–	301	Q-hexoside monoacetate
48	32.0	344, 270	594	593	–	285	K-coumaroyl hexoside
49	32.5		478	477	–	433, 315	Isorhamnetin hexoside
50	32.9	333, 267	434	433	–	301	Ellagic acid pentoside
51	33.5		550	549	–	399, 285	K-conjugate
52	33.7		464	463	–	301	Q-hexoside
53	34.5		448	447	–	301	K-hexoside
54	34.7		432	431	–	269	Apigenin hexoside
55	35.9		490	489	–	285	K-hexoside monoacetate
56	36.1		418	417	–	285	K-pentoside

(*Continued*)

Table 2. Continued.

Peak	Rt (min)	λ max (nm)	MW	[M + H]+ or [M – H]−	+/– ions	MS/MS	Tentative identification
57	36.3	517, 280	818	817	+	655, 449, 369, 287	Cyanidin hexoside derivative
58	43.1–43.2		286	285	–		K
59	43.5		302	301	–	178, 151	Q

K, Kaempferol; Q, Quercetin; Myr, Myricetin.
[1]According to Clifford et al. (2003).

with a pseudomolecular ion at *m/z* 341 and neutral loss of 162 amu, were assigned as caffeic acid hexosides. Both compounds differ either in the identity of the hexose or in the place of attachment of caffeic acid in the sugar moiety. The compound **2** with an UV spectrum compatible with a caffeoylquinic acid derivative shows a pseudomolecular ion of *m/z* 729 amu and fragments at 353 and 179 amu, compatible with a caffeoylquinic acid derivative. Compounds **11** and **12**, with a $[M - H]^-$ of 367 amu showed the neutral loss of 174 amu, leading to deprotonated ferulic acid and were assigned as feruloylquinic acid isomers. The coumaroyl hexoside pentoside derivative **21** was tentatively identified on the basis of the loss of 308 amu from the a $[M - H]^-$ pseudomolecular ion at 775 amu, leading to further fragments at 467, 313, and 163 amu, compatible with a conjugate of coumaric acid.

Four caffeoylquinic acid isomers, caffeoyl hexoside, two coumaroylquinic acids and two feruloylquinic acids were detected in a southern Chile (Patagonia) collection of *R. magellanicum* (Ruiz et al. 2015). The samples investigated in our work showed caffoylquinic acid as a main phenolic and 11 hydroxycinnamic acid derivatives, most of them related to caffeic acid.

Flavonol derivatives

The UV spectra of the main flavonoids in the samples shows maxima at 352-353 nm for compounds **20, 26,** and **34** and 344–348 nm for compounds **38, 41,** and **48,** suggesting the occurrence of glycosides of quercetin (Q) and quercetin or kaempferol (K), respectively.

Selected ion chromatograms and MS/MS experiments led to a base peak at *m/z* 301 or *m/z* 285, allowing the identification of the compounds into derivatives of Q or K, respectively. In the samples, 38 flavonoids were tentatively identified based on the MS data and fragmentation patterns. Compounds **13–16, 22, 40, 41, 43–45, 48, 51, 53, 55, 56** were assigned as K conjugates and **58** was identified as the aglycone K. The K derivatives **13, 14, 16, 41, 43, 44, 45, 53, 55,** and **56** differ in the number and identity of the conjugate. Compounds **13, 41,** and **53** show neutral loss of a hexose, **14** presents the consecutive losses of rhamnose and hexose, **16** a hexose and a rhamnose, **43** shows neutral loss of a pentose and a hexose, **44** losses a rhamnose and a hexose, **45** losses two hexoses, **55** an acetate and a hexose and **56** a pentose, leading to K. The compounds were assigned as K-hexoside, K-rhamnoside hexoside, K-hexoside rhamnoside, K-pentosidehexoside, K-rhamnosidehexoside, and K-dihexoside, respectively. Compounds **15** and **22** show neutral loss of a 180 amu and 164 amu fragment, respectively, whereas **51** loss 264 amu leading to the *m/z* peak at 285 amu of K. Compound **40** losses three hexoses and an additional fragment and were assigned as K -hexoside and K-trihexoside conjugate. The compound **48** showing the loss of a coumaroyl and hexose was assigned as K-coumaroylhexoside. Compounds **9, 20, 23, 25–27, 31, 34, 37–39, 42, 46, 47, 52** were tentatively identified as Q glycosides and **59** was identified as Q. All of them showed the characteristic ion of Q at *m/z* 301, which further fragmented to the diagnostic peaks at 178 and 151 amu in the MS^2 spectra. The identity of the sugars was determined by the neutral loss of hexose (162 amu), pentose (132 amu), or rhamnose (146 amu). The Q glycosides comprised a triglycoside (dihexosylrhamnoside **20**), several disaccharides including: dihexosides (**23** and **27**), hexosiderhamnoside (**26, 34, 39**), rhamnoside hexoside (**31**), dipentoside (**38**), monosaccharides (hexoside **9, 37, 42,** and **52**), a hexoside monoacetate (**47**), and the Q conjugate **46**. Four myricetin derivatives were found in *R. magellanicum*, including the dipentoside **24**, hexosylpentoside **28**, hexoside **29,** and pentoside **35**. Ruiz et al. (2015) reported 11 flavonoid glycosides from a single collection of *R. magellanicum* from Magallanes, Chilean Patagonia. The glycosides included quercetin derivatives (seven compounds), kaempferol, and myricetin rutinoside and hexoside. This new study offers a much broader array of compounds, including 38 flavonol conjugates distributed into quercetin (16), kaempferol (16), myricetin (4), isorhamnetin (1), and apigenin (1) derivatives.

Quantification of main anthocyanins, hydroxycinnamic acids, and flavonols

Phenolic metabolites in plants are greatly influenced by environmental conditions, and their composition and content defines the quality and flavor characteristics of fruits (Mikulic-Petkovsek et al. 2015). The location and year of collection has been shown to be an important factor affecting the composition of phenolic compounds in *Ribes nigrum* (Anttonen and Karjalainen 2006; Vagiri et al. 2013). Several strategies are reported in literature to quantify the main phenolic compounds, including the use of suitable calibration curves or the addition of an internal standard (Gros et al. 2006). We used the external calibration curve and internal standards in order to quantify the main hydroxycinnamic acids, flavonols, and anthocyanins in the studied samples. Differences between both methodologies were found, and the results are summarized in Table 3 for external calibration and Table 4 for internal standard.

Ripe fruits from Argentina presented a higher content of cyanidin-3-glucoside (**18**), whereas in the ripe sample from Chile the rutinoside (**17**) was the main anthocyanin (Table 3 and 4, Fig. 5). Arena & Coronel studied fruit growth and chemical properties of *R. magellanicum* from Ushuaia, Tierra del Fuego, Argentina (Arena and Coronel 2011). Authors described a total anthocyanin content ranging from 0.05 to 2.40 g kg^{-1} fresh fruit weight, increasing during the ripening period. Ruiz et al. (2013) reported a total of 2.44 ± 0.09 μmol of monomeric anthocyanins g^{-1} fresh fruit, whereas by HPLC-DAD the value was of 5.08 ± 0.01 μmol total anthocyanins g^{-1} fresh fruit. In the red variety of black currants (*Ribes nigrum x pallidum* cv. Red Dutch) only cyanidin derivatives were found in low amounts, whereas in the black variety (*Ribes nigrum* cv. Öjebyn), the main anthocyanins were cyanidin-3-rutinoside and delphinidin-3-rutinoside (Määttä et al. 2003). The anthocyanin content of the unripe sample from Villa La Angostura, Argentina was below our detection limits. In berries, anthocyanins begin to appear at onset of the ripening stage due to the increase in the expression of genes from the anthocyanin biosynthesis, thus explaining the low amount of anthocyanins in this sample (Ribera et al. 2010; Zhang et al. 2013; Mikulic-Petkovsek et al. 2015; Veberic et al. 2015). The level of anthocyanins variation has also been related to season, varieties and growing conditions (Bizjak et al. 2013). In *Ribes nigrum* cv. Vertti and *Ribes nigrum x pallidum* cv. White Dutch, the green and white varieties, respectively, anthocyanins were also not detected (Määttä et al. 2003).

Table 3. Content of main hydroxycinnamic acid (HCA) derivatives, anthocyanins, and flavonol derivatives in *Ribes magellanicum* PEEs (in mg kg^{-1} PEE) quantified by external calibration curve.

	Argentina		Chile	
Compound (peak)	Arroyo Casa de Piedra	Laguna Verde, Villa La Angostura	Parque Nacional Conguillio	Reserva Nacional Malalcahuello
HCA derivatives				
3[1]	1826.7 ± 0.9	1602.7 ± 9.5	594.6 ± 0.7	177.8 ± 0.3
4[1]	36.0 ± 0.0	129.4 ± 5.0	ND	ND
8[1]	34.7 ± 0.0	54.0 ± 1.4	33.4 ± 0.9	4.2 ± 0.1
11[1]	99.6 ± 0.2	749.4 ± 17.9	20.3 ± 0.0	86.4 ± 0.3
Anthocyanins				
17[2]	157.5 ± 0.6	ND	275.8 ± 2.3	6.8 ± 0.7
18[3]	241.1 ± 1.0	ND	125.4 ± 0.7	23.1 ± 0.6
19[3]	20.5 ± 0.1	ND	22.0 ± 0.1	ND
32[3]	20.4 ± 0.0	ND	33.0 ± 0.0	ND
33[2]	1.2 ± 0.3	ND	ND	ND
Flavonol derivatives				
20[4]	10.4 ± 0.1	6.3 ± 0.0	5.2 ± 0.0	4.5 ± 0.0
22[5]	105.1 ± 0.0	15.7 ± 0.0	6.2 ± 0.0	6.7 ± 0.0
37[4]	211.9 ± 0.1	76.3 ± 0.1	13.2 ± 0.5	13.6 ± 0.1
41–43[5]	358.4 ± 0.4	97.2 ± 0.0	34.9 ± 0.5	33.3 ± 0.1
53[5]	14.3 ± 0.1	7.0 ± 0.0	5.2 ± 0.1	7.7 ± 0.1
54[5]	44.9 ± 0.2	11.4 ± 0.1	7.1 ± 0.1	7.6 ± 0.1
56[5]	35.7 ± 0.2	18.9 ± 0.1	8.9 ± 0.6	5.7 ± 0.0

PEE, phenolic enriched extract; nd, below quantification limit.
[1]Expressed as chlorogenic acid equivalents.
[2]Expressed as cyanidin-3-rutinoside equivalent.
[3]Expressed as cyanidin-3-glucoside equivalent.
[4]Expressed as quercetin-3-glucoside equivalent.
[5]Expressed as kaempferol-3-glucoside equivalent.

Table 4. Content of main hydroxycinnamic acid (HCA) derivatives, anthocyanins, and flavonol derivatives in *Ribes magellanicum* PEEs (in mg kg^{-1} PEE) quantified by internal standard method.

	Argentina		Chile	
Compound (peak)	Arroyo Casa de Piedra	Laguna Verde, Villa La Angostura	Parque Nacional Conguillio	Reserva Nacional Malalcahuello
HCA derivatives[1]				
3	1864.0 ± 7.8	1592.5 ± 2.0	670.3 ± 28.1	190.2 ± 1.2
4	51.6 ± 0.5	183.8 ± 3.5	47.3 ± 2.2	ND
8	26.4 ± 1.2	68.3 ± 0.9	53.6 ± 2.4	19.3 ± 0.3
11	87.3 ± 0.7	752.7 ± 12.2	44.5 ± 2.4	100.3 ± 0.5
Anthocyanins[2]				
17	93.6 ± 1.8	ND	147.7 ± 1.3	9.6 ± 0.3
18	199.0 ± 2.3	ND	90.9 ± 0.0	7.9 ± 0.4
19	6.6 ± 0.0	ND	8.0 ± 0.1	ND
32	6.2 ± 0.0	ND	5.6 ± 0.1	ND
33	6.3 ± 0.0	ND	ND	ND
Flavonol derivatives[3]				
20	10.2 ± 0.3	5.6 ± 0.1	4.4 ± 0.1	3.5 ± 0.0
22	90.4 ± 2.2	13.1 ± 0.2	4.9 ± 0.1	5.3 ± 0.1
37	236.8 ± 6.1	82.8 ± 0.3	13.3 ± 0.4	13.8 ± 0.2
41–43	309.4 ± 8.2	83.5 ± 0.8	29.7 ± 0.3	28.3 ± 0.8
53	11.9 ± 0.2	5.6 ± 0.0	4.1 ± 0.1	6.2 ± 0.0
54	38.3 ± 0.7	9.4 ± 0.3	4.8 ± 0.0	6.1 ± 0.0
56	30.2 ± 0.6	15.8 ± 0.3	4.6 ± 0.1	4.5 ± 0.0

PEE, phenolic enriched extract; ND, below quantification limit.
[1]Expressed as *trans*-caffeic acid equivalents.
[2]Expressed as delphinidin-3-glucoside equivalents.
[3]Expressed as quercetin-3-glucuronide equivalents.

Several hydroxycinnamic acids (HCA) have been detected in *Ribes* species (Määttä et al. 2003; Mikulic-Petkovsek et al. 2015; Ruiz et al. 2015). HCA in *R. magellanicum* fruits from Argentina were about three times higher than in samples from Chile according to both quantification methodologies (Table 3, 4). The main HCA, 3-caffeoylquinic acid (**3**), was almost 10 times higher in the sample from Arroyo Casa de Piedra compared to the sample collected in the Reserva Nacional Malalcahuello (Table 3 and 4). The different varieties of *R. nigrum* presented as main compounds caffeoyl hexosides derivatives, followed by coumaric acid and ferulic acid derivatives (Määttä et al. 2003). In our analysis the main compounds found were only caffeoylquinic acid derivatives (>90%), followed by lower levels of feruloyl quinic acid and coumaroylquinic acid derivatives. In black currant varieties, 3-coumaroylquinic acid represented almost 70–80% of total HCA (Mikulic-Petkovsek et al. 2015). The levels of HCA, as for anthocyanins, vary according to the ripeness stage of the fruit. In apples, Bizjak et al. (2013). demonstrated a decrease by 27% during ripening, whereas MacLean et al. (2006) reported an increase in the level of hydroxycinnamic acids as the fruit maturity progressed. Mikulic-Petkovsek et al. (2015) proposed that the content levels of individual phenolics groups can be used to predict the optimal ripeness of *Ribes* fruits for harvest. In our samples, the HCA content showed differences between the degree of ripeness and collection place. While in the samples from Argentina the unripe fruit presented higher content than the ripe sample, the ripe fruits from Chile presented higher content than the unripe fruits. However, the results in Argentinean samples are strongly influenced by the particularly high content of feruloylquinic acid (**11**) in the unripe sample.

The main flavonols in *Ribes magellanicum* were quercetin-3-glucoside (**37**) and the mixture of quercetin-hexoside/kaempferol hexoside (**41, 42,** and **43**), in agreement with previous reports (Ruiz 2015). In black currants the major flavonoids are quercetin-3-rutinoside, myricetin-3-rutinoside, quercetin-3-glucoside, and myricetin-acetylhexoside (Mikulic-Petkovsek et al. 2015). The samples from Argentina presented higher levels of these compounds (Table 3 and 4). The TF content in *R. magellanicum*, determined by HPLC, was previously reported as 0.68 ± 0.00 μmol g^{-1} fresh fruit (Ruiz et al. 2015).

In food chemistry, the development of chemometrics and multivariate analysis has proven to be a powerful tool in the analysis of a large amount of data (Arvanitoyannis et al. 1999). The multivariate analysis generates mathematical-statistical models based on quantitative and qualitative information about the natural constituents to obtain characteristic fingerprints of each sample (Geana et al. 2016). The Spearman's rank correlation coefficient was calculated setting the concentration of the identified compounds as the independent variable and the antioxidant activity (DPPH and FRAP) as the dependent variable. Results are presented in Table 5. The most significant correlation was found for compounds **3**, **20,** and **41–43** and both antioxidant assays. Interestingly, no significant correlation was found among individual anthocyanins and the antioxidant activity. In a study on the correlation of antioxidant capacity (measured as ORAC) and the total phenolic and anthocyanin content in *Vaccinium* species, the authors found that the anthocyanin content of the different blueberry samples was linearly related to the ORAC measurement; however, a better correlation was found among total phenolics and ORAC (Prior et al. 1998). In a study of 26 different berries species, the correlation between the antioxidant activity with flavonols and hydroxycinnamic acids only explained a 31% of total antioxidant activity (Kähkönen et al. 2001). In this study, hydroxycinnamic acid and flavonols seem to be responsible for the antioxidant activity of the *Ribes magellanicum* samples. Nevertheless, according to Liu (2003) this activity is more likely attributed to a synergistic and additive effect of all compounds.

Table 5. Correlation coefficients for antioxidant activity (DPPH, FRAP) and the concentration of individual compounds identified in *Ribes magellanicum* samples from Argentina and Chile.

	DPPH		FRAP	
Compound	Spearman coefficient	*P* value	Spearman coefficient	*P* value
HCA derivatives				
3	−0.958042	0.000001	0.930070	0.000012
4	−0.720340	0.008232	0.705411	0.010383
8	−0.727273	0.007355	0.769231	0.003446
11	−0.580420	0.047856	0.580420	0.047856
Anthocyanins				
17	0.070424	0.827831	0.021127	0.948038
18	−0.330994	0.293298	0.401418	0.195884
19	0.021279	0.947666	−0.014186	0.965099
32				
33	−0.734316	0.006538	0.752674	0.004728
Flavonol derivatives				
20	−0.930070	0.000012	0.930070	0.000012
22	−0.797203	0.001900	0.727273	0.007355
37	−0.825175	0.000951	0.769231	0.003446
41–43	−0.916084	0.000028	0.944056	0.000004
53	−0.412587	0.182564	0.363636	0.245265
54	−0.762238	0.003950		
56	−0.916084	0.000028		

Among other chemometric tools, principal component analysis (PCA) is commonly used for discrimination, classification, modeling, and correlation (Di Paola-Naranjo et al. 2011). As presented in Figure 6, the samples were classified into three clearly separated groups. The first

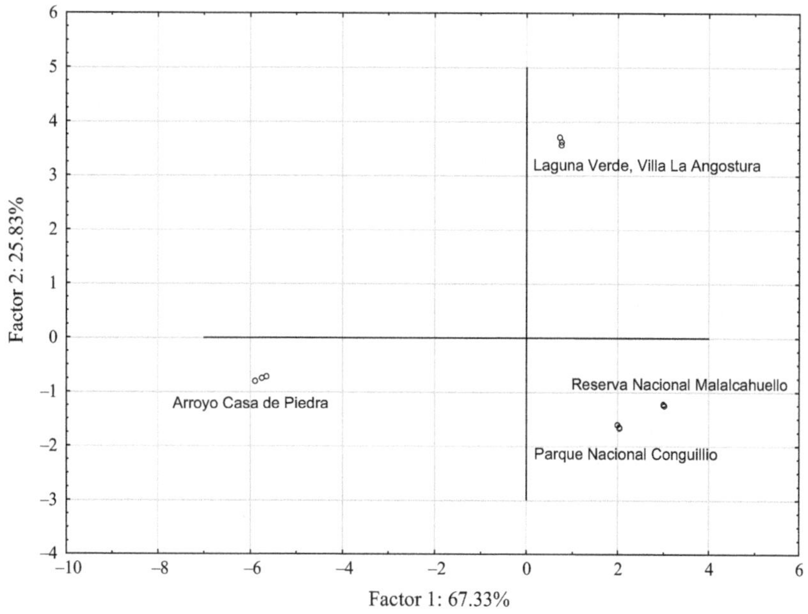

Figure 6. Scatter plot of the first and second discriminating factors showing differences between Argentinean (Laguna Verde, Villa La Angostura, and Arroyo Casa de Piedra) and Chilean (Reserva Nacional Malalcahuello and Parque Nacional Conguillio) *Ribes magellanicum* samples.

discriminating factor accounts for 67.33% of the variability and the second discriminating factor for 25.83% of the variability. The TF (−0.9966), FRAP (−0.9994), and compounds **33** (−0.9600), **20** (−0.9983), **22** (−0.9868), **37** (−0.9888), **41–43** (−0.9950), **54** (−0.9874), and **56** (−0.9788) showed negative correlation and influenced more significantly the first discriminating factor. On the other hand, compounds **11** (0.9975), **4** (0.9865), and **19** (−0.9899) exerted more effect on the second discriminating factor. This distinction between Chilean and Argentinean *Ribes magellanicum* fruits (Fig. 6) can be considered a first approach; however, more samples are needed in order to obtain a more complete picture.

Ribes berries are good sources of anthocyanins, hydroxycinnamic acids, flavonols, and flavan-3-ol (Milivojevic et al. 2012), with known biological properties, including in vitro inhibition of enzymes involved in metabolic syndrome, hyperglycemia, and hypertension. Several biological activities have been reported for polyphenols occurring in berries and can explain, at least in part, their positive effect on diet. Inhibition of starch digestion and glucose absorption are some of the possible action mechanisms of polyphenols occurring in foods. Polyphenols inhibit digestive enzymes including α-amylase, maltase, and sucrase. The inhibition of both enzymes in vitro is a method used in studies on the potential beneficial effect of dietary polyphenols. Boath et al. (2012) reported the effect of PEE from black currants (*Ribes nigrum* L. var. 8982-6) and rowanberry (*Sorbus aucuparia* var. Sahharnaja) on α-glucosidase activity. Both PEEs potentiated the inhibitory effect of acarbose on α-glucosidase and suggest the potential of PEEs from native berries as a complementary dietary mean to control glycemia. The reduction in carbonyl stress and advanced glycation end products has been suggested as a strategy to alleviate diabetic-related complications. In a recent article by Chen et al. (2014) a *R. nigrum* extract with high anthocyanin content was assessed for its ability to scavenge methylglyoxal (MGO). The blackcurrant had a high content of anthocyanins; both the extract as well as the individual main anthocyanins were able to form MGO adducts. The results suggest that anthocyanin-rich food sources might prevent diabetic-related complications through decreasing reactive precursors of α-dicarbonyl/advanced glycation products (Chen et al. 2014). Obesity is a major worldwide problem and changes in diet can contribute to reduction in the intake of fats. The effect of extracts from the berries *Ribes nigrum*, *Vaccinium corymbosum*, *Rubus chamaemorus*, *Rubus stellatus x R. arcticus*, *Vaccinium vitis-idaea*, *Sorbus aucuparia*, *Fragaria x ananassa* var. Elsanta and *Rubus idaeus* var. Glen Ample on pancreatic lipase was investigated (McDougall et al. 2009). The inhibitory effect of these berries on pancreatic lipase may reduce the rate in which triglycerides are split into absorbable glycerol and fatty acids (de la Garza et al. 2011; Sosnowska et al. 2015). The most active samples as pancreatic lipase inhibitors were *R. stellatus x R. arcticus*, *R. chamaemorus*, *F. x ananassa*, and *R. idaeus*, reducing up to >85% the activity of the enzyme at 50 mg GAE L^{-1}. The most active was the raspberry extract with inhibitions up to >95% at the concentration mentioned. Recently, it was reported that anthocyanins from *R. nigrum* were able to attenuate weight gain and improve glucose metabolism in diet-induced obese mice (Esposito et al. 2015). The results of our study can be useful for further works on *R. magellanicum* fruits from Argentina and Chile, including studies on the inhibition of certain metabolic enzymes that may have potential beneficial health effects.

Conclusion

In summary, in vitro antioxidant assays showed a higher capacity to scavenge radicals of ripe Argentinean fruits PEE. The most significant cytoprotective effect against oxidative stress-induced by H_2O_2 was found in the sample from Arroyo Casa de Piedra. The Spearman's correlation coefficient pointed out HCA and flavonols as the responsible compounds for the antioxidant activity of the samples. The PCA allowed a preliminary insight about the differences between the Chilean and Argentinean samples. The phenolic compounds identified in the Patagonian currant *Ribes magellanicum* can explain the antioxidant effect found in the samples and suggest further nutraceutical potential for this South American berry.

Acknowledgments

Financial support from FONDECYT Project N° 1120096 and CONICYT-PCHA/Doctorado Nacional/2013-21130048 (F. Jiménez-Aspee) and CONICYT-PCHA/Doctorado Nacional/2013-63130042 (S. Thomas- Valdés) are kindly acknowledged. Ayla Schulz thanks DAAD-RISE for a fellowship. We would like to express our gratitude to Prof. Dr. Daniel A. Wunderlin from Universidad Nacional de Córdoba (Argentina) for his advice in the statistical analysis and critical reading of the manuscript. We also thank the Academic Writing Center at Programa de Idiomas at Universidad de Talca (Mrs. Rachael Lange) for the English corrections and to the Corporación Nacional Forestal (CONAF, Chile) for the permission to collect plant material in protected areas and national parks.

Conflict of Interest

None declared.

References

Anttonen, M. J., and R. O. Karjalainen. 2006. High-performance liquid chromatography analysis of black currant (*Ribes nigrum* L.) fruit phenolics grown either conventionally or organically. J. Agric. Food Chem. 54:7530–7538.

Arena, M. E., and L. J. Coronel. 2011. Fruit growth and chemical properties of *Ribes magellanicum* "parrilla". Scientia Hortic. 127:325–329.

Arvanitoyannis, I. S., M. N. Katsota, E. P. Psarra, E. H. Soufleros, and S. Kallithraka. 1999. Application of quality control methods for assessing wine authenticity: use of multivariate analysis (chemometrics). Trends Food Sci. Technol. 10:321–336.

Benvenuti, S., F. Pellati, M. Melegari, and D. Bertelli. 2004. Polyphenols, anthocyanins, ascorbic acid, and radical scavenging activity of *Rubus*, *Ribes* and *Aronia*. J. Food Sci. 69:164–169.

Bizjak, J., M. Mikulic-Petkovsek, F. Stampar, and R. Veberic. 2013. Changes in primary metabolites and polyphenols in the peel of "Braeburn" apples (*Malus domestica* Borkh.) during advanced maturation. J. Agric. Food Chem. 61:10283–10292.

Boath, A. S., D. Stewart, and G. J. McDougall. 2012. Berry components inhibit α-glucosidase in vitro: synergies between acarbose and polyphenols from black currant and rowanberry. Food Chem. 135:929–936.

Boeing, H., A. Bechthold, A. Bub, S. Ellinger, D. Haller, A. Kroke, et al. 2012. Critical review: vegetables and fruit in the prevention of chronic diseases. Eur. J. Nutr. 51:637–663.

Borges, G., A. Degeneve, W. Mullen, and A. Crozier. 2010. Identification of flavonoid and phenolic antioxidants in black currants, blueberries, raspberries, red currants, and cranberries. J. Agric. Chem. 58:3901–3909.

Burin, V. M., S. G. Arcari, L. L. Costa, and M. T. Bordignon-Luiz. 2011. Determination of some phenolic compounds in red wine by RP-HPLC: method development and validation. J. Chromatogr. Sci. 49:647–651.

Cheli, F., and A. Baldi. 2011. Nutrition based health: cell-based bioassays for food antioxidant activity evaluation. J. Food Sci. 76:197–205.

Chen, X.-Y., I.-M. Huang, L. S. Hwang, C.-T. Ho, S. Li, and C.-Y. Lo. 2014. Anthocyanins in backcurrants effectively prevent the formation of advanced glycation end products by trapping methylglyoxal. J. Funct. Foods 8:259–268.

Clifford, M. N., K. L. Johnston, S. Knight, and N. Kuhnert. 2003. Hierarchical scheme for LC-MS^n identification of chlorogenic acids. J. Agric. Food Chem. 51:2900–2911.

Di Paola-Naranjo, R. D., M. V. Baroni, N. S. Podio, H. R. Rubinstein, M. P. Fabani, R. G. Badini, et al. 2011. Fingerprints for main varieties of Argentinian wines: terroir differentiation by inorganic, organic, and stable isotopic analysis coupled to chemometrics. J. Agric. Food Chem. 59:7854–7865.

Djordevic, B., K. Savikin, G. Zdunic, T. Jankovic, T. Vulic, C. Oparnica, et al. 2010. Biochemical properties of red currant varieties in relation to storage. Plants Foods Hum. Nutr. 65:326–332.

Esposito, D., T. Damsud, M. Wilson, M. H. Grace, R. Strauch, X. Li, et al. 2015. Black currant anthocyanins attenuate weight gain and improve glucose metabolism in diet-induced obese mice with intact, but not disrupted, gut microbiome. J. Agric. Food Chem. 63:6172–6180.

Eyssartier, C., A. H. Ladio, M. Lozada. 2011. Traditional horticultural knowledge change in a rural population of the Patagonian steppe. J. Arid Environ. 75:78–86.

de la Garza, A. L., F. I. Milagro, N. Boque, J. Campión, and J. A. Martínez. 2011. Natural inhibitors of pancreatic lipase as new players in obesity treatment. Planta Med. 77:773–785.

Gavrilova, V., M. Kajdzanoska, V. Gjamovski, and M. Stefova. 2011. Separation, characterization and quantification of phenolic compounds in blueberries and red and black currants by HPLC-DAD-ESI-MSn. J. Agric. Food Chem. 59:4009–4018.

Geana, E. I., R. Popescu, D. Costinel, O. R. Dinca, R. E. Ionete, I. Stefanescu, et al. 2016. Classification of red wines using suitable markers coupled with multivariate statistical analysis. Food Chem. 192:1015–1024.

Ghosh, D., T. K. McGhie, J. Zhang, A. Adaim, and M. Skinner. 2006. Effects of anthocyanins and other phenolics of boysenberry and blackcurrant as inhibitors of oxidative stress and damage to cellular DNA in SH-SY5Y and HL-60 cells. J. Sci. Food Agric. 86:678–686.

González-Castejón, M., and A. Rodriguez-Casado. 2011. Dietary phytochemicals and their potential effects on obesity: a review. Pharmacol. Res. 64:438–455.

Gros, M., M. Petrovic, and D. Barceló. 2006. Development of a multi-residue analytical methodology based on liquid chromatography-tandem mass spectrometry (LC-MS/MS) for screening and trace level determination of pharmaceuticals in Surface and wastewaters. Talanta 70:678–690.

Halliwell, B. 1994. Free radicals and antioxidants: a personal view. Nutr. Rev. 52:253–265.

Halliwell, B., J. Gutteridge, and C. Cross. 1992. Free radicals, antioxidants, and human disease: where are we now? J. Lab. Clin. Med. 119:598.

Halliwell, B., J. Rafter, and A. Jenner. 2005. Health promotion by flavonoids, tocopherols, tocotrienols and other phenols: direct or indirect effects? Antioxidant or not? Am. J. Clin. Nutr. 81:268–276.

Heo, H. J., S. J. Choi, S. G. Choi, D. H. Shin, J. M. Lee, and C. Y. Lee. 2008. Effects of banana, orange, and apple on oxidative stress-induced neurotoxicity in PC12 cells. J. Food Sci. 73:28–32.

Hollman, P. C. H. 2001. Evidence for health benefits of plant phenols: local or systemic effects. J. Sci. Food Agric. 81:842–852.

Im, S. E., T. G. Nam, H. Lee, M. W. Han, H. J. Heo, S. Koo, et al. 2013. Anthocyanins in the ripe fruits of *Rubus coreanus* Miquel and their protective effect on neuronal PC-12 cells. Food Chem. 139:604–610.

Jia, N., T. Li, X. Diao, and B. Kong. 2014. Protective effects of black currant (*Ribes nigrum* L.) extract on hydrogen peroxide-induced damage in lung fibroblast MRC-5 cells in relation to the antioxidant activity. J. Funct. Foods 11:142–151.

Jimenez-Aspee, F., C. Theoduloz, F. Ávila, S. Thomas-Valdés, C. Mardones, D. von Baer, et al. 2016. The Chilean wild raspberry (*Rubus geoides* Sm.) increases intracellular GSH content and protects against H_2O_2 and methylglyoxal-induced damage in AGS cells. Food Chem. 194:908–919.

Jiménez-Aspee, F., C. Quispe, M. D. P. C. Soriano, J. Fuentes, E. Hüneke, C. Theoduloz, et al. 2014. Antioxidant activity and characterization of constituents in Copao fruits (*Eulychnia acida* Phil., Cactaceae) by HPLC-DAD-MS/MS^n. Food Res. Int. 62:286–298.

Kähkönen, M. P., A. I. Hopla, and M. Heinonen. 2001. Berry phenolics and their antioxidant activity. J. Agric. Food Chem. 49:4076–4082.

Kapasakalidis, P. G., R. A. Rastall, and M. H. Gordon. 2009. Effect of a cellulase treatment on extraction of antioxidant phenols from black currant (*Ribes nigrum* L.) pomace. J. Agric. Food Chem. 57:4342–4351.

Ladio, A., M. Lozada, and M. C. Weigandt. 2007. Comparison of traditional wild plant knowledge between aboriginal communities inhabiting arid and forest environments in Patagonia, Argentina. J. Arid Environ. 69:695–715.

Liu, R. H. 2003. Health benefits of fruit and vegetables are from additive and synergistic combinations of phytochemicals. Am. J. Clin. Nutr. 78:517S–520S.

Määttä, K. R., A. Kamal-Eldin, and R. Törrönen. 2003. High-performance liquid chromatography (HPLC) analysis of phenolic compounds in berries with diode array and electrospray ionization mass spectrometric (MS) detection: *Ribes* species. J. Agric. Food Chem. 51:6736–6744.

MacLean, D. D., D. P. Murr, J. R. DeEll, and C. R. Horvath. 2006. Post-harvest variation in apple (*Malus domestica* Borkh.) flavonoids following harvest, storage, and 1-MCP treatment. J. Agric. Food Chem. 54:870–878.

McDougall, G. J., N. N. Kulkarni, and D. Stewart. 2009. Berry polyphenols inhibit pancreatic lipase activity in vitro. Food Chem. 115:193–199.

Mikulic-Petkovsek, M., J. Rescic, V. Schmitzer, F. Stampar, A. Slatnar, D. Koron, et al. 2015. Changes in fruit quality parameters of four *Ribes* species during ripening. Food Chem. 173:363–374.

Milivojevic, J., A. Slatnar, M. Mikulic-Petkovsek, F. Stampar, M. Nikolic, and R. Veberic. 2012. The influence of early yield on the accumulation of major taste and health related compounds in black and red currant cultivars (*Ribes* spp.). J. Agric. Food Chem. 60:2682–2691.

Molares, S., and A. Ladio. 2012. Mapuche perceptions and conservation of Andean *Nothofagus* forests and their medicinal plants: a case study from a rural community in Patagonia, Argentina. Biodivers. Conserv. 21:1079–1093.

Moskaug, J. Ø., H. Carlsen, M. C. Myhrstad, and R. Blomhoff. 2005. Polyphenols and gluthatione synthesis regulation. Am. J. Clin. Nutr. 81:277S–283S.

Nenadis, N., L. F. Wang, M. Tsimidou, and H. Y. Zhang. 2004. Estimation of scavenging activity of phenolic compounds using the ABTS ($^{*+}$) assay. J. Agric. Food Chem. 52:4669–4674.

Pinto, M. S., Y.-I. Kwon, E. Apostolidis, F. M. Lajolo, M. I. Genovese, and K. Shetty. 2010. Evaluation of red currants (*Ribes rubrum* l.), black currants (*Ribes nigrum* l.), red and green gooseberries (*Ribes uva-crispa*) for potential management of type 2 diabetes and hypertension using in vitro models. J. Food Biochem. 34:639–660.

Prior, R. L., G. Cao, A. Martin, E. Sofic, J. McEwen, C. O'Brien, et al. 1998. Antioxidant capacity as influenced by total phenolic and anthocyanin content, maturity, and variety of *Vaccinium* species. J. Agric. Food Chem. 46:2686–2693.

Rapoport, E., and A. Ladio. 1999. The Andean Patagonian forests as a source of food. Bosque 20:55–64.

Ribera, A. E., M. Reyes-Díaz, M. Alberdi, G. E. Zuñiga, and M. L. Mora. 2010. Antioxidant compounds in skin and pulp of fruits change among genotypes and maturity stages in highbush blueberry (*Vaccinium corymbosum* L.) grown in southern Chile. J. Soil Sci. Plant Nutr. 10:509–536.

Ruiz, A., I. Hermosín-Gutiérrez, C. Vergara, D. von Baer, M. Zapata, A. Hitschfeld, et al. 2013. Anthocyanin profiles in south Patagonian wild berries by HPLC-DAD-ESI-MS/MS. Food Res. Int. 51:706–713.

Ruiz, A., L. Bustamante, C. Vergara, D. von Baer, I. Hermosín-Gutiérrez, L. Obando, et al. 2015. Hydroxycinnamic acids and flavonols in native edible berries of South Patagonia. Food Chem. 167:84–90.

Schreckinger, M. E., J. Lotton, M. A. Lila, and E. Gonzalez de Mejia. 2010. Berries from South America: a comprehensive review on chemistry, health potential, and commercialization. J. Med. Food 13:233–246.

Shukitt-Hale, B., F. C. Lau, and J. A. Joseph. 2008. Berry fruit supplementation and the aging brain. J. Agric. Food Chem. 56:636–641.

Simirgiotis, M. J., J. Bórquez, and G. Schmeda-Hirschmann. 2013. Antioxidant capacity, polyphenolic content and tandem HPLC-DAD-ESI/MS profiling of phenolic compounds from South American berries *Luma apiculata* and *L. chequén*. Food Chem. 139:289–299.

Slimestad, R., and H. Solheim. 2002. Anthocyanins from black currants (*Ribes nigrum* L.). J. Agric. Food Chem. 50:3228–3231.

Sosnowska, D., A. Podsędek, M. Redzynia, and D. Żyżelewicz. 2015. Effects of fruit extracts on pancreatic lipase activity in lipid emulsions. Plants Foods Hum. Nutr. 70:344–350.

Sparre, B. 1984. Grossulariaceae. Pp. 19–26 *in* M. N. Correa, ed. Flora Patagonica, parte IV-B. Instituto Nacional de Tecnologia Agropecuaria, INTA, Buenos Aires, Argentina.

Vagiri, M., A. Ekholm, E. Öberg, E. Johansson, S. C. Andersson, and K. Rumpunen. 2013. Phenols and ascorbic acid in black currants (*Ribes nigrum* L.): variation due to genotype, location and year. J. Agric. Food Chem. 61:9298–9306.

Veberic, R., A. Slatnar, J. Bizjak, F. Stampar, and M. Mikulic-Petkovsek. 2015. Anthocyanin composition of different wild and cultivated berry species. LWT Food Sci. Technol. 60:509–517.

Zafra-Stone, S., T. Yasmin, M. Bagchi, A. Chatterjee, J. A. Vinson, and D. Bagchi. 2007. Berry anthocyanins as novel antioxidants in human health and disease prevention. Mol. Nutr. Food Res. 51:675–683.

Zhang, D., M. J. Qian, B. Yu, and Y. W. Teng. 2013. Effect of fruit maturity on UV-B-induced post-harvest anthocyanin accumulation in red Chinese sand pear. Acta Physiol. Plant 35:2857–2866.

Zheng, J., B. Yang, V. Ruusunen, O. Laaksonen, R. Tahvonen, J. Hellsten, et al. 2012. Compositional differences of phenolic compounds between black currant (*Ribes nigrum* L.) cultivars and their response to latitude and weather conditions. J. Agric. Food Chem. 60:6581–6593.

4

Multivariate modeling of settling depth of apple fruit (Red Delicious variety) in water

Kamran Kheiralipour & Farshid Marzbani

Mechanical Engineering of Biosystems Department, Ilam University, Ilam, Iran

Keywords

Hydraulic handling, multivariate modeling, physical characteristics, settling depth

Correspondence

Kamran Kheiralipour, Mechanical Engineering of Biosystems Department, Ilam University, Ilam, Iran 69315-516.

E-mail: kamrankheiralipour@gmail.com

Funding Information

The authors thank Ilam University for the support to this research.

Abstract

Settling depth of targets, with a density lower than the density of water, is a distance between water surface and a depth that the target reaches after drop-ping from a height. In this research, settling depth of apple was determined by a water column and a digital camera and then was experimentally modeled using multivariate regression program coded in MATLAB software. The con-sidered parameters in multivariate modeling were physical characteristics (density, mass, and volume) and dropping height of the target. The characteristics were determined by standard methods. The best models were based on the density, dropping height and volume/mass with coefficient of determination (R^2), and mean square error (MSE) of 0.90 and 4.08, respectively.

Introduction

Engineering properties of agricultural materials are important information required to design handling, cleaning, conveying, grading, packaging, and storage systems (Tabatabaeefar 2003). Settling depth of fruits and vegetables in water is of the hydrodynamic properties defined for targets with density lower than the density of water. It is a depth that a target dropped from a height will reaches to that and returns to the water surface. Settling depth of fruits and vegetables is necessary for determining the depth of water in channel to avoid the fruit contact with channel bottom (Mohsenin 1986).

Kheiralipour (2014) theoretically modeled the settling depth of fruits and vegetables with the density lower than the density of water, $\rho_f < \rho_w$, as following formula:

$$d = \frac{2d_0\left(\rho_f - \rho_a\right)V^{\frac{n+1}{3}}}{\left(\rho_w - \rho_f\right)V^{\frac{n+1}{3}} + K\mu_w^n\rho_w^{1-n}S_h\left(2gd_0\left(1-\frac{\rho_a}{\rho_f}\right)\right)^{\frac{2-n}{2}}} \quad (1)$$

where d is settling depth of fruit, d_0 is dropping height, ρ_f is target density, ρ_a is air density, V is target volume, ρ_w is water density, μ_w is the static viscosity of water, S_h is shape factor, g is acceleration of gravity, and k and n are constant factors. The more important effec-tive parameters on settling depth are dropping height, density, mass, and volume of target (Kheiralipour 2014).

In the world, the total production of apple fruit (*Malus domestica* Borkh L.) is around 76.38 million tons. China is the first apple producer in the world with 37 million tons annual production. After United States, Turkey, Poland, India, and Italy, Islamic Republic of Iran with production of 17.00 million tons is ranked as the seventh producer country (FAOSTAT, 2012). In the literature, physical characteristics of apple fruit were investigated and reported (Tabatabaeefar and Rajabipour 2005; Kheiralipour et al. 2008; Jalali et al. 2013) but there is no information about settling depth of apple fruit. So, the decision in this research was to develop experimental model of apple settling depth based on its physical properties. The set-tling depth of apple, Red Delicious variety, was determined and modeled considering theoretical model developed by Kheiralipour (2014) and multivariate regression procedure.

Materials and Methods

Theory

In this research, equation (1) was considered for experimental modeling of settling of targets in water. By reversing *d*, equation (1) is changes to:

$$\frac{1}{d} = \frac{\left(\rho_w - \rho_f\right) V^{\frac{n+1}{3}} + K\mu_w^n \rho_w^{1-n} S_h \left(2gd_0\left(1-\frac{\rho_a}{\rho_f}\right)\right)^{\frac{2-n}{2}}}{2d_0\left(\rho_f - \rho_a\right) V^{\frac{n+1}{3}}} \quad (2)$$

Equation (2) can be broken as following:

$$\frac{1}{d} = \frac{\left(\rho_w - \rho_f\right) V^{\frac{n+1}{3}}}{2d_0\left(\rho_f - \rho_a\right) V^{\frac{n+1}{3}}} + \frac{K\mu_w^n \rho_w^{1-n} S_h \left(2gd_0\left(1-\frac{\rho_a}{\rho_f}\right)\right)^{\frac{2-n}{2}}}{2d_0\left(\rho_f - \rho_a\right) V^{\frac{n+1}{3}}} \quad (3)$$

After simplification, equation (3) would be changed as following:

$$\frac{1}{d} = \frac{1}{2d_0}\frac{\left(\rho_w - \rho_f\right)}{\left(\rho_f - \rho_a\right)} + \frac{K\mu_w^n \rho_w^{1-n} S_h \left(2gd_0\right)^{\frac{2-n}{2}}}{2d_0}\frac{\left(\rho_f - \rho_a\right)^{-n} V^{-\frac{n+1}{3}}}{\rho_f} \quad (4)$$

The parameters $\frac{1}{2d_0}$ and $\frac{K\mu_w^n \rho_w^{1-n}(2g)^{\frac{2-n}{2}}}{2}$ in equation (4) are replaced by K_2 and K_3. So equation (5) can be:

$$\frac{1}{d} = K_2 d_0^{-1}\frac{\left(\rho_w - \rho_f\right)}{\left(\rho_f - \rho_a\right)} + K_3 S_h d_0^{-n}\frac{\left(\rho_f - \rho_a\right)^{-n} V^{-\frac{n+1}{3}}}{\rho_f} \quad (5)$$

The air density (ρ_a) can be neglected in previous equation and $K_2\ \rho_w = K_1$, so:

$$\frac{1}{d} = K_1 d_0^{-1}\rho_f^{-1} - K_2 d_0^{-1} + K_3 S_h d_0^{-n}\rho_f^{-1-n} V^{-\frac{n+1}{3}} \quad (6)$$

The volume in the equation 6 can be replaced by target mass, *m*, as following:

$$\frac{1}{d} = K_1 d_0^{-1}\rho_f^{-1} - K_2 d_0^{-1} + K_3 S_h d_0^{-n}\rho_f^{\frac{-2n-2}{3}} m^{-\frac{n+1}{3}} \quad (7)$$

So, descent depth of target can be modeled using equations (8) or (9):

$$\frac{1}{d} = Ad_0^{-1}\rho_f^{-1} + BS_h d_0^{C}\rho_f^{D} V^{E} + Fd_0^{-1} + G \quad (8)$$

$$\frac{1}{d} = Ad_0^{-1}\rho_f^{-1} + BS_h d_0^{C}\rho_f^{D} m^{E} + Fd_0^{-1} + G \quad (9)$$

where *A*, *B*, *C*, *D*, *E*, *F*, and *G* are constant factors. The constant coefficient *G* was added to the end of the equations (8) and (9) as an error in experimental modeling. The difference between equations (8) and (9) is volume and mass, only.

Experiments

The targets in this research were apple fruit from Red Delicious variety. Target mass was determined by Precisa electronic balance (Model: 3100c) with accuracy of 0.1 g. Volume and density of the targets were determined by the water displacement method (Mohsenin 1986).

A water column (35 × 35 × 90 cm^3) was constructed by glass with thickness of 8 mm. It was filled by water to a height of 80 cm. Each target was placed on a specific height (dropping height = 10, 25, and 50 cm) on top of the water surface, so that the largest areas of them were parallel to the surface of the water column. In order to determine settling depth of the targets a digital camera (Sony, Model) with 25 frames per second recorded the moving of them from the dropping height point to the end of the target's settling depth in water column. Each fruit was tested three times in each dropping height. In order to correctly determine the settling depth of the fruits, Video to Frame Software was used to change each video film to corresponding images (Fig. 1).

Multivariate modeling

The obtained data were considered for modeling of settling depth of apples using equation (8) and (9). In the present research, the projected area of the targets was not determined due to low effect on the terminal velocity (Jordan and Clark 2004; Kheiralipour et al. 2010). So, the equations (8) and (9) can be changed to:

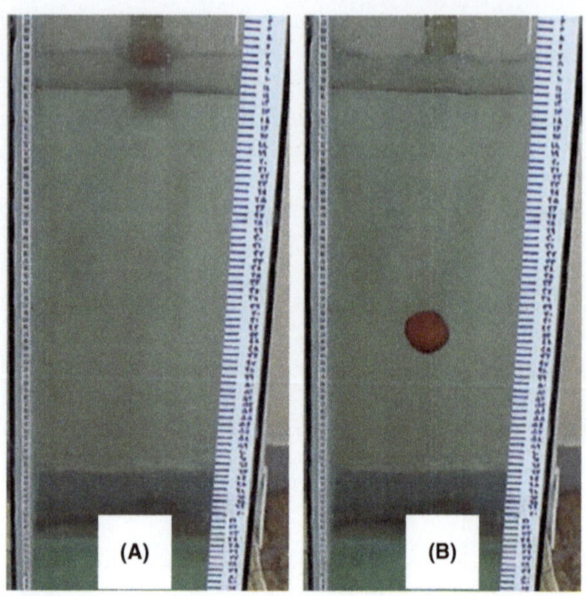

Figure 1. Traveling a target from (A) water surface to (B) its settling depth.

$$\frac{1}{d} = Ad_0^{-1}\rho_f^{-1} + Hd_0^{\,C}\rho_f^{\,D}V^E + Fd_0^{-1} + G \quad (10)$$

$$\frac{1}{d} = Ad_0^{-1}\rho_f^{-1} + Hd_0^{\,C}\rho_f^{\,D}m^E + Fd_0^{-1} + G \quad (11)$$

where, H is a new constant factor instead of BS_h.

The multivariate regression method was used for modeling settling depth of the targets. For this, a program was coded in MATLAB Software. The program was applied "nlinfit" command in the software. The program was able to calculate determination coefficient (R^2) and mean square error (MSE) of each model.

Results and Discussions

Some physical properties of the targets were presented in Table 1. In this table, besides density, volume and mass, settling depth of the targets when dropping from the different heights of 10 cm (d_{10}), 25 cm (d_{25}), and 50 cm (d_{50}) were listed.

Settling depth of all experimented targets was plotted in Figure 2. As shown in this figure, by increasing the dropping height from 10–50 cm, the settling depth was increased. As can be seen in this figure, the settling depth of all targets was not uniformly increased. This is due to effect of other parameters of target on the settling depth.

As can be seen in this figure, most of the lines to show the relations between settling depth and physical attributes of the fruit have increasing trend by the increase in target mass, volume, and density. This trend is more detectable for Figure 2A. Also by comparing all parts of Figure 2, it is observed that the effect of dropping height is higher than that of mass, volume, and density of the target.

Multivariate models of settling depth of the targets were done based on equations (10) and (11) for each dropping height individually. The models were shown in Tables 2–4 for dropping height of 10, 25, and 50 cm, respectively.

Table 1. Some physical properties of the targets.

	Minimum	Mean	Maximum	Standard deviation
Density (g/cm^3)	0.82	0.86	0.88	0.02
Volume (cm^3)	123.78	162.64	211.00	25.84
Mass (g)	104.44	139.40	171.94	20.32
d_{10} (cm)[1]	25.7	30.3	34.0	2.2
d_{25} (cm)[1]	33.9	38.0	42.0	2.0
d_{50} (cm)[1]	39.0	44.6	51.0	3.4

[1] d_{10}, d_{20} and d_{50} are settling depth of the targets when dropping from a height of d_0 = 10, 25 and 50 cm, respectively.

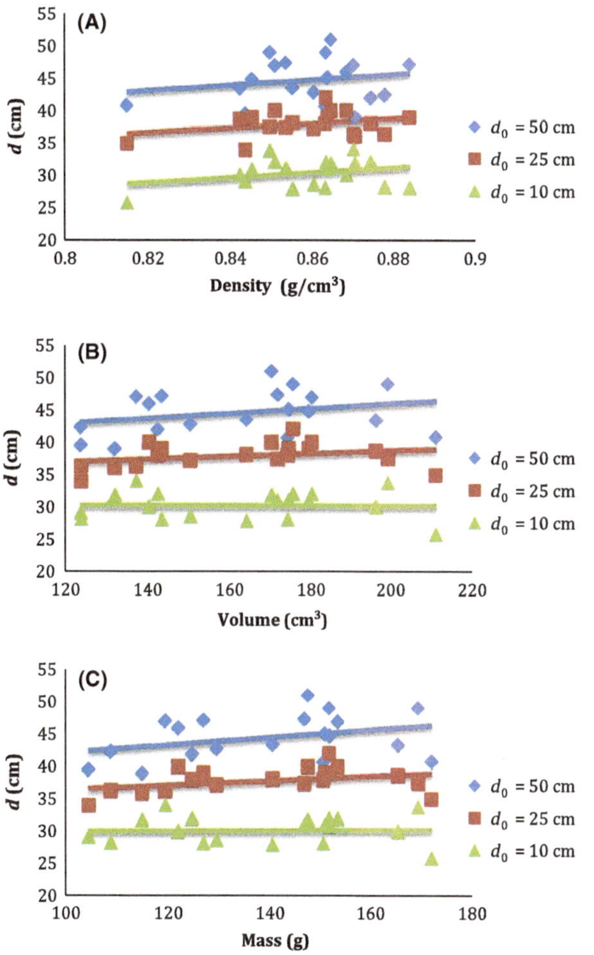

Figure 2. The settling depth of targets versus (A) fruit density, (B) volume, and (C) fruit mass. d is settling depth and d_0 is dropping height.

In Table 2, model No. 1, 2, and 3 (single-variate) with R^2 = 0.1021, 0.0199, and 0.0090, respectively, show that density, volume, and mass of the targets cannot individually model the settling depth from 10 cm dropping height. Also other models which are multivariate, with a coefficient determination of 0.3358–0.3994 cannot strongly predict the settling depth with 10 cm dropping height.

Models No. 1, 2, and 3 in Table 3, are same as those in Table 2. The other models in Table 3 have the determination coefficients higher than the corresponding values of Table 2.

Also, Models No. 1, 2, and 3 in Table 4 have low determination coefficient same as corresponding values in Tables 2 and 3. The other models show that settling depth of apple dropped from height of 25 cm can be better modeled than the settling depth of targets dropped from the height of 10 cm (Table 2).

Table 2. Multivariate models of the settling depth of the targets with dropping height of 10 cm.

Model No.	Model	MSE	R^2
1	$\frac{1}{d}=0.0362\rho_f^{-1}-0.0090$	5.2246×10^{-6}	0.1021
2	$\frac{1}{d}=6.9800 \times 10^{-15}V^{4.87}+0.033$	5.7015×10^{-6}	0.0199
3	$\frac{1}{d}=8.2200 \times 10^{9}m^{-6.43}+0.033$	5.7650×10^{-6}	0.0090
4	$\frac{1}{d}=341.2355\rho_f^{-163.8828}V^{-8.3104}+0.0323$	3.8646×10^{-6}	0.3358
5	$\frac{1}{d}=344.6594\rho_f^{-155.6381}m^{-8.3149}+0.0328$	3.8645×10^{-6}	0.3358
6	$\frac{1}{d}=-0.2955\rho_f^{-1}+0.0067\rho_f^{-13.4032}V^{-0.1310}+0.03502$	3.5561×10^{-6}	0.3994
7	$\frac{1}{d}=-0.2955\rho_f^{-1}+0.0067\rho_f^{-13.4032}m^{-0.1310}+0.3502$	3.5561×10^{-6}	0.3994

Table 3. Multivariate models of the settling depth of apple with dropping height of 25 cm.

Model No	Model	MSE	R^2
1	$\frac{1}{d}=0.0205\rho_f^{-1}+0.0025$	1.6152×10^{-6}	0.1057
2	$\frac{1}{d}=2.9694\times 10^{10}V^{-6.2481}+0.0257$	1.2514×10^{-6}	0.3068
3	$\frac{1}{d}=1.7067\times 10^{10}m^{-6.3113}+0.0256$	1.1576×10^{-6}	0.3588
4	$\frac{1}{d}=0.2515\rho_f^{-0.3194}V^{-0.0373}-0.1920$	6.7594×10^{-6}	0.6256
5	$\frac{1}{d}=0.2020\rho_f^{-0.3658}m^{-0.0484}-0.1419$	6.8423×10^{-6}	0.6256
6	$\frac{1}{d}=0.0631\rho_f^{-1}+2.2925\times 10^{4}\rho_f^{6.7748}V^{-2.9721}-0.0498$	5.5090×10^{-6}	0.6948
7	$\frac{1}{d}=0.1172\rho_f^{-1}+0.7941\rho_f^{6.0461}m^{-0.6364}-0.1228$	5.9653×10^{-6}	0.6699

Table 4. Multivariate models of the settling depth of the targets with dropping height of 50 cm.

Model No	Model	MSE	R^2
1	$\frac{1}{d}=0.0159\rho_f^{-1}+0.0040$	2.7568×10^{-6}	0.0398
2	$\frac{1}{d}=1.0505\times 10^{10}V^{6.0249}+0.0218$	2.2829×10^{-6}	0.2048
3	$\frac{1}{d}=1.3282\times 10^{10}m^{-6.2536}+0.0217$	2.2035×10^{-6}	0.2324
4	$\frac{1}{d}=1.0841\rho_f^{-0.0631}V^{-0.0081}-1.0299$	1.7423×10^{-6}	0.3942
5	$\frac{1}{d}=1.7559\rho_f^{-0.0385}m^{-0.0049}-1.6999$	1.7409×10^{-6}	0.3942
6	$\frac{1}{d}=0.0977\rho_f^{-1}+1.4534\rho_f^{5.6407}V^{-0.8112}-0.1015$	1.6627×10^{-6}	0.4211
7	$\frac{1}{d}=0.0977\rho_f^{-1}+1.4536\rho_f^{5.6409}m^{-0.8112}-0.1015$	1.6625×10^{-6}	0.4211

Table 5. Final multivariate models of settling depth of apple.

Model No	Model	MSE	R^2
1	$\frac{1}{d}=-234.4133d_0^{-1}\rho_f^{-1}+0.0019d_0^{0.7568}\rho_f^{10.9868}V^{1.4870}-209.6996d_0^{-1}+32.7118$	4.0752	0.9004
2	$\frac{1}{d}=-234.4135d_0^{-1}\rho_f^{-1}+0.0019d_0^{0.7568}\rho_f^{9.4998}m^{1.4870}-209.6996d_0^{-1}+32.7118$	4.0752	0.9004

Settling depth of the targets was modeled based on equations (10) and (11) but with considering all dropping heights (Table 5).

As can be seen in Table 5, the coefficient of determination and mean square error of the two models is same and equal to 0.9004 and 4.0752, respectively. By this result it can be told that both parameter groups ([1] dropping height, density and volume and [2] dropping height density and mass) can model the settling depth with same ability. Also, these models have higher coefficient of determination compare with the models in Tables 2–4.

The models in Table 5 can be used to predict the settling depth of apple, Red Delicious variety. For hydraulic handling and transporting of apple when dropped from a specific height, the settling depth can be predicted to avoid the fruit impact, for example, with channel bottom.

Conclusions

Some physical characteristics, density, volume, and mass of apple variety were determined. The settling depth of the dropped target from different heights of 10, 25, and 50 cm was determined using a water column and a digital camera. The settling depth was experimentally modeled based on the determined parameters. Based on the best model, R^2 = 0.9004 and MSE = 4.0752.

Acknowledgments

The authors thank Ilam University for the support to this research.

Conflict of Interest

None declared.

References

FAOSTAT, 2012. Available at: http://faostat.fao.org/site/339/default.aspx.

Jalali, A., H. Ghaffari, S. Lotfi, and V. Akhunipour. 2013. Some physical and chemical properties of four apple varieties of North-West Iran. Int. J. Agric. Crop Sci. 5:559–564.

Jordan, R. B., and C. J. Clark. 2004. Sorting of kiwifruit for quality using drop velocity in water. ASAE 47:1991–1998.

Kheiralipour, K. 2014. Theoretical modeling of fruit settling depth in water. Int. J. Food Prop. 17:2361–2366.

Kheiralipour, K., A. Tabatabaeefar, H. Mobli, S. Rafiee, M. Sharifi, A. Jafari, et al. 2008. Some physical and hydrodynamic properties of two varieties of apple (*Malus domestica* Borkh L.). Int. Agrophysics 22:225–229.

Kheiralipour, K., A. Tabatabaeefar, H. Mobli, S. S. Mohtasebi, S. Rafiee, A. Rajabipour, et al. 2010. Terminal velocity and its relationship to physical characteristics of apple (*Malus domestica* Borkh L.). IJFP 13:261–271.

Mohsenin, N. N. 1986. Physical properties of plant and animal materials, 2nd ed. Gordon and Breach Science Publishers, New York.

Tabatabaeefar, A. 2003. Moisture-dependent physical properties of wheat. Int. Agrophysics 17:207–211.

Tabatabaeefar, A., and A. Rajabipour. 2005. Modeling the mass of apples by geometrical attributes. Sci. Hortic. 105:373–382.

5

Maillard reaction products and potatoes: have the benefits been clearly assessed?

DeAnn J. Liska[1], Chad M. Cook[1], Ding Ding Wang[2] & John Szpylka[3]

[1]Biofortis Research, 211 E. Lake St., Addison, Illinois 60101
[2]D&V Systematic Consulting, 1945 Eastchester Rd., Apt 26D, Bronx, New York 10461
[3]Silliker, a Mérieux NutriSciences Company, Chicago, Illinois 60601

Keywords
Advanced glycation end products, browning reaction, fiber, potassium, *Solanum tuberosum*

Correspondence
DeAnn J. Liska, Senior Director Nutrition & Scientific Affairs, Biofortis Research, 211 Lake Street, Addison, IL 60101.

E-mail: deann.liska@mxns.com

Funding Information
Funding provided by the Frozen Potato Products Institute.

Abstract

Cooking foods affords numerous food safety benefits. During heating, Maillard reaction products (MRPs) are formed. MRPs contribute sensory aspects to food, including color, taste, and texture. One MRP, acrylamide, has been implicated in negative health outcomes; however, emerging data suggests MRPs may also deliver certain health benefits. The food industry has taken steps to decrease acrylamide formation, but the perception that high levels of acrylamide compromise the nutritional benefit of certain foods has continued. Potatoes are susceptible to MRP formation during cooking but also are considered an affordable, high nutrient content food. In particular, potatoes contribute significantly to fiber and potassium intakes in the U.S. population, two nutrients of need. How, then, should potatoes be judged for effects on health? A structured evidence assessment was conducted to identify literature, specifically clinical trials, on MRPs from potatoes and health, as well as nutritional contribution of potatoes. The results indicate limited human clinical data are available on negative health outcomes of potato-based MRPs, whereas potatoes are important contributors of key nutrients, such as fiber and potassium. Therefore, a balanced benefit-risk approach is warranted in order to assure that decreasing consumption of certain foods, like potatoes, does not lead to unintended consequences of nutrition inadequacies.

Introduction

Cooking food is considered to be the most effective food safety measure to reduce contaminants. The Maillard reaction, or nonenzymatic browning [reviewed in detail elsewhere (Birlouez-Aragon et al. 2010a; Van Lancker et al. 2011; Parker 2013)], occurs in foods during heating, and results in literally hundreds of different intermediates and end products, called Maillard reaction products (MRPs). Some MRPs have been shown to have in vitro antioxidant activity and/or deter oxidation of unsaturated fatty acids in foods. It is estimated that a person eating a Western diet may consume from ~1 to 10 g or higher of MRPs per day, mainly in the forms of N-ε-(6)-Carboxymethyllysine (CML) and pyrraline, although the actual intakes are not known (Ames 2007; Fogliano and Morales 2011).

Many MRPs are large polymers and it is estimated that up to 80% escape digestion. Emerging science suggests these large molecules may be fermented by bacteria in the colon, leading to potentially bioactive metabolites. In particular, the class of MRPs known as melanoidins, high molecular weight, brown-colored MRP end products found in roasted coffee or bread crusts, has obtained the most interest (Delgado-Andrade 2014). Overall, the data support that the polysaccharide-rich melanoidins found in coffee and cereal grains may be preferentially metabolized by bifidobacteria, whereas protein-rich melanoidins may be substrates for potentially harmful protein metabolizing bacteria that are predominantly present in the descending tract of the colon (Tuohy et al. 2006; Mills et al. 2008; Summa et al. 2008; Moreira et al. 2012). Evidence with melanoidins also suggests they may have chemopreventive activities, antioxidant activities, and anti-hypertensive actions (Chen and Kitts 2011a,b; Zeng et al. 2011; Moreira et al. 2012; Vitaglione et al. 2012; Delgado-Andrade 2014; Kanzler et al. 2014).

Some of the small molecule MRPs, such as CML, acrylamide, and pyrraline are generally thought to be bioavailable, although the majority appear to be rapidly excreted (Ames 2007). One MRP, acrylamide, has been implicated in negative health effects and has gained much attention (Pruser and Flynn 2011) but less information is available on health impacts of other MRPs in humans. Additionally, although in vitro and animal studies on MRPs suggest potentially beneficial effects on various health outcomes, the effects may not translate to humans. Therefore, assessment of data in humans is necessary to understand the actual impact of MRPs on health outcomes.

Potatoes, a food susceptible to MRP formation during cooking, have been a staple food in populations across the world for over 10,000 years (Camire et al. 2009). Potatoes are an affordable food option and are unique amongst vegetables in that they are a carbohydrate-rich food, but also provide beneficial fats (MUFA and PUFA), and are particularly noted for their contribution of key nutrients such as fiber and potassium (Freedman and Keast 2011; Weaver and Marr 2013). Despite the potential benefits associated with consumption of nutrients found in potatoes, the role of potatoes in a healthy diet is controversial (King and Slavin 2013; Ouhtit et al. 2014). In particular, diets such as the "meat and potatoes" diet, and diets that include specific processed forms of potato products such as chips or French fries, are called out as representing unhealthy dietary patterns (King and Slavin 2013; Ouhtit et al. 2014). It remains unclear from discussions to date, however, whether the issue relates specifically to potatoes. Thus, this review was conducted using an evidence mapping approach to understand the balance of science available for assessing benefit versus risk specifically related to MRPs and potatoes. To our knowledge, this is the first attempt to characterize the breadth and scope of human clinical research on this topic.

Methods

We employed evidence mapping techniques using a bottom-up approach, in which we started with a broad question and search strategy to identify all published literature. Study designs, populations, interventions, and outcomes were collected to provide a better understanding of the existing studies. The literature was then categorized and characterized.

The structured literature reviews on human health outcomes related to MRPs and/or potatoes were conducted essentially as outlined in the Institute of Medicine's Standards for Systematic Reviews (Moher et al. 2009). Literature searches were conducted in Medline® (January 1994 to April 2014) and Scopus® databases. Studies published in English language were screened to identify articles relevant to the inclusion/exclusion criteria. Reference lists of selected reviews were also screened for additional publications. No gray literature or unpublished data were included.

The assessment of MRPs and human health outcomes was conducted as a systematic literature search. The detailed methodology and the evidence map tables can be found in the Appendix S1. Search terms included "MRPs", "maillard reaction", "advanced glycation end products", "CML", "melanoidins", "pentosidine", and "pyrraline", as well as terms representing health outcomes. In addition, studies were included if they had a randomized controlled trial (RCT), cohort, case report, or cross-sectional design, and included an assessment of MRPs or a food with MRPs. Only studies with both an MRP-related term and a health outcome were selected for abstract review. Studies specifically on acrylamide were included in the search and initial review, but generally excluded from this report due to the availability of numerous recent reviews. The exception was if the study was a clinical trial and/or included assessment of other MRPs with acrylamide.

The potato evidence assessment included a general review of the literature on potatoes and nutrition as well as a systematic review of literature specific to potato MRPs and human health. The general review on potatoes and nutrition was conducted using the search terms "potato(es)" and "white vegetables" singly and in combination with "nutrient intakes". Studies were included if they were conducted in humans and contained an assessment of dietary intake of potatoes. Reviews and primary literature were included. A systematic search (Appendix S1) was also performed to identify human studies on MRPs from potato(es). For this search, methods followed those for the systematic review of MRPs and health outcomes with the additional search terms of "potato(es)" and "*Solanum tuberosum*". In addition, only studies that reported a dietary assessment were included.

Results

MRPs and health outcomes

The literature search for MRPs and health outcomes generated numerous studies on analytical systems from foods and in vitro or food safety and quality effects of MRPs. With respect to studies on the putative benefits and risks to human health from MRPs in foods, the literature was more limited. Eighteen publications (Vlassara et al. 2002;

Uribarri et al. 2003, 2011; Vesper et al. 2005; Seiquer et al. 2006; Negrean et al. 2007; Abramsson-Zetterberg et al. 2008; Stirban et al. 2008, 2013; Garcia et al. 2009; Mesias et al. 2009; Naruszewicz et al. 2009; Birlouez-Aragon et al. 2010b; Delgado-Andrade et al. 2011, 2012; Harcourt et al. 2011; Vikstrom et al. 2011; Correa et al. 2012) on clinical trials that included a health outcome and dietary MRP were identified, with six of these considered duplicate publications (Stirban et al. 2008; Garcia et al. 2009; Mesias et al. 2009; Delgado-Andrade et al. 2011, 2012; Vikstrom et al. 2011) (Table 1). The majority of the clinical trials were conducted on mixed diets that altered the cooking conditions, with 4 reporting potatoes in both the test diet and control diet (Seiquer et al. 2006; Negrean et al. 2007; Abramsson-Zetterberg et al. 2008; Naruszewicz et al. 2009). Two studies examined the effects of beverages containing differing amounts of MRPs on health outcomes; one was conducted on differing roasts of coffee (Correa et al. 2012) and one was on a purified protein (beta-lactalbumin) (Stirban et al. 2013).

The primary focus of research on health impacts of food-based MRPs related to acrylamide and cancer risk. Acrylamide has been classified as a 'probable carcinogen,' and when administered at very high levels is a causative agent for nervous system damage. Acrylamide was first reported as present in some processed foods in 2002, which led to a worldwide effort to decrease its formation during cooking (Fleck 2002; Granda et al. 2004; Pruser and Flynn 2011; Halford et al. 2012; Lineback et al. 2012; Arvanitoyannis and Dionisopoulou 2014; Xu et al. 2014). Three recent reviews have summarized the epidemiological evidence on association of acrylamide with risk of certain cancers (Hogervorst et al. 2010; Pelucchi et al. 2011; Tessier and Birlouez-Aragon 2012). In addition, Lipworth et al. (2012) published a qualitative review using more restrictive criteria. Our evidence mapping found the same cohorts and cross-sectional studies (with the exclusion of infant studies), as included in these reviews. In addition, we identified the U.K. Women's Cohort study (Burley et al. 2010), the Baltimore Longitudinal Study of Aging (Semba et al. 2009), and a case–control study in Taiwanese subjects (Chao et al. 2010) (Appendix S1). We did not include some of the earlier publications [from Mucci et al. (case–control studies) and Wilson et al. (Nurses' Health Study II, Sweden Prostate Cancer Cohort)], which are referenced in previous reviews (Lipworth et al. 2012). Furthermore, it should be noted that several expert panel reports on acrylamide [e.g., HEATOX (2007)] are available, but were not specifically identified in our general review of the peer-reviewed scientific literature. The vast majority of these reports do not include discussions of MRPs beyond acrylamide, and a detailed discussion of acrylamide is beyond the scope of our assessment.

In general, the human studies reporting a relationship between dietary acrylamide and increased risk of cancer are controversial (Hogervorst et al. 2010; Pelucchi et al. 2011). Hogervort et al. (2010) reported that most of the case–control studies did not observe associations between dietary acrylamide intake and increased risk of several cancer types (Hogervorst et al. 2010). However, data from some prospective cohorts suggested dietary acrylamide exposure may be associated with increased risk of post-menopausal endometrial and ovarian cancers, with weaker evidence for renal cell cancer, estrogen (and progesterone) receptor-positive breast cancer, and oral cavity cancer. Interestingly, these authors also noted acrylamide intake was associated with a reduced risk of many other cancers including lung and bladder cancers in women, and prostate and oro- and hypopharynx cancers in men. In contrast, Pelucchi et al. (2011) failed to find an increased risk for most types of cancer from exposure to acrylamide (Pelucchi et al. 2011). The divergent findings of these two review papers, which essentially analyzed the same evidence, suggests the need for more prospective cohort studies that are adequately controlled for confounding and have a sensitive measure to assess dietary acrylamide intakes.

Challenges have been reported in accurately identifying the MRP content of foods, particularly acrylamide, due to the effect that variable food preparation methods has on the type and amount of MRPs formed. The studies discussed above commonly assessed mixed diets with differences in cooking processes (frying and/or baking vs. steaming, boiling, and/or raw foods) (Hogervorst et al. 2010; Pelucchi et al. 2011). Additionally, dietary assessment methods and MRP food databases used may vary considerably and exposure measurement can be imprecise (Dybing et al. 2005; Birlouez-Aragon et al. 2010a). As noted by Freisling et al. 2013; in an analysis of 24-h diet recall data, these instruments are not typically designed to gather information related to food processing, such as cooking methods and extent of cooking (Freisling et al. 2013). In addition, it is difficult to quantify the confounding by acrylamide from cigarette smoking and other environmental sources, which contribute higher levels than found in the diet (Pruser and Flynn 2011). Therefore, data on MRP intakes across populations likely do not accurately reflect intakes when dietary self-report is the primary assessment tool. Furthermore, quantifying dietary acrylamide intakes in large population studies and comparing dietary acrylamide intake estimates from one analysis to another is not reliable, if not unwarranted.

Another complication in assessing the literature on food-based MRPs and health is the presence of nonenzymatic, chemical modification of in vivo proteins by sugars. The products resulting from this reaction are called advanced glycation end products (AGEs). The first

Table 1. Clinical trials on MRPs and potential health outcomes published from January 1994 to April 2014.

Citation	Study design	Sample size, population, country	%F	Age (y)	Test Food/Diet	Control Food/Diet	Duration	Findings
Mixed Diets Containing Potatoes								
Seiquer, et al. AJCN. 2006;83: 1082–1088	RCT X-over Controlled diet	• $N = 18$ • Healthy children • Spain	0%	12.4 ± 0.34	Brown diet (BD) MRP enriched (fried & breaded foods, corn flakes, chocolates, baked products)	White diet (WD) Similar foods and energy/nutrient contents as brown diet. Free as much as possible of MRPs	2 week/diet 40–days washout	Nutrient bioavailability study. Significantly lower absorption and higher fecal excretion of nitrogen, although modest effect. Suggests some impact on protein availability from heat treatment. No significant effects on plasma protein profile, however, suggesting no effect on protein metabolism. Comments: Potatoes on both diets (boiled/baked vs. fried) and differences in the food forms. Although diets matched as much as possible, some differences in nutrient composition (e.g., protein lower (not significant) and fat higher ($P < 0.05$) for BD compared to WD)

Four studies were a re-analysis of data from Seiquer, 2006 (above) and each cross-referenced Seiqer, 2006 as the primary study (see above for caveats)

1. Garcia, et al. Mol Nutr Food Res. 2009;53:1551–60
   - Findings: Iron intakes similar between BD and WD, but significantly lower apparent iron absorption and retention and higher excretion on BD compared to WD. Suggests MRPs can affect iron bioavailability.
2. Delgado-Andrade, et al. Nutrition. 2011;27:86–91
   - Findings: Phosphate intakes similar between BD and WD and were higher than dietary recommendations. Non significant increase in fecal phosphate excretion, with significant decrease in apparent absorption, however, no differences in phosphate-related serum parameters between diets.
3. Mesias, et al. J Agric Food Chem. 2009;57:9532–38.
   - Findings: Calcium intakes essentially the same for BD and WD. No significant differences in calcium utilization or biochemical indices of bone metabolism except deoxypyridinoline, which may be related to adolescent bone development (e.g., inconclusive).
4. Delgado-Andrade, et al. Amino Acids. 2012;43:595–602.
   - Findings: CML intake ~2× higher, and fecal excretion ~3× more with BD than WD. Considering fecal and urinary excretion together, both WD and BD resulted in similar proportional excretion, at 45.1% and 49.7%, respectively. Results suggest ~50% of ingested CML may be metabolized (e.g., microbiota) and/or absorbed.

(Continued)

Table 1. Continued.

Citation	Study design	Sample size, population, country	%F	Age (y)	Test Food/Diet	Control Food/Diet	Duration	Findings
Negrean, et al. AJCN. 2007;85:1236–1243	RCT Single-blind X-over	• $N = 20$ • Hospital inpatients with T2DM • Germany	30%	55.4 ± 2.2	High MRP meal (580 kcal) • Food was fried or broiled: ○ 200 g chicken ○ 150 g potatoes ○ 100 g carrots ○ 200 g tomatoes ○ 15 g vegetable oil	Low MRP meal (580 kcal): • Same foods as high MRP prepared by steaming or boiling	6-days standardized diabetes diet. Test diets on day 4 and 6	Flow-mediated dilation (FMD) decreased on both diets, although significantly more after high MRP diet ($P < 0.01$). No significant differences in glucose or insulin. Comments: Heating can affect other factors (vitamins, antioxidants) that have been shown to influence FMD. Potatoes included in both diets.
One study was a possible duplicate publication with Negrean, 2007 (above) that used the same study design and diet intervention, and which cross-referenced Negrean, 2007. However, the study population and demographic/disease characteristics were nearly identical, with apparent differences in one subject per study (e.g., Negrean reported 14 men and 6 women; whereas Stirban reported 13 men and 7 women). 1. Stirban, et al. Ann NY Acad Sci. 2008;1126:276–79. ○ Findings: increased excretion of urinary CML, while serum adiponectin and leptin significantly decreased, and vascular cell adhesion molecule 1 increased ($P < 0.05$).								
Vesper et al. Adv Exp Med Biol. 2005;561:89–96	CT Single arm	• $N = 6$ • Healthy, nonsmokers • USA	NR	≥18	3 oz potato chips/d (21 oz total)	None	7 days	MRP bioavailability study. Exposure to acrylamide was 1.9 μg/kg/day, which is higher than FDA estimated average of 0.4 μg/kg/day. Acrylamide and glycindamide adducts could be detected in serum, but none reached the level expected from high exposure to tobacco smoke. High intra and inter-subject variability compared to signal. Comments: Substudy of a larger Center for Disease Control (CDC) study that only assessed biomarkers; no health outcomes. Potato chip intake ~3× higher than average consumption, and acrylamide content of potato chips also ~3× higher than average. Therefore, exposure does not reflect average exposure.

(Continued)

Table 1. Continued.

Citation	Study design	Sample size, population, country	%F	Age (y)	Test Food/Diet	Control Food/Diet	Duration	Findings
Abramsson-Zetterberg, et al. Mutation Res. 2008;653:50–56	RCT Parallel	• $N = 24$ • Healthy • Sweden	58%	24–60	High-heated food diet (HHF) Subjects counseled to choose fried foods; supplied with French fries, potato crisps, biscuits, and crisp bread.	Low-heated food diet (LHF) Subjects counseled to minimize heated foods; supplied with fresh potatoes, buns, and white bread.	4 d	Significant increase in frequency of micronucleated transferring-positive reticulocytes after HHF diet. Differences in macronutrient content of the diets, particularly fat, which was higher in the HHF diet.
Naruszewicz, et al. AJCN. 2009; 89:733–777	CT Single arm	• $N = 14$ • Healthy • Sweden or Poland	57%	22–56	160 g Potato Chips (PC) 878 kcal 1374 mg sodium 157 mcg acrylamide	400 g Boiled Potatoes (BP) With fat and salt in amounts found in potato chips diet; subjects instructed to avoid potato chips	2 week run-in on boiled potatoes; 28-days on PC, then 28-days on BP	Increased oxidized LDL, hs IL-6, hsCRP, and γ-glutamyltransferase with PC diet. Transient effect with no significant changes at the end of study. Smokers ($n = 6$) assessed separately from nonsmokers ($n = 8$) and showed larger responses. Comments; Not randomized.
As stated by study authors, one publication was a re-analysis of a combined subset of data from two clinical trials Abramsson-Zetterberg, 2008 (Study 1) and Naruszewicz (Study 2) and was considered a duplicate publication in the evidence map								
1. Vikström, et al. Toxicol Sci. 2011;119(1):41–49.								
o Findings: This study compared AUC values of acrylamide and glycidamide Hb adducts in humans after high (11 lg/kg bw) or medium (2.5 lg/kg) acrylamide intake from food with similar values from rodent carcinogenicity tests. This biomarker study suggests Hb adducts of acrylamide and glycidamide in humans may be a useful marker of exposure to dietary AA.								
Mixed Diets – Potatoes Not Included or Not Reported/Unknown								
Birlouez-Aragon, et al. AJCN. 2010b;91:1220–1226	RCT X-over	• $N = 62$ • Healthy • France	50%	18–24	Standard diet (STD) rich in MRP (coffee, grilled/roasted foods, corn flakes, dry cookies, well-baked bread)	Steamed diet (STMD) low in MRP (raw foods, team, mildly baked bread, sponge cake, steamed corn flakes)	1 week/diet 10-days washout	Significantly higher total and HDL cholesterol on STD, no difference in LDL cholesterol. HOMA score significantly higher on STD. Comment: Significant differences in total kcal, carbohydrates, fats, and vitamin C on the different diets. Change in body weights not provided.

(Continued)

Table 1. Continued.

Citation	Study design	Sample size, population, country	%F	Age (y)	Test Food/Diet	Control Food/Diet	Duration	Findings
Harcourt, et al. Kidney Intl. 2011;80:190–198	RCT X-over	• *N* = 11 • Generally healthy overweight & obese • NR	0%	30 ± 9	High MRP meal • Food prepared by frying, toasting, heating	Low MRP meal • Matched in kcal and foods to high MRP meal; preparations changed to steaming, poaching, fresh/raw	2 week/diet 4 week washout	No differences in total cholesterol or fasting glucose. Significantly higher urine 8-isoprostane and plasma monocyte chemotactic protein-1, and lower macrophage inhibitory factor on high MRP. Comments: Relatively short-term intakes.
Uribarri, et al. J Am Soc Nephrol. 2003;14:728–731	RCT Parallel	• *N* = 18 • Stable renal failure patients; nondiabetic • USA	67%	NR	High MRP diet Patients instructed to roast, broil, and oven fry foods	Low MRP diet Patients instructed to boil, poach, steam, stew foods and avoid fried foods	4 week	MRP bioavailability study. Higher serum CML associated with the high MRP diet period, as well as serum AGE levels, suggesting dietary MRPs can contribute to serum AGE in renal failure patients. Comments: Several differences in diet changes from baseline between the two interventions, including total energy, fat, carbohydrate, and protein.
Vlassara, et al. Proc NatlAcad Sci USA. 2002; 99:15596–15601.	Study 1 RCT X-over Study 2 RCT Parallel Controlled diet	Study 1: • *N* = 11 Study 2: • *N* = 13 Both studies: • Nonsmoking T1DM & T2DM adults • USA	NR	1: 52 ± 2 2: ~62	High MRP diet Foods prepared with high cooking times; followed NCEP Step 1 & AHA plans for weight maintenance; MRP content $16.3 \pm 3.7\times10^6$ U/day	Low MRP diet Comparable foods to high MRP diet with lower cooking times; MRP content $3.7 \pm 1.2 \times 10^6$ U/day	Study 1: 2 week/diet 1–2 week washout Study 2: 6 week	Significantly higher serum CML during high MRP diet. Changes in blood inflammatory markers suggested pro-inflammatory response during high MRP diet. No differences in lipids, although significantly more AGE-modified LDL components during high MRP diet. Comments Meals appeared to vary in food type, and thus likely varied in fat, protein, etc. Study did control for energy intake per subject for weight maintenance.

(Continued)

Table 1. Continued.

Citation	Study design	Sample size, population, country	%F	Age (y)	Test Food/Diet	Control Food/Diet	Duration	Findings
Uribarri, et al. Diabetes Care. 2011; 34:1610–1616.	RCT	• $N = 36$ • T2DM (16) and health (16); age-matched • USA	78%	>60	High MRP diet $n = 6$ T2DM; Subjects' usual diet rich in MRP (dietary MRP intake ≥20 AGE Eq/day)	MRP-restricted diet $n = 12$ T2DM and 16 healthy; isocaloric to high MRP diet; boil, poach, stew, or steam food; limited MRP intake by ~40–50% of usual diet	4 month	No significant changes in healthy controls for any markers except lower serum CML and urinary 8-isoprostane with the MRP-restricted diet. Differences were identified with diabetic subjects, including decreased HOMA scores, leptin levels, and plasma insulin, however, adiponectin was ~2× higher with MRP-restricted diet. Comments: Diets not well described.
Beverages (not Potato-Based)								
Corrêa et al. Plant Foods Hum Nutr. 2012;67:277–282	RCT X-over	• $N = 20$ Healthy, usual coffee drinkers • Age 49 ± 9 • Brazil	70%	49 ± 9	Higher MRP medium roast coffee (~482 mL/ day)	Lower MRP medium light roast coffee (~482 mL/day)	1 week run-in 4 week/diet No washout	Both coffees resulted in significant increases in plasma total antioxidant capacity, ORAC, and several other antioxidant markers. The lower MRP roast delivered more chlorogenic acid and less caffeine than the higher MRP roast.
Stirban, et al. Diabetes Care. 2013;36:1278–1282.	RCT Double-blind X-over	• $N = 19$ • T2DM patients • Germany	NR	36–66	MRP beverage • Beta-lactoglobulin and dextrose heated beverage • 120,000 U CML/ serve	Control beverage • Prepared the same as test beverage but without dextrose • 19,400 U CML/serve	One day – single dose 7-days washout	Significantly lower flow-mediated dilation and plasma CML concentration at 90 min post consumption but not at 180 min for MRP beverage. Comments: Single dose in patients with frank diabetes.

AHA, American Heart Association; AJCN, Am J Clin Nutr; BD, brown diet; Ca, calcium; CML, N-ε-carboxymethyl-lysine; CT; controlled trial; d, day; Eq, equivalents; g, gram; HHF, high-heated food; HOMA, homeostasis model assessment; kcal, kilocalorie; LDL, low-density lipoprotein; LHF, low-heated food; mcg, microgram; mg, milligram; mo, month; MRP, Maillard reaction product; NCEP, National Cholesterol Education Program; NR, not reported; ORAC, Oxygen Radical Absorbance Capacity; RCT, randomized clinical trial; STD, standard diet; STMD, steamed diet; T1DM, T2DM, type 1 or 2 diabetes mellitus; U, units; wk, week(s); WD, white diet; X-over, crossover; y, years.

Many of the clinical trials referred to diets as containing advanced glycation end-products (AGEs). For consistency in terminology, AGEs was changed to MRPs in our evidence map.

Table 2. Major reviews and/or meta-analyses relevant to potatoes and potato nutrition.

Citation	Comments
Literature Reviews	
Camire, et al. Potatoes and Human Health. Crit Rev Food Sci Nutr. 2009; 49:823–840.	Review of potatoes in the food supply, including potato nutrition, varieties, cooking effect on nutrients, contaminants, and health relationships
Weaver & Marr. White Vegetables: A forgotten source of nutrients. Purdue roundtable executive summary. Adv. Nutr. 2013; 4:318S–326S.	Nine reviews of nutrients provided by white vegetables, with some specific to potatoes, including mineral nutrition, fiber, and glycemic response and diabetes
Yoshimatsu, et al. [Current status in the commercialization and application of genetically modified plants and their effects on human and livestock health and photoremediation]. Yakugaku Zasshi. 2012; 132 (5):629–274.	Summary of developments with genetically modified plants, such as use for nutraceuticals, medical curatives, and for production of oral vaccines
Zaheer & Akhtar. Recent advances in potato production, usage, nutrition – a review. Crit Rev Food Sci Nutr. June 2012.	General summary of potato nutrition, generation and mitigation of acrylamide, and other risks from potato consumption (e.g., allergies, alkaloids). Some health benefit-related studies referenced
Systematic Reviews	
Al-Khudairy, et al. Dietary factors and type 2 diabetes in the Middle East: what is the evidence for an association? Nutrients. 2013; Sep 26; 5(10): 3871–3897.	Identified 17 studies, mainly observational, examining association between dietary factors with T2DM. Only 2 studies (case–control and cross-sectional) reported a significant positive association between potatoes and T2DM risk
Vlachojannis, et al. Medicinal uses of potato-derived products: a systematic review. Phytother Res. 2010; 24 (2): 159–162.	Identified 5 clinical trials on medical use of potato extracts (e.g., oralfor dyspepsia, topical for perianal dermatitis). Only one RCT, which suggested an oral potato proteinase inhibitor may reduce food intake at subsequent meals
Yusof, et al. Dietary patterns and risk of colorectal cancer: A systematic review of cohort studies (2000–2011). Asian Pac J Cancer Prev. 2012; 13(9): 4713–4717.	Concluded a Western dietary pattern was associated with increased risk of colorectal cancer, whereas a prudent diet was not. Although Western diet was referenced as meat and potatoes, no specific data on potato intake was provided in most studies
Meta-Analyses	
Mozaffarian, et al. Changes in diet and lifestyle and long-term weight gain in women and men. N Engl J Med. 2011; 364 (25):2392–2404.	Dietary factors with the largest positive association with 4-year weight gain in three large US cohorts included potato chips and potatoes
Nettleton, et al. Meta-analysis investigating associations between healthy diet and fasting glucose and insulin levels and modification by loci associated with glucose homeostasis in data from 15 cohorts. Am J Epidemiol. 2013; 177 (2):103–115.	Utilized data from 15 US and European cohort studies to construct a diet score, with fried potatoes a component of an unfavorable score. Excluded baked, boiled, or mashed white potatoes in the assessment, although the cohort data included these foods

observation of AGEs occurred with the discovery of glycated hemoglobin (HbA_{1c}), which is used today as a marker for diabetes (Henle et al. 1996). A relationship has been established between increases in AGEs and presence of age-related diseases, such as diabetes and cardiovascular disease (Delgado-Andrade 2014). However, the investigation into whether food-based AGEs demonstrate similar associations with disease conditions is still in its infancy. Only a handful of studies that clearly identified specific food-based MRPs have been conducted in human subjects. Thus, the role of food-based MRPs in health is still an emerging science.

Potatoes and nutrition

The nutritional contribution of potatoes has been recently thoroughly reviewed, and a summary of reviews on potatoes and nutrient intakes is provided in Table 2. In general, potatoes have been reported to provide more nutrients per calorie than most other staple foods (Freedman and Keast 2011). It is also notable that potato products deliver most of their fat in the form of MUFA and PUFA. Fried potatoes contribute only ~2.0% to the average saturated fatty acid intake of the U.S. population, and are not among the top 10 contributors to saturated fatty acid intake (U.S. Department of Agriculture and U.S. Department of Health and Human Services, 2010). In addition, frozen potato products have been shown to contain <0.5 g/serving of *trans* fat (Doell et al. 2012).

Freedman and Keast (2011) assessed the contribution of white potatoes, French fries, and oven-baked potatoes in the diets of children. Potatoes accounted for between 7.7% and 9.2% of daily energy intakes in children, and provided a higher average contribution of dietary fiber, vitamin B6, magnesium, copper, potassium, and MUFA than calories, and less sodium and saturated fats (Fig. 1A

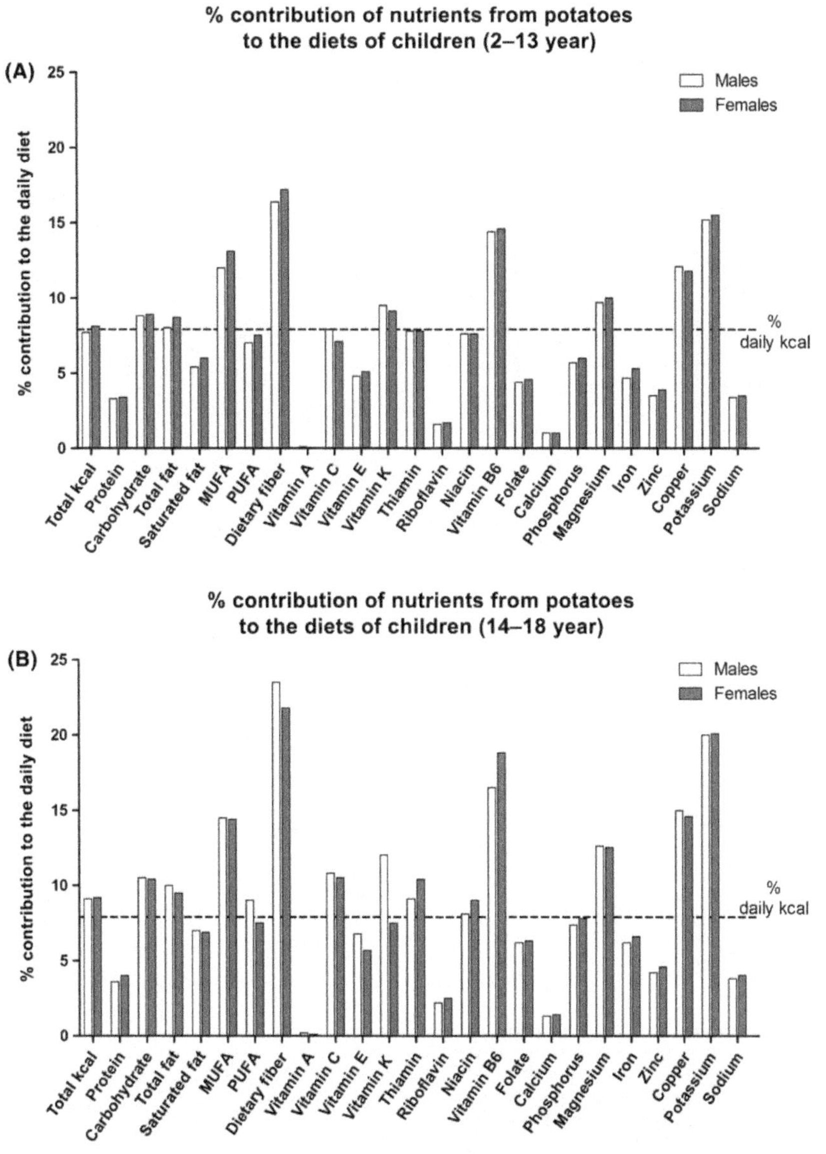

Figure 1. Percent contribution of nutrients from white potatoes, French fries, and oven-baked fries compared to total calories for children age 2–13 years (A) and 14–18 years (B) using National Health and Nutrition Examination Survey (NHANES) 2003–2006 (Freedman and Keast 2011). Intakes for males and females are shown in solid white and gray bars, respectively. Percent total calories provided by potato foods is shown in the first column and represented by the horizontal dotted line.

and B). In particular, potatoes delivered between 16.4% and 23.5% daily intakes of dietary fiber and between 15.2% and 20.1% of potassium to children's diets, two nutrients of concern in the U.S. population. Similar to the findings in children, studies with adults using National Health and Nutrition Examination Survey (NHANES) 2003–2006 (Freedman and Keast 2012) and 2009–2010 (Storey and Anderson 2013) have shown that potatoes and potato products provided more fiber, vitamin B6, and potassium than the corresponding energy contribution. Potatoes also provided substantial vitamin C, MUFA, and PUFA.

King and Slavin (2013) reviewed the role of the white potato in meeting dietary recommendations and noted that only ~1/3 of the total fat in white potatoes is in the form of saturated fatty acids (King and Slavin 2013). Moreover, potatoes have less lipid than that found in rice (0.2%) and pasta (0.9%), and have a higher biological value of protein than soybeans or legumes. Drewnowski 2013; reviewed the nutrient contribution of potatoes with respect to cost using the Affordable Nutrition Index, and report that, of the foods evaluated only white potatoes (boiled and baked) and carrots provide the three key characteristics of nutrient density, affordability, and consumer acceptance (Drewnowski 2013).

Potatoes are generally considered a high glycemic index (GI) food; however, in a recent review it was reported that the actual GI for potatoes commonly consumed in North America ranges from 56 to 94, indicating that not all potato preparations have a high GI (Anderson et al. 2013). The highest GI values are noted for mashed potatoes, although reported values vary considerably, with baked potatoes, French fries, and potato crisps generally having GI values in the medium range. The role of GI in health outcomes is controversial: recent assessments indicate there is only a moderate body of inconsistent evidence to support the relationship between high GI and type 2 diabetes; and that the amount of evidence regarding a link between GI and cardiovascular disease has not been conclusive (U.S. Department of Agriculture and U.S. Department of Health and Human Services, 2010).

Epidemiological evidence has shown an association between higher intakes of potato products and weight gain (Mozaffarian et al. 2011), but these studies have not separated the effect of potato consumption from the effect of components added during cooking/processing, such as fat, or other foods consumed with the potato. In our literature assessment, only one RCT that attempted to evaluate the specific role of potatoes as part of a weight-loss diet was identified (Randolph et al. 2014). In that study, 90 overweight men and women were randomly assigned to one of three 12-week interventions: (1) low GI energy reduced (−500 kcal/day) diet; (2) high GI energy reduced (−500 kcal/day) diet; or (3) habitual diet (control). All subjects were counseled to consume 5–7 servings of potatoes per week from a provided allotment of 6 russet and 3 red potato varieties weekly. All groups lost a modest, but statistically significant, amount of weight (average of −1.5 to 2.3 kg). As a result of these findings, the authors suggest potatoes do not interfere with weight loss or cause weight gain as part of a usual diet.

Several studies have investigated the effects of potato chips on markers of appetite/satiety, which are often linked to weight management. Potato chips were compared to other snack options on short-term appetite and energy intake in 26 normal-weight children, 8–11 years, and reported to lead to increased cumulative food intake compared with raisins or grapes, but lower than cookies (Patel et al. 2013). In another study, children who ate a snack of cheese and vegetables consumed ~72% fewer calories compared to children provided with potato chips in a short-term assessment (Wansink et al. 2013). Tey et al. (2012) demonstrated that habitual consumption of energy-dense snack foods (hazelnuts, chocolate milk, or salted potato chips) resulted in a decrease in sensory-specific satiety over a 12-week consumption period (Tey et al. 2012). These effects were not specific to potato chips alone, and results were compared to a control group that did not receive snack foods. Therefore, the effect of potato chip consumption as a snack on long-term energy intake has not been thoroughly explored.

Potato MRPs and health outcomes

The systematic literature search on MRPs from potato(es) and health outcomes yielded few studies. Vesper et al. (2005) conducted a pilot validation study in six generally healthy, nonsmoking adults to determine if acrylamide exposure from consumption of 3 ounces of potato chips daily over the course of a week increased the concentration of proposed biomarkers of acrylamide intake (Hb-acrylamide and Hb-glycidamide adducts) (Vesper et al. 2005). Adduct levels were detected in all subjects with increases of up to 46% for Hb-acrylamide and 79% for glycidamide. The authors noted that the concentrations were within the range of background levels observed in previous studies (not specific to potato chip consumption). No results on health outcomes were reported.

In the only RCT identified that specifically examined dietary acrylamide exposure from potato, Naruszewicz et al. (2009) found that daily consumption of 160 g of potato chips (157 mg acrylamide) over four weeks induced a proinflammatory metabolic profile (increased blood concentrations of oxidized LDL-C, interleukin-6, and high sensitive C-reactive protein) in generally healthy adults (Naruszewicz et al. 2009). Changes in these inflammatory biomarkers are potentially important because increased levels have been associated with risk for developing atherosclerosis. These results should be interpreted with caution, as the acrylamide intake level in this study was approximately three times higher than estimated intakes from a Western diet (~50 μg/day) (Hagmar et al. 2005).

One observation study included in the evidence map was an analysis of a series of hospital-based case–control studies in Italy and Switzerland (Bosetti et al. 2002). These studies were designed to describe the relationship between dietary intake of fried and baked potatoes and risk of developing various types of cancer (oral cavity/pharynx, esophagus, larynx, colon, rectum, breast, and ovary). The main findings from this study suggested a lack of an association between consumption of baked/fried potatoes and risk of cancer at several anatomical sites. This study was conducted in southern European populations that use different cooking processes than most population groups in the United States, which should be considered in translating the findings.

Three additional clinical trials of potatoes, MRPs, and health outcomes were identified in this literature review, but were not adequately designed to examine the effect of MRPs specifically from potatoes on health outcomes (Seiquer et al. 2006; Negrean et al. 2007; Abramsson-Zetterberg et al. 2008). Two of these studies included potatoes in both dietary intervention groups using different methods of cooking (Seiquer et al. 2006; Negrean et al. 2007), and one included potatoes (French fries and potato chips) as part of a high-fat diet (Abramsson-Zetterberg et al. 2008). Further research is needed to characterize the MRP profile of potato and potato products. Additional research on the effect of different potato cooking methods on health outcomes is also needed, including prospective study designs that control for potential confounding of high-protein foods (e.g., protein-based melanoidins vs. starch-based melanoidins).

Benefits-risk of potatoes and MRPs

The traditional approach to risk assessment has been described as a scientific endeavor that follows a defined pathway: (1) hazard identification, (2) hazard characterization, (3) exposure assessment, and (4) risk characterization (European Food Safety Authority (EFSA), 2006; Tijhuis et al. 2012). The approach is primarily based on studies in animals with defined components used in subchronic or chronic dose–response studies. Historically, the risk from specific foods and food components has been assessed separately from benefits, and has been the domain of the toxicology experts. More recently, scientists and public health officials have recognized that the health-related benefits from foods need to be considered as well as part of a risk assessment (Tijhuis et al. 2012).

The most notable summary of benefit-risk is that of Seal et al. (2008), who published three case studies on acrylamide showing an approach to including benefit along with a risk assessment (Seal et al. 2008). These authors used potatoes as one of the case studies, summarizing its benefits as provision of energy, vitamins C and B6, magnesium, and fiber (particularly when skins remain intact). However, the authors did not address potassium, a nutrient of need in the U.S. diet, or importance of potatoes in fiber nutriture even when skins are not attached. Increased potassium intake is thought to be the largest explanation for the decrease in blood pressure that occurs with consumption of the Dietary Approaches to Stop Hypertension (DASH) dietary pattern, and it has been estimated that an average increase of 1.6 g/day of potassium could lead to a 21% decreased risk of stroke in the U.S. population, independent of blood pressure benefits (D'Elia et al. 2014). Furthermore, in adults, dietary fiber has been shown to be associated with decreased risk for chronic diseases (e.g., obesity and diabetes) (Liu et al. 2015). Clearly, assessment of the impact of decreased consumption of potatoes on potassium and fiber, and potential increases in health issues, is warranted in order to balance the assessment of risk from acrylamide. Seal et al. (2008) also commented on the relatively high GI of potatoes and potato products when eaten hot, and suggested a relationship between high GI foods and adverse health outcomes, but as described previously in this document, the role of GI and health outcomes is controversial and not strongly supported by current science.

The review by Seal et al. (2008) did note a specific benefit of commercial production of potatoes as compared to home cooking from their literature assessment, indicating that: "*In general terms, it can be stated that industrial cooking leads to a much better control of desired and undesired changes than home cooking.*" Studies analyzing for markers of MRP formation in home cooked foods have shown wide ranges in the types of MRPs. It is interesting to speculate that MRPs may be less variable in processed foods due to consistent manufacturing practices. This point is particularly important in relation to mitigation efforts on acrylamide, which have resulted in substantial decreases of this MRP in foods that are manufactured.

Although not directly included in benefit-risk assessments, which generally define benefit in terms of a nutrition or health outcome that can be defined and quantified, another important 'benefit' associated with food is the sensory attributes that impact consumer acceptability. For example, fried and baked potatoes are well accepted by consumers from a sensory perspective (Tijhuis et al. 2012), thus supporting the consumption of the nutrients, potassium and fiber.

Conclusions

To our knowledge, this is the first attempt to characterize the breadth and scope of human clinical research on potato MRPs and health outcomes. The available studies have primarily focused on the formation of acrylamide and not other MRPs. There appears to be a major gap in the current understanding of the impact of MRPs, and specifically MRPs from potatoes, on human health. Indeed, much of the information on potential human health effects of MRPs, both positive and negative, has been extrapolated from in vitro and animal studies. For example, Muscat and colleagues, in a series of in vitro experiments, have shown that MRPs are cytotoxic (i.e., toxic to living cells) (Muscat et al. 2009) and can generate reactive oxygen species (e.g., H_2O_2) that may be important in immune and inflammatory reactions (Muscat et al. 2007), although these findings have not been confirmed in human clinical studies.

In our assessment, we found the majority of studies on potatoes conducted to date have either been confounded by inclusion of other nonpotato foods, or have focused on specific forms of potatoes (e.g., potato chips). For example, only one study has been conducted associating daily consumption of a large quantity of potato chips with risk of developing atherosclerosis, but this study does not definitively prove a link between potato consumption and cardiovascular disease. In addition, some studies have used colored potatoes (e.g., purple), which contain phytochemicals that may confer health benefits not typically associated white/yellow potatoes; however, these varieties are not commonly consumed in the average Western diet. Many of the limitations of observational evidence should be taken into consideration as well when interpreting the data for public health messages around MRPs, such as acrylamide, and potato intake. Furthermore, the focus on a specific individual compound may not be the optimal approach to evaluating a class of compounds (e.g., dietary MRPs), which may have differing health outcomes in the context of food (e.g., potato) that provides nutritional benefit.

Maillard reaction products gained attention in 2002 with the identification of acrylamide occurring in foods high in reducing sugars and asparagine after heating (e.g., via the Maillard Reaction). Because acrylamide has been classified as a 'probable carcinogen' and a causative agent in damage to the nervous system when administered at very high levels, a worldwide effort was initiated to decrease acrylamide in foods [reviewed in (Pruser and Flynn 2011)]. Several recent in-depth reviews on the occurrence, mitigation efforts, and risk from acrylamide have been published (HEATOX 2007; Lineback et al. 2012; Arvanitoyannis and Dionisopoulou 2014). While associations between acrylamide at high intake levels and chronic health disease risks (primarily cancer) have been shown, few, if any, human studies using acrylamide intakes representative of current consumption patterns have been conducted.

Potatoes and potato products play a significant role in providing nutrients. Specifically, fiber and potassium are nutrients of concern in the U.S. population, with nearly all Americans, both adults and children falling short of meeting their daily recommendations for intakes (Hornick et al. 2011; King et al. 2012; Weaver and Marr 2013). Consideration of the impact of decreased potato consumption on intake of nutrients, particularly fiber and potassium and the potential subsequent health effects, should be included in a benefit-risk assessment. Given the predominance of potatoes in providing the nutrients to the diets of U.S. adults and children, further research is warranted before conclusions on benefit-risk of potato consumption can be made.

1. Understanding the current acrylamide intake from potatoes given the substantial mitigation efforts.
2. Include assessments of decreased potassium and fiber consumption when modeling changes in potato consumption.
3. Better identify the MRPs in potatoes, specifically the melanoidins, and understand whether in vitro effects as antioxidants and modulators of microbiota translate to health outcomes in humans.

Acknowledgments

Funding provided by the Frozen Potato Products Institute.

Conflict of Interest

Biofortis Research, Addison, IL received financial support for the evidence mapping project from the Frozen Potato Products Institute. The views expressed in this article are those of the authors and were developed independent of the funding agency.

References

Abramsson-Zetterberg, L., A. C. Vikstrom, M. Tornqvist, and K. E. Hellenas. 2008. Differences in the frequency of micronucleated erythrocytes in humans in relation to consumption of fried carbohydrate-rich food. Mutat. Res. 653:50–56.

Al-Khudairy, L., S. Stranges, S. Kumar, N. Al-Daghri, and K. Rees. 2013. Dietary factors and type 2 diabetes in the Middle East: what is the evidence for an association?–a systematic review. Nutrients. 5:3871–3897.

Ames, J. M. 2007. Evidence against dietary advanced glycation endproducts being a risk to human health. Mol. Nutr. Food Res. 51:1085–1090.

Anderson, G. H., C. D. Soeandy, and C. E. Smith. 2013. White vegetables: glycemia and satiety. Adv. Nutr. 4:356S–367S.

Arvanitoyannis, I. S., and N. Dionisopoulou. 2014. Acrylamide: formation, occurrence in food products, detection methods, and legislation. Crit. Rev. Food Sci. Nutr. 54:708–733.

Birlouez-Aragon, I., F. Morales, V. Fogliano, and J. P. Pain. 2010a. The health and technological implications of a better control of neoformed contaminants by the food industry. Pathol. Biol. (Paris) 58:232–238.

Birlouez-Aragon, I., G. Saavedra, F. J. Tessier, A. Galinier, L. Ait-Ameur, F. Lacoste, et al. 2010b. A diet based on high-heat-treated foods promotes risk factors for diabetes mellitus and cardiovascular diseases. Am. J. Clin. Nutr. 91:1220–1226.

Bosetti, C., R. Talamini, F. Levi, E. Negri, S. Franceschi, L. Airoldi, et al. 2002. Fried foods: a risk factor for laryngeal cancer? Br. J. Cancer 87:1230–1233.

Burley, V. J., D. C. Greenwood, S. J. Hepworth, L. K. Fraser, T. M. de Kok, S. G. van Breda, et al. 2010. Dietary acrylamide intake and risk of breast cancer in the UK women's cohort. Br. J. Cancer 103:1749–1754.

Camire, M. E., S. Kubow, and D. J. Donnelly. 2009. Potatoes and human health. Crit. Rev. Food Sci. Nutr. 49:823–840.

Chao, P. C., C. N. Huang, C. C. Hsu, M. C. Yin, and Y. R. Guo. 2010. Association of dietary AGEs with circulating AGEs, glycated LDL, IL-1alpha and MCP-1 levels in type 2 diabetic patients. Eur. J. Nutr. 49:429–434.

Chen, X. M., and D. D. Kitts. 2011a. Correlating changes that occur in chemical properties with the generation of antioxidant capacity in different sugar-amino acid Maillard reaction models. J. Food Sci. 76:C831–C837.

Chen, X. M., and D. D. Kitts. 2011b. Antioxidant and anti-inflammatory activities of Maillard reaction products isolated from sugar-amino acid model systems. J. Agric. Food Chem. 59:11294–11303.

Correa, T. A., M. P. Monteiro, T. M. Mendes, D. M. Oliveira, M. M. Rogero, C. I. Benites, et al. 2012. Medium light and medium roast paper-filtered coffee increased antioxidant capacity in healthy volunteers: results of a randomized trial. Plant Foods Hum. Nutr. 67:277–282.

Delgado-Andrade, C. 2014. Maillard reaction products: some considerations on their health effects. Clin. Chem. Lab. Med. 52:53–60.

Delgado-Andrade, C., I. Seiquer, M. M. Garcia, G. Galdo, and M. P. Navarro. 2011. Increased Maillard reaction products intake reduces phosphorus digestibility in male adolescents. Nutrition 27:86–91.

Delgado-Andrade, C., F. J. Tessier, C. Niquet-Leridon, I. Seiquer, and M. Pilar Navarro. 2012. Study of the urinary and faecal excretion of Nepsilon-carboxymethyllysine in young human volunteers. Amino Acids 43:595–602.

D'Elia, L., C. Iannotta, P. Sabino, and R. Ippolito. 2014. Potassium-rich diet and risk of stroke: updated meta-analysis. Nutr. Metab. Cardiovasc. Dis. 24:585–587.

Doell, D., D. Folmer, H. Lee, M. Honigfort, and S. Carberry. 2012. Updated estimate of trans fat intake by the US population. Food Addit. Contam. Part A Chem. Anal. Control Expo. Risk Assess 29:861–874.

Drewnowski, A. 2013. New metrics of affordable nutrition: which vegetables provide most nutrients for least cost? J. Acad. Nutr. Diet. 113:1182–1187.

Dybing, E., P. B. Farmer, M. Andersen, T. R. Fennell, S. P. Lalljie, D. J. Muller, et al. 2005. Human exposure and internal dose assessments of acrylamide in food. Food Chem. Toxicol. 43:365–410.

European Food Safety Authority (EFSA). 2006. Risk-benefit analysis of foods: Methods and approaches. Summary Report of EFSA Scientific Colloquium. 10155.

Fleck, F. 2002. Experts launch action on acrylamide in staple foods. BMJ 325:120.

Fogliano, V., and F. J. Morales. 2011. Estimation of dietary intake of melanoidins from coffee and bread. Food. Funct. 2:117–123.

Freedman, M. R., and D. R. Keast. 2011. White potatoes, including french fries, contribute shortfall nutrients to children's and adolescents' diets. Nutr. Res. 31:270–277.

Freedman, M. R., and D. R. Keast. 2012. Potatoes, including French fries, contribute key nutrients to diets of U.S. Adults: NHANES 2003–2006. J. Nutr. Ther. 1:1–11.

Freisling, H., A. Moskal, P. Ferrari, G. Nicolas, V. Knaze, F. Clavel-Chapelon, et al. 2013. Dietary acrylamide intake of adults in the European Prospective Investigation into Cancer and Nutrition differs greatly according to geographical region. Eur. J. Nutr. 52:1369–1380.

Garcia, M. M., I. Seiquer, C. Delgado-Andrade, G. Galdo, and M. P. Navarro. 2009. Intake of Maillard reaction products reduces iron bioavailability in male adolescents. Mol. Nutr. Food Res. 53:1551–1560.

Granda, C., R. G. Moreira, and S. E. Tichy. 2004. Reduction of acrylamide formation in potato chips by low-temperature vacuum frying. J. Food Sci. 69:E405–E411.

Hagmar, L., E. Wirfalt, B. Paulsson, and M. Tornqvist. 2005. Differences in hemoglobin adduct levels of acrylamide in the general population with respect to dietary intake, smoking habits and gender. Mutat. Res. 580:157–165.

Halford, N. G., T. Y. Curtis, N. Muttucumaru, J. Postles, J. S. Elmore, and D. S. Mottram. 2012. The acrylamide problem: a plant and agronomic science issue. J. Exp. Bot. 63:2841–2851.

Harcourt, B. E., K. C. Sourris, M. T. Coughlan, K. Z. Walker, S. L. Dougherty, S. Andrikopoulos, et al. 2011. Targeted reduction of advanced glycation improves renal function in obesity. Kidney Int. 80:190–198.

Heat-generated food toxicants: Identification, Characterisation and Risk Minimisation (HEATOX). 2007. http://www.heatox.org and http://cordis.europa.eu/result/rcn/51664_en.html (accessed 9 July 2015).

Henle, T., R. Deppisch, and E. Ritz. 1996. The Maillard reaction–from food chemistry to uraemia research. Nephrol. Dial. Transplant. 11:1718–1722.

Hogervorst, J. G., B. J. Baars, L. J. Schouten, E. J. Konings, R. A. Goldbohm, and P. A. van den Brandt. 2010. The carcinogenicity of dietary acrylamide intake: a comparative discussion of epidemiological and experimental animal research. Crit. Rev. Toxicol. 40:485–512.

Kanzler, C., P. T. Haase, and L. W. Kroh. 2014. Antioxidant capacity of 1-deoxy-D-erythro-hexo-2,3-diulose and D-arabino-hexo-2-ulose. J. Agric. Food Chem. 62:2837–2844.

King, J. C., and J. L. Slavin. 2013. White potatoes, human health, and dietary guidance. Adv. Nutr. 4:393S–401S.

King, D. E., A. G. 3rd Mainous, and C. A. Lambourne. 2012. Trends in dietary fiber intake in the United States, 1999–2008. J. Acad. Nutr. Diet. 112:642–648.

Lineback, D. R., J. R. Coughlin, and R. H. Stadler. 2012. Acrylamide in foods: a review of the science and future considerations. Annu. Rev. Food. Sci. Technol. 3:15–35.

Lipworth, L., J. S. Sonderman, R. E. Tarone, and J. K. McLaughlin. 2012. Review of epidemiologic studies of dietary acrylamide intake and the risk of cancer. Eur. J. Cancer Prev. 21:375–386.

Liu, L., S. Wang, and J. Liu. 2015. Fiber consumption and all-cause, cardiovascular, and cancer mortalities: a systematic review and meta-analysis of cohort studies. Mol. Nutr. Food Res. 59:139–146.

Mesias, M., I. Seiquer, and M. P. Navarro. 2009. Influence of diets rich in Maillard reaction products on calcium bioavailability. Assays in male adolescents and in Caco-2 cells. J. Agric. Food Chem. 57:9532–9538.

Mills, D. J., K. M. Tuohy, J. Booth, M. Buck, M. J. Crabbe, G. R. Gibson, et al. 2008. Dietary glycated protein modulates the colonic microbiota towards a more detrimental composition in ulcerative colitis patients and non-ulcerative colitis subjects. J. Appl. Microbiol. 105:706–714.

Moher, D., A. Liberati, J. Tetzlaff, D. G. Altman, and Group, P. 2009. Preferred reporting items for systematic reviews and meta-analyses: the PRISMA statement. PLoS Med. 6:e1000097.

Moreira, A. S., F. M. Nunes, M. R. Domingues, and M. A. Coimbra. 2012. Coffee melanoidins: structures, mechanisms of formation and potential health impacts. Food. Funct. 3:903–915.

Mozaffarian, D., T. Hao, E. B. Rimm, W. C. Willett, and F. B. Hu. 2011. Changes in diet and lifestyle and long-term weight gain in women and men. N. Engl. J. Med. 364:2392–2404.

Muscat, S., J. Pelka, J. Hegele, B. Weigle, G. Munch, and M. Pischetsrieder. 2007. Coffee and Maillard products activate NF-kappaB in macrophages via H_2O_2 production. Mol. Nutr. Food Res. 51:525–535.

Muscat, S., M. Pischetsrieder, A. Maczurek, S. Rothemund, and G. Munch. 2009. Cytotoxicity of Maillard reaction products determined with a peptide spot library. Mol. Nutr. Food Res. 53:1019–1029.

Naruszewicz, M., D. Zapolska-Downar, A. Kosmider, G. Nowicka, M. Kozlowska-Wojciechowska, A. S. Vikstrom, et al. 2009. Chronic intake of potato chips in humans increases the production of reactive oxygen radicals by leukocytes and increases plasma C-reactive protein: a pilot study. Am. J. Clin. Nutr. 89:773–777.

Negrean, M., A. Stirban, B. Stratmann, T. Gawlowski, T. Horstmann, C. Gotting, et al. 2007. Effects of low- and high-advanced glycation endproduct meals on macro- and microvascular endothelial function and oxidative stress in patients with type 2 diabetes mellitus. Am. J. Clin. Nutr. 85:1236–1243.

Nettleton, J. A., M. F. Hivert, R. N. Lemaitre, N. M. McKeown, D. Mozaffarian, T. Tanaka, et al. 2013. Meta-analysis investigating associations between healthy diet and fasting glucose and insulin levels and modification by loci associated with glucose homeostasis in data from 15 cohorts. Am. J. Epidemiol. 177:103–115.

Ouhtit, A., M. Al-Sharbati, I. Gupta, and Y. Al-Farsi. 2014. Potato chips and childhood: what does the science say? An unrecognized threat? Nutrition 30:1110–1112.

Parker, J. K. 2013. The kinetics of thermal generation of flavour. J. Sci. Food Agric. 93:197–208.

Patel, B. P., N. Bellissimo, B. Luhovyy, L. J. Bennett, E. Hurton, J. E. Painter, et al. 2013. An after-school snack of raisins lowers cumulative food intake in young children. J. Food Sci. 78:A5–A10.

Pelucchi, C., C. La Vecchia, C. Bosetti, P. Boyle, and P. Boffetta. 2011. Exposure to acrylamide and human cancer–a review and meta-analysis of epidemiologic studies. Ann. Oncol. 22:1487–1499.

Pruser, K. N., and N. E. Flynn. 2011. Acrylamide in health and disease. Front. Biosci. (Schol Ed) 3:41–51.

Randolph, J. M., I. Edirisinghe, A. M. Masoni, T. Kappagoda, and B. Burton-Freeman. 2014. Potatoes, glycemic index, and weight loss in free-living individuals: practical implications. J. Am. Coll. Nutr. 33:375–384.

Seal, C. J., A. de Mul, G. Eisenbrand, A. J. Haverkort, K. Franke, S. P. Lalljie, et al. 2008. Risk-benefit considerations of mitigation measures on acrylamide content of foods–a case study on potatoes, cereals and coffee. Br. J. Nutr. 99(Suppl 2):S1–S46.

Seiquer, I., J. Diaz-Alguacil, C. Delgado-Andrade, M. Lopez-Frias, A. Munoz Hoyos, G. Galdo, et al. 2006. Diets rich in Maillard reaction products affect protein digestibility in adolescent males aged 11–14 y. Am. J. Clin. Nutr. 83:1082–1088.

Semba, R. D., S. S. Najjar, K. Sun, E. G. Lakatta, and L. Ferrucci. 2009. Serum carboxymethyl-lysine, an advanced glycation end product, is associated with increased aortic pulse wave velocity in adults. Am. J. Hypertens. 22:74–79.

Stirban, A., M. Negrean, C. Gotting, J. Uribarri, T. Gawlowski, B. Stratmann, et al. 2008. Dietary advanced glycation endproducts and oxidative stress: in vivo effects on endothelial function and adipokines. Ann. N. Y. Acad. Sci. 1126:276–279.

Stirban, A., P. Kotsi, K. Franke, U. Strijowski, W. Cai, C. Gotting, et al. 2013. Acute macrovascular dysfunction in patients with type 2 diabetes induced by ingestion of advanced glycated beta-lactoglobulins. Diabetes Care 36:1278–1282.

Storey, M. L., and P. A. Anderson. 2013. Contributions of white vegetables to nutrient intake: NHANES 2009–2010. Adv. Nutr. 4:335S–344S.

Summa, C., J. McCourt, B. Cammerer, A. Fiala, M. Probst, S. Kun, et al. 2008. Radical scavenging activity, anti-bacterial and mutagenic effects of cocoa bean Maillard reaction products with degree of roasting. Mol. Nutr. Food Res. 52:342–351.

Tessier, F. J., and I. Birlouez-Aragon. 2012. Health effects of dietary Maillard reaction products: the results of ICARE and other studies. Amino Acids 42:1119–1131.

Tey, S. L., R. C. Brown, A. R. Gray, A. W. Chisholm, and C. M. Delahunty. 2012. Long-term consumption of high energy-dense snack foods on sensory-specific satiety and intake. Am. J. Clin. Nutr. 95:1038–1047.

Tijhuis, M. J., N. de Jong, M. V. Pohjola, H. Gunnlaugsdottir, M. Hendriksen, J. Hoekstra, et al. 2012. State of the art in benefit-risk analysis: food and nutrition. Food Chem. Toxicol. 50:5–25.

Tuohy, K. M., D. J. Hinton, S. J. Davies, M. J. Crabbe, G. R. Gibson, and J. M. Ames. 2006. Metabolism of Maillard reaction products by the human gut microbiota–implications for health. Mol. Nutr. Food Res. 50:847–857.

Uribarri, J., M. Peppa, W. Cai, T. Goldberg, M. Lu, C. He, et al. 2003. Restriction of dietary glycotoxins reduces excessive advanced glycation end products in renal failure patients. J. Am. Soc. Nephrol. 14:728–731.

Uribarri, J., W. Cai, M. Ramdas, S. Goodman, R. Pyzik, X. Chen, et al. 2011. Restriction of advanced glycation end products improves insulin resistance in human type 2 diabetes: potential role of AGER1 and SIRT1. Diabetes Care 34:1610–1616.

U.S. Department of Agriculture and U.S. Department of Health and Human Services. 2010. Dietary guidelines for Americans, 7th ed. U.S. Government Printing Office, Washington, DC.

Van Lancker, F., A. Adams, and N. De Kimpe. 2011. Chemical modifications of peptides and their impact on food properties. Chem. Rev. 111:7876–7903.

Vesper, H. W., H. Licea-Perez, T. Meyers, M. Ospina, and G. L. Myers. 2005. Pilot study on the impact of potato chips consumption on biomarkers of acrylamide exposure. Adv. Exp. Med. Biol. 561:89–96.

Vikstrom, A. C., L. Abramsson-Zetterberg, M. Naruszewicz, I. Athanassiadis, F. N. Granath, and M. A. Tornqvist. 2011. In vivo doses of acrylamide and glycidamide in humans after intake of acrylamide-rich food. Toxicol. Sci. 119:41–49.

Vitaglione, P., V. Fogliano, and N. Pellegrini. 2012. Coffee, colon function and colorectal cancer. Food Funct. 3:916–922.

Vlachojannis, J. E., M. Cameron, and S. Chrubasik. 2010. Medicinal use of potato-derived products: a systematic review. Phytother. Res. 24:159–162.

Vlassara, H., W. Cai, J. Crandall, T. Goldberg, R. Oberstein, V. Dardaine, et al. 2002. Inflammatory mediators are induced by dietary glycotoxins, a major risk factor for diabetic angiopathy. Proc. Natl Acad. Sci. USA 99:15596–15601.

Wansink, B., M. Shimizu, and A. Brumberg. 2013. Association of nutrient-dense snack combinations with calories and vegetable intake. Pediatrics 131:22–29.

Weaver, C., and E. T. Marr. 2013. White vegetables: a forgotten source of nutrients: Purdue roundtable executive summary. Adv. Nutr. 4:318S–326S.

Xu, Y., B. Cui, R. Ran, Y. Liu, H. Chen, G. Kai, et al. 2014. Risk assessment, formation, and mitigation of dietary acrylamide: current status and future prospects. Food Chem. Toxicol. 69:1–12.

Yoshimatsu, K., N. Kawano, N. Kawahara, H. Akiyama, R. Teshima, and M. Nishijima. 2012. Current status in the commercialization and application of genetically modified plants and their effects on human and livestock health and phytoremediation. Yakugaku Zasshi 132:629–674.

Yusof, A. S., Z. M. Isa, and S. A. Shah. 2012. Dietary patterns and risk of colorectal cancer: a systematic review of cohort studies (2000–2011). Asian Pac. J. Cancer Prev. 13:4713–4717.

Zeng, Y., X. Zhang, Y. Guan, and Y. Sun. 2011. Characteristics and antioxidant activity of Maillard reaction products from psicose-lysine and fructose-lysine model systems. J. Food Sci. 76:C398–C403.

Zhang, Y., and Y. Zhang. 2007. Formation and reduction of acrylamide in Maillard reaction: a review based on the current state of knowledge. Crit. Rev. Food Sci. Nutr. 47:521–542.

6

Rapid methods for extracting and quantifying phenolic compounds in citrus rinds

Lembe Samukelo Magwaza[1], Umezuruike Linus Opara[2,3], Paul J. R. Cronje[4], Sandra Landahl[5], Jose Ordaz Ortiz[5] & Leon A. Terry[5]

[1]Department of Crop Science, School of Agricultural, Earth and Environmental Sciences, University of KwaZulu-Natal, Private Bag X01, Scottsville 3209, Pietermaritzburg, South Africa
[2]Postharvest Technology Research Laboratory, Department of Horticultural Science, Stellenbosch University, Stellenbosch 7602, South Africa
[3]Postharvest Technology Research Laboratory, Department of Food Science, South African Research Chair in Postharvest Technology, Stellenbosch University, Stellenbosch 7602, South Africa
[4]Citrus Research International, Department of Horticultural Science, Stellenbosch University, Stellenbosch 7602, South Africa
[5]Plant Science Laboratory, Cranfield University, Bedfordshire, MK43 0AL, UK

Keywords
Extraction method, flavanone glycosides, phenolic acids, phenolics

Correspondence
Lembe Samukelo Magwaza, Department of Crop Science, School of Agricultural Earth and Environmental Sciences, University of KwaZulu-Natal, Private Bag X01, Scottsville 3209, Pietermaritzburg, South Africa.

E-mail: magwazal@ukzn.ac.za; lembe.magwaza@gmail.com

Funding Information
Postharvest Innovation Fund of the Department of Science and Technology. Citrus Research International. National Research Foundation. Flanders Research Cooperation Programme (Project UID: 73936). Commonwealth Scholarship Commission of the United Kingdom.

Abstract

Conventional methods for extracting and quantifying phenolic compounds in citrus rinds are time consuming. Rapid methods for extracting and quantifying phenolic compounds were developed by comparing three extraction solvent combinations (80:20 v/v ethanol:H_2O; 70:29.5:0.5 v/v/v methanol:H_2O:HCl; and 50:50 v/v dimethyl sulfoxide (DMSO):methanol) for effectiveness. Freeze-dried, rind powder was extracted in an ultrasonic water bath at 35°C for 10, 20, and 30 min. Phenolic compound quantification was done with a high-performance liquid chromatography (HPLC) equipped with diode array detector. Extracting with methanol:H_2O:HCl for 30 min resulted in the optimum yield of targeted phenolic acids. Seven phenolic acids and three flavanone glycosides (FGs) were quantified. The dominant phenolic compound was hesperidin, with concentrations ranging from 7500 to 32,000 μg/g DW. The highest yield of FGs was observed in samples extracted, using DMSO:methanol for 10 min. Compared to other extraction methods, methanol:H_2O:HCl was efficient in optimum extraction of phenolic acids. The limit of detection and quantification for all analytes were small, ranging from 1.35 to 5.02 and 4.51 to 16.72 μg/g DW, respectively, demonstrating HPLC quantification method sensitivity. The extraction and quantification methods developed in this study are faster and more efficient. Where speed and effectiveness are required, these methods are recommended.

Introduction

Citrus fruit has a high concentration of natural bioactive compounds with a positive influence on antioxidant capacity (Xu et al. 2008a,b; Tomas-Barberan and Andres-Lacueva 2012). As an effective bioactive compound source, rinds of citrus fruit can be explored for health promoting food product values. The phenolic compound profile and concentration in citrus fruit rind has received scientific interest in recent years, due to antioxidant capacity (Manthey and Grohmann 1996; Li et al. 2006; Xu et al. 2008b; Khan et al. 2010; Sun et al. 2010).

The phenolic profile of citrus fruit rinds consists of numerous compounds such as coumarins, psoralens, phenolic acids, and flavonoids (Benavente-García et al. 1998; Bocco et al. 1998). Flavonoids in citrus rinds are represented by two classes of compounds referred to as flavanone glycosides (FGs) and polymethoxylated flavones (Benavente-García et al. 1998). These two classes of flavonoids are found only in citrus fruit, and their presence or absence is specific for each species and therefore could be used as taxonomic markers and be related to postharvest physiology (Manthey and Grohmann 1996; Tomás-Barberán et al. 2003; Mathur et al. 2011). The polymethoxylated flavones occur in relatively lower concentrations but exhibit higher biological activity than phenolic acids and FGs, which are the main primary groups of phenolic compounds in citrus rinds (Benavente-García et al. 1998; Ma et al. 2008; Simonne and Ritenour 2011; Ye et al. 2011).

An Abundant flavonoid group found in different parts of citrus fruit are FGs including hesperidin, neohesperidin, naringin, narirutin, and didymin (Khan et al. 2010; Jabri-Karoui and Marzouk 2013). FGs are unique to citrus and are characteristic of some species and varieties (Tomás-Barberán et al. 2003). A classic example is hesperidin which is a major component in rind tissues of oranges and mandarins. Naringin on the other hand is a predominant FG in grapefruit (Kalt et al. 1999). The concentrations of FGs may differ due to differences in fruit maturity, environmental conditions during growth and development, postharvest treatments, and storage conditions (Abad-García et al. 2012). Thus, these compounds have a potential to be used as biochemical indicators of fruit origin, species and cultivar.

The health-related beneficial characteristics of some phenolic compounds have led to a number of studies to develop better extraction, identification, and quantification methods. Many analytical methods are widely used to determine and quantify phenolic compounds in citrus fruit (Ahmad et al. 2006). High-performance liquid chromatography (HPLC) is the most used technique for analysis of individual compounds (Li et al. 2006).

Extraction of compounds from plant materials is one of the most important steps prior to their determination by HPLC. Conventional extractions are usually time consuming and require relatively large quantities of solvents. It is also well known that the complexity of phenolic compounds in plant matrixes makes extraction difficult (Manthey and Grohmann 1996). In recent years, some novel extraction methods of phenolic compounds have been developed including enzyme-assisted extraction methods (Li et al. 2006), ultrasound-assisted extraction (Khan et al. 2010), ultrasonic extraction (Ma et al. 2008), microwave-assisted extraction (Ahmad et al. 2006), and the use of solvents like dimethyl sulfoxide (DMSO), methanol-DMSO mixtures, and dimethylformamide (Manthey and Grohmann 1996).

A major trend in modern HPLC is the reduction in particle size and column length to allow very fast separations with greater resolution (Gritti and Guiochon 2012). The use of smaller particles in packed-column LC to provide increased efficiencies is currently the most prevalent method employed in liquid phase separation (de Villiers et al. 2006). As a result of this new leap forward in column technology, manufacturers began to produce and commercialize shorter columns, down to between 50 and 150 mm, which are as or more efficient than longer columns (Omamogho et al. 2011). This study was therefore conducted to develop a fast faster extraction method and rapid HPLC method for the quantification of phenolic compounds in 'Nules Clementine' mandarin rind tissues.

Materials and Methods

Chemicals

All chemicals were of analytical grade. Polyphenols (ρ-hydroxybenzoic acid, chlorogenic acid, vanillic acid, caffeic acid, ρ-coumaric acid, ferulic acid, sinapic acid, naringin, and hesperidin) standards were purchased from Sigma Aldrich (Dorset, UK). Narirutin and didymin standards were purchased from Extrasynthese (Lyon, France). Acetonitrile, methanol, and formic acid were all of HPLC grade, dimethyl sulfoxide (DMSO) was analytical grade, and purchased from Fisher Scientific Chemicals (Leics., UK). Solutions and solvents were prepared with Milli-Q water (Milipore Inc. (Molsheim, France); σ = 18 mol/L Ω/cm).

Plant material and sample preparation

A total of 20 "Nules Clementine" mandarin (*Citrus reticulata* Blanco) fruit were harvested in 2012 from an orchard at Stellenbosch University experimental farm, Western Cape Province, South Africa (33°53′04.56″S, 18°37′36.84″ E). These fruit were selected, weighed, peeled, and the rind snap-frozen in liquid nitrogen and stored at ultra-low temperature of −80°C. Fresh frozen samples were then freeze-dried in a Labogene ScanVac CoolSafe Freeze Dryer System (CS55-4, Lynge, Denmark) for 7 days at 0.015 kPA and −55°C. Lyophilized samples were ground using a pestle and mortar into fine powder. To achieve standard particle size, the ground material was sieved through a 1-mm metal sieve. Large particles remaining on the sieve were further ground until all the material passed through the sieve. Ground samples were returned into the freezer until extraction and further analysis.

Polyphenol extraction method

Three different extraction solvent combinations and three extraction times were compared for effectiveness. The extraction solvents included aqueous ethanol [80:20; v/v, ethanol:H_2O] (Xu et al. 2008a), acidic aqueous methanol

[70:29.5:0.5; v/v/v, methanol:H_2O:HCl] (Crespo et al. 2010), and 50:50; v/v dimethyl sulfoxide (DMSO) as described elsewhere (Manthey and Grohmann 1996; Xu et al. 2008b). Freeze-dried citrus rind powder (150 ± 0.5 mg) was added into 5 mL solvent following the optimum solvent to solid ratio of citrus fruit prescribed elsewhere (Sun et al. 2010) and put into an ultrasonic water bath (Ma et al. 2008) at 35°C for 10, 20, or 30 min. Samples were agitated for 30 sec every 5 min, centrifuged at 16,000 g force for 10 min before the flocculate was filtered through a 0.2 μm syringe-driven filter (Millipore corporation, Billerica, MA).

Extraction recovery and preparation of standard solution

The recovery of different phenolic compounds was evaluated using a pooled rind sample extracted as above. Briefly, freeze-dried samples were prepared, spiked with specific concentration of naringin and cinnamic acid (16 μg/mL) and extracted in triplicates. The recoveries were calculated based on a method described elsewhere (Chang et al. 1997). The recovery of these phenolic compounds ranged from 94.3% to 103.7%. A mixed standard solution (5 mg/mL) was prepared by transferring all measured phenolic compounds into the extraction solvent. Eight concentration levels of the mixed standard solution were prepared by serial dilution of the stock solution. Concentrations of phenolic acids were determined from linear standard calibration curves (R^2 = 0.99).

HPLC quantification of polyphenols

Quantification of phenolic compounds was executed in triplicate on an Agilent 1200 series HPLC equipped with an Agilent DA G1315B/G1365G diode array detector. (DAD) with multiple wavelength detector, degasser and cooled autosampler (Agilent Technologies, Berks, UK). The system was operated by Windows NT-based ChemStation© software (Agilent Technologies), which was also used for data processing. Citrus rind extracts (20 μL) were injected into a Poroshell 120 column (4.6 × 150 mm and 2.7 μm particle size, Agilent), which was held at 40°C. The flow rate of the mobile phase was set at 1 mL/min. The mobile phases consisted of two solvents, 0.1% (v/v) formic acid: water (A) and 80% (v/v) acetonitrile:water (B). The DAD UV detection of all phenolic acids and FGs was carried out at 280 nm. The solvent gradient conditions for phenolic acids in volume ratios were as follows: 0–5% B during 5 min, 5–10% B up to 10 min; 10–12% B up to 16 min, 12–15% up to 25 min, 15–100% B up to 27 min. For FGs, the solvent gradient conditions were 0–15% during 5 min, 15–20% up to 10 min, 20–60% up to 25 min, and 60–100% up to 27 min. FGs were quantified using naringin (an FG not present in "Nules Clementine" mandarin) as an internal standard. The identification of phenolic compounds was accomplished by comparing the retention times and HPLC spectra of each compound of the peaks in the sample to those of the phenolic compound standards.

Limit of detection and limit of quantification

The limit of detection (LOD) and limit of quantification (LOQ) for phenolic compounds were calculated by repeatedly (n = 10) injecting known concentration of a mixture of standard solution. The LOD and LOQ values were calculated as the amount of each individual phenolic compound required to give the signal to noise ratio of 3:1 and 10:1, respectively (Bressolle et al. 1996).

Statistical analysis

Statistical analyses were carried out using SPSS 10.0 for Windows (SPSS Inc. Chicago, IL). Data were subjected to analysis of variance (ANOVA). Duncan's multiple-range tests were used to compare the significant differences in the mean values ($P \leq 0.05$).

Results and Discussion

Development of polyphenols extraction method

Dry powder samples of mandarin rind were extracted with 80:20 (v/v) aqueous ethanol compared to acidic aqueous methanol 70:29.5:0.5 (v/v/v; methanol:H_2O:HCl) and 50:50 (v/v; DMSO:methanol) to determine the efficacy of the extraction procedure for optimum phenolic acid and flavanones yield. Extraction solvent and extraction time were the two main parameters that affected the yield of phenolic compounds (Table 1). The concentration of phenolic acids increased with an increase in ultrasonic extraction time, while flavanones stayed the same. Results showed that an extraction period of 30 min using 70:29.5:0.5 (v/v/v; methanol:H_2O:HCl) was sufficient to extract phenolic acids. For example, the concentration of ferulic acid after extraction using acidic methanol for 10, 20, and 30 min, gradually increased (12.43, 13.37, 25.19 μ/g DM), respectively. The same trend was observed for sinapic acid, where the corresponding concentrations were 41.35, 61.23, and 64.87 μ/g DM. In general, phenolic acids yield was higher in samples extracted for 30 min using aqueous methanol. For flavanones, the highest yield was observed in samples extracted using 50:50 (v/v; DMSO:methanol) for 10 min. However,

Table 1. Composition of phenolic compounds in rind extracts using different extraction solvents and time combination. Means with different letters in the three rows (solvent) and three columns (extraction times) corresponding to the same compound are significantly different ($P < 0.05$).

		Concentration (μg/g DW)		
Phenolic compound	Extraction solvent	10 min	20 min	30 min
Hydroxybenzoic acids				
p-Hydroxybenzoic acid	Methanol	22.08 ± 0.6^{ab}*	19.78 ± 0.7^{a}	21.02 ± 3.1^{ab}
	DMSO	92.85 ± 1.5^{e}	87.75 ± 5.6^{d}	86.66 ± 1.9^{d}
	Ethanol	29.26 ± 3.5^{c}	25.32 ± 1.5^{bc}	29.29 ± 0.3^{c}
Vanillic acid	Methanol	17.82 ± 0.2^{c}	12.69 ± 0.6^{b}	24.47 ± 2.7^{d}
	DMSO	nd	nd	nd
	Ethanol	8.86 ± 0.8^{a}	7.11 ± 1.1^{a}	17.25 ± 1.9^{c}
Hydroxycinnamic acids				
Chlorogenic acid	Methanol	15.37 ± 0.4^{c}	25.91 ± 0.5^{e}	43.25 ± 1.2^{h}
	DMSO	5.98 ± 1.1^{a}	11.89 ± 0.3^{b}	33.89 ± 4.4^{g}
	Ethanol	18.76 ± 0.9^{d}	11.06 ± 0.7^{b}	29.85 ± 0.4^{f}
Caffeic acid	Methanol	28.21 ± 0.7^{e}	23.57 ± 0.5^{d}	39.81 ± 3.9^{f}
	DMSO	11.95 ± 0.9^{a}	12.44 ± 0.2^{a}	23.33 ± 1.9^{d}
	Ethanol	15.49 ± 1.7^{b}	11.94 ± 0.6^{a}	19.70 ± 0.8^{c}
p-Coumaric acid	Methanol	9.63 ± 0.1^{c}	14.55 ± 1.8^{e}	6.94 ± 0.1^{b}
	DMSO	5.63 ± 0.4^{ab}	5.35 ± 1.1^{a}	9.80 ± 1.3^{c}
	Ethanol	4.49 ± 0.2^{a}	10.43 ± 0.1^{c}	12.53 ± 0.2^{d}
Ferulic acid	Methanol	12.43 ± 0.8^{b}	13.37 ± 0.8^{b}	25.19 ± 4.9^{d}
	DMSO	7.92 ± 1.2^{a}	6.28 ± 2.5^{a}	13.50 ± 1.1^{b}
	Ethanol	17.81 ± 0.3^{c}	15.81 ± 0.1^{bc}	40.55 ± 0.5^{e}
Sinapic acid	Methanol	41.35 ± 0.5^{e}	61.23 ± 3.8^{d}	64.87 ± 2.8^{e}
	DMSO	15.19 ± 1.6^{a}	23.52 ± 2.4^{c}	23.58 ± 2.8^{c}
	Ethanol	19.45 ± 4.3^{b}	24.99 ± 0.8^{c}	39.45 ± 1.1^{d}
Flavanones				
Narirutin	Methanol	737 ± 1.4^{b}	738 ± 7.9^{b}	690 ± 14.4^{b}
	DMSO	1370 ± 29.6^{d}	1299 ± 140^{d}	1151 ± 23.1^{c}
	Ethanol	396 ± 30.7^{a}	355 ± 11.2^{a}	408 ± 12.6^{a}
Hesperidin	Methanol	8005 ± 529^{cd}	8628 ± 269^{d}	7553 ± 290^{c}
	DMSO	32,008 ± 373^{e}	31,179 ± 1181^{e}	32,019 ± 866^{e}
	Ethanol	5456 ± 389^{b}	4329 ± 439^{a}	3966 ± 161^{a}
Didymin	Methanol	268 ± 4.6^{d}	246 ± 23.6^{bc}	257 ± 11.1^{cd}
	DMSO	402 ± 7.2^{e}	402 ± 9.5^{e}	404 ± 4.5^{e}
	Ethanol	238 ± 5.1^{ab}	224 ± 7.4^{a}	232 ± 3.2^{ab}

nd, non detectable; *Mean ± SD of three samples.

phenolic acids yield was lower using this extraction combination. The concentrations of phenolic acids are similar to those reported by Xu et al. (2008a,b). Therefore, acidic aqueous methanol extraction in ultrasonic bath for 30 min is suitable to extract phenolic acids and 50:50 (v/v; DMSO: methanol) for 10 min was ideal to extract flavanones. By using these methods, extraction time was reduced significantly from 1, 3, 24, and 72 h reported by Xu et al. (2008a), Li et al. (2006), Manthey and Grohmann (1996), and Mathur et al. (2011), respectively.

Development of HPLC quantification for polyphenols

A typical chromatogram with phenolic compounds separation obtained using conditions described earlier is portrayed in Figure 1. A total of seven phenolic acids, including three hydroxybenzoic acids (*ρ*-hydroxybezoic and vanillic), and five hydroxycinnamic acids (chlorogenic, caffeic, *ρ*-coumaric, ferulic, and sinapic) as well as three flavanones (narirutin, hesperidin and didymin) were identified and quantified. The method separated 10 phenolic compounds faster (50 min) than 120 min previously reported (Li et al. 2006; Kelebek 2010; Kelebek and Selli 2011). Hesperidin was the dominant compound ranging from 31,179 to 32,019 μg/g DM in samples extracted using DMSO (Table 1). These results are similar to those previously observed by Xu et al. (2008a,b), who reported a total of seven phenolic acids and four flavanones. The flavanones profile was similar to that reported by Ye et al. (2011) who reported hesperidin as the major flavanone in mandarin fruit.

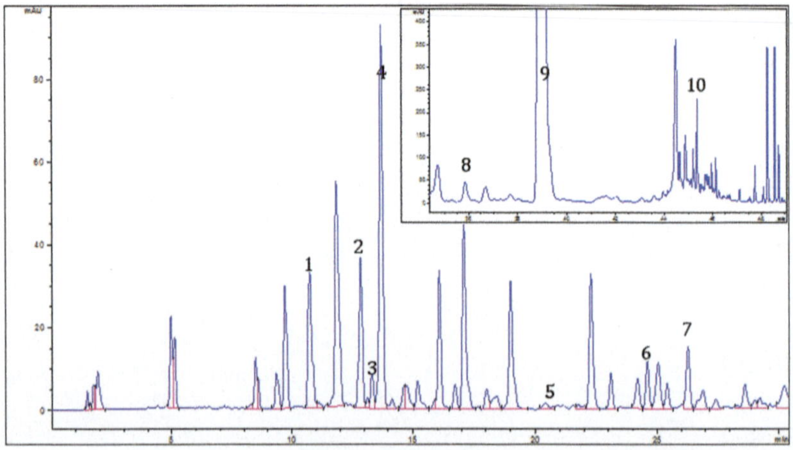

Figure 1. Typical HPLC-DAD chromatogram at 280 nm showing separation of phenolic compounds in the rind sample (1, ρ-Hydroxybezoic acid; 2, Vanillic acid; 3, Chlorogenic acid; 4, Caffeic acid; 5, ρ-Coumaric acid; 6, Ferulic acid; 7, Sinapic acid; 8, Narirutin; 9, Hesperidin, and 10, Didymin, respectively.

Table 2. Response characteristics of phenolic compound standards using HPLC. In the regression equation, *x* represents concentration of phenolic compounds and *y* represents the peak area. The linear standard concentration range was between 5 and 150 μg/mL (5, 16, 20, 60, 100, 150). The presented values LOQ, LOD, and RSD were measured with repeated injections ($n = 10$) of standard mixture at a concentration of 10 μg/mL each.

Phenolic compound	Retention time	Regression equation	R^2	LOD (μg/mL)	LOQ (μg/mL)	R.S.D (%)
Hydroxybenzoic acids						
ρ-Hydroxybenzoic acid	11.5	$y = 23.45x$	0.9997	1.48	4.92	0.49
Vanillic acid	14.1	$y = 30.62x$	0.9995	1.39	4.62	0.46
Hydroxycinnamic acids						
Chlorogenic acid	14.4	$y = 33.83x$	0.9997	1.48	4.92	0.49
Caffeic acid	14.9	$y = 62.73x$	0.9995	1.35	4.51	0.45
ρ-Coumaric acid	20.2	$y = 96.81x$	0.9997	1.45	4.84	0.48
Ferulic acid	25.0	$y = 60.076x$	0.9997	1.42	4.74	0.47
Sinapic acid	26.9	$y = 27.45x$	0.9990	2.32	7.73	0.77
Flavanones*						
Narirutin	17.0	$y = 30.83x$	0.9994	1.50	3.01	0.50
Didymin	24.8	$y = 31.13x$	0.9994	1.32	4.23	0.45
Hesperidin	21.0	$y = 30.84x$	0.9994	5.02	16.72	1.67

*Flavanones were determined on a different HPLC run.

Table 2 summarizes the concentration range, retention times, regression equation ($y = mx$), coefficient of determination (R^2), LOD, LOQ, and the relative standard deviation (RSD) for each compound. The reproducibility of the retention time of phenolic compounds under selected HPLC conditions was executed by doing repeated injections ($n = 10$) of the mixture of the 10 standards at the concentration of 10.0 μg/mL. The regression equation, LOD, LOQ, and RSD were calculated for each identified phenolic compound using only the best extraction method, which in this case was acidic methanol. The LOD, defined as the smallest concentration that the analytical procedure can reliably distinguish from the noise levels and LOQ for all analytes were very small, ranging from 1.35 to 5.02 and 4.51–16.72 μg/mL, respectively. The RSD values for all retention times ranged from 0.45 to 1.67 indicating good stability and adequate performance of the method investigated.

Conclusions

Rapid and efficient methods for extracting and quantifying phenolic compounds in citrus rinds were successfully developed. Aqueous acidic methanol and 50:50 (v/v; DMSO:methanol, respectively) extract phenolic acids and flavanone glycosides rapidly and efficiently. The HPLC method developed in this study separated faster than methods previously described. Phenolic compounds can be extracted rapidly and efficiently from citrus rind tissue.

Acknowledgments

This work is supported by the Postharvest Innovation Fund of Department of Science and Technology, Citrus Research International, National Research Foundation and the Flanders Research Cooperation Programme (Project UID: 73936). We are grateful to contributions made by Dr Katherine Cools, Dr Maria Del Carmen Alamar Gavidia, Dr Jose Ordaz Ortiz, and Ms Rosemary Burns, for technical research support.

Conflict of Interest

None declared.

References

Abad-García, B., L. A. Berrueta, S. Garmón-Lobato, A. Urkaregi, B. Gallo, and F. Vicente. 2012. Chemometric characterization of fruit juices from Spanish cultivars according to their phenolic compound contents: I. citrus fruits. J. Agric. Food Chem. 60:3635–3644.

Ahmad, M. M., S.-R. Rehman, F. M. Anjum, and E. E. Bajwa. 2006. Comparative physical examination of various citrus peel essential oils. Int. J. Agric. and Biol. 8:186–190.

Benavente-García, O., J. Castillo, F. R. Marin, A. Ortunõ, and J. A. Del Río. 1998. Uses and properties of citrus flavonoids. J. Agric. Food Chem. 45:4505–4515.

Bocco, A., M. Cuvelier, H. Richard, and C. Berset. 1998. Antioxidant activity and phenolic composition of citrus peel and seed extracts. J. Agric. Food Chem. 46:2123–2129.

Bressolle, F., M. Bromet-Petit, and M. Audran. 1996. Validation of liquid chromatographic and gas chromatographic methods, applications to pharnacokinetics. J. Chromatogr. B 686:3–10.

Chang, C. W., S. L. Hsiu, P. P. Wu, S. C. Kuo, and P. D. L. Chao. 1997. HPLC Assay of naringin and hesperidin in Chinese herbs and serum. J. Food Drug Anal. 5:111–120.

Crespo, P., J. Giné Bordonaba, L. A. Terry, and C. Carlen. 2010. Characterisation of major taste and health-related compounds of four strawberry genotypes grown at different Swiss production sites. Food Chem. 122:16–24.

Gritti, F., and G. Guiochon. 2012. The current revolution in column technology: how it began, where is it going? J. Chromatogr. A 1228:2–19.

Jabri-Karoui, I., and B. Marzouk. 2013. Characterization of bioactive compounds in Tunisian bitter orange (*Citrus aurantium* L.) peel and juice and determination of their antioxidant activities. BioMed. Res. Int. http://dx.doi.org/10.1155/2013/345415.

Kalt, W., C. F. Forney, A. Martin, and R. Prior. 1999. Antioxidant capacity, vitamin C, phenolics, and anthocyanin after fresh storage of small fruit. J. Agric. Food Chem. 47:4638–4644.

Kelebek, H. 2010. Sugars, organic acids, phenolic compositions and antioxidant activity of Grapefruit (*Citrus paradisi*) cultivars grown in Turkey. Ind. Crops Prod. 32:269–274.

Kelebek, H., and S. Selli. 2011. Determination of volatile, phenolic, organic acid and sugar components in a Turkish cv. Dortyol (*Citrus Sinesis* L. Osbeck). J. Sci. Food Agric. 91:1855–1862.

Khan, M. K., M. Albert-Vian, A. Fabiano-Tixier, O. Dangles, and F. Chemat. 2010. Ultrasound-assisted extraction of polyphenols (flavanone glycosides from orange (*Citrus sinensis* L.)) peel. Food Chem. 119:851–858.

Li, B. B., B. Smith, and M. M. Hossain. 2006. Extraction of phenolics from citrus peels II. Enzyme-assisted extraction method. Sep. Purific. Technol. 48:189–196.

Ma, Y.-Q., X.-Q. Ye, Z.-X. Fang, J.-C. Chen, G.-H. Xu, and D. H. Liu. 2008. Phenolic compounds and antioxidant activity of extracts from ultrasonic treatment of Satsuma mandarin (*Citrus unshiu* Marc.) peels. J. Agric. Food Chem. 56:5682–5690.

Manthey, J. A., and K. Grohmann. 1996. Concentration of hesperidin and other orange peel flavonoids in citrus processing byproducts. J. Agric. Food Chem. 44:811–814.

Mathur, A., S. K. Verma, R. Purohit, V. Gupta, V. K. Dua, G. B. K. S. Prasad, et al. 2011. Evaluation of in vitro antimicrobial and antioxidant activities of peel and pulp of some citrus fruits. IJPI's J. Biotechnol. Biotherapeutics 1:1–17.

Omamogho, J. O., J. P. Hanrahan, J. Tobin, and J. D. Glennon. 2011. Structural variation of solid core and thickness of porous shell of 1.7 m core–shell silica particles on chromatographic performance: narrow bore columns. J. Chromatogr. A 1218:1942–1953.

Simonne, A. H., and M. A. Ritenour. 2011. Citrus (Orange, Lemon, Mandarin, Grapefruit, Lime and Other citrus fruits). Pp. 90–117 *in* L. A. Terry, ed. Health-promoting properties of fruits and vegetables. CAB International, Oxfordshire, U.K.

Sun, Y., J. Wang, S. Gu, Z. Liu, Y. Zhang, and X. Zhang. 2010. Simultaneous determination of flavonoids in different parts of *Citrus reticulate* 'Chachi' fruit by high performance liquid chromatography-photodiode array detection. Molecules 15:5378–5388.

Tomas-Barberan, F. A., and C. Andres-Lacueva. 2012. Polyphenols and health: current state and progress. J. Agric. Food Chem. 60:8773–8775.

Tomás-Barberán, F. A., A. Gil-Izquierdo, F. Ferreres, and M. I. Gil. 2003. Analysis and purification of flavanones, chalcones and dihydrochalcones. Pp. 359–371 *in* C. Santos-Buelga and C. Williamson, eds. Methods in polyphenol analysis. The Royal Society of Chemistry, Cambridge.

de Villiers, A., H. Lauer, R. Szucs, S. Goodall, and P. Sandra. 2006. Influence of frictional heating on temperature gradients in ultra-high-pressure liquid chromatography on 2.1 mm I.D. columns. J. Chromatogr. A 1113:84–91.

Xu, G. H., J. C. Chen, D. H. Liu, Y. H. Zhang, P. Jiang, and X. Q. Ye. 2008a. Minerals, phenolic compounds, and antioxidant capacity of citrus peel extract by hot water. J. Food Sci. 73:C11–C18.

Xu, G. H., X. Q. Ye, D. H. Liu, Y. Q. Ma, and J. C. Chen. 2008b. Composition and distribution of phenolic acids in Ponkan (*Citrus poonensis* Hort. ex Tanaka) and Hoyou (*Citrus paradisi* Macf. Changshanhuyou) during maturity. J. Food Comp. Anal. 21:382–389.

Ye, X. Q., J. C. Chen, D. H. Liu, P. Jiang, J. Shi, S. Xue, et al. 2011. Identification of bioactive composition and antioxidant activity in young mandarin fruits. Food Chem. 124:1561–1566.

7

Change in carbohydrate and enzymes from harvest to sprouting in garlic

Kambiz Mashayekhi[1], Siamak Mohammadi Chiane[1], Manizheh Mianabadi[2], Farshid Ghaderifar[3] & Seyyed Javad Mousavizadeh[1]

[1]Department of Horticultural Science, Gorgan University of Agricultural Sciences and Natural Resources, Gorgan, Iran
[2]Department of Biology, Faculty of Sciences, University of Golestan, Gorgan, Iran
[3]Department of Agronomy, Gorgan University of Agricultural Sciences and Natural Resources, Gorgan, Iran

Keywords
Carbohydrate, chlorophyll, enzyme, sprouting, storage

Correspondence
Seyyed Javad Mousavizadeh, Department of Horticultural Science, Gorgan University of Agricultural Sciences and Natural Resources, Gorgan, I.R. Iran.

E-mail: mousavizadeh@ut.ac.ir

Funding Information
No funding information provided.

Abstract

Changes in carbohydrates, enzymes, and pigments were investigated in the Red Garlic (*Allium sativum* L.) cv. Azarshahr bulbs in storage from harvest to sprouting. For storage period, garlic cloves of the same diameter with 3–4 g weight were arranged in dark condition and exposed to 4 and 21°C, separately. Soluble sugar, total sugar, glucose, sucrose, fructose, starch, chlorophyll a, b, ab, carotenoid, anthocyanin, lipase, α-amylase, and protease were measured every 2 weeks up to sprouting time. Result revealed that starch, lipase, and protease levels declined at the end of storage when clove sprouting started at both 4 and 21°C storage temperature. Starch, glucose, chlorophyll a, b, ab, and carotenoid content during the first 14 days and sucrose at 42 days showed a decreasing trend. Anthocyanin showed an increasing trend 14 and 42 days after harvesting and then decreased at the end of storage (when sprouting began) at both 4 and 21°C storage periods. Finally, starch, glucose, and sucrose measurement can be used as a criterion to predict sprouting time of garlic, due to the decrease in the levels of starch, lipase, and protease, and increase in the levels of α-amylase, glucose, and sucrose in garlic cloves under storage.

Introduction

Garlic (*Allium sativum* L.), a plant of the Liliaceae family, plays an important role in human nutrition and has medicinal value (Rubatzky and Yamaguchi 1997). Plants store sugars usually as large molecules of starch which are required to produce energy; plants are required to break them into smaller molecules (Hapkins 1999).

Previous reports indicated that garlic dormancy ends by storage at low temperatures (Cantwell et al. 2003 and Vazquez-Barrios et al. 2006). Arguello et al. (2001) reported that cold treatment at 4°C and Gibberellic Acid (GA3) initiated the garlic sprouting process. During cold storage, due to hydrolysis of starch, carbohydrates in onion tissues acquire mobility (Fulton et al. 2001). Carbohydrate macromolecules such as starch are converted into simple sugars such as sucrose, glucose, and fructose, making this process possible. Transport and accumulation of these substances (sugars) that are source of energy, are used in cellular metabolism, and produce the energy needed for plant growth (Langens-Grrits et al. 2003). In addition to energy transfer in plants, carbohydrates are also involved in the regulation of gene expression (Gupta and Kaur 2005; Iraqi et al. 2005).

Despite the large-scale production of garlic in Iran, research into the changes in garlic carbohydrates from harvest to sprouting is scarce. We believe the changes in garlic carbohydrates play an important role from dormancy to sprouting. This study aimed to understand the physiological changes in carbohydrates of garlic from dormancy to sprouting. Understanding these changes create optimal conditions for clove sprouting, plant growth, and ultimately increases in yield.

Materials and Methods

Plant materials

Red garlic (*A. sativum* L.) cv. Azarshahr bulbs were collected from local fields in Azarshahr when they were fully ripe and their leaves began browning. Four thousand bulbs with the same diameter were selected. Pieces of garlic were arranged in plastic trays enclosed in aluminum foils in order to avoid light.

Storage condition and sprout treatment

Garlic cloves of the same diameter and weighing 3–4 g were taken in plateaus and arranged in a dark enclosure to avoid light and treated in two ways: (1) at 21°C with 45% humidity (common condition) and (2) at 4°C with 60% humidity, the latter of which is the most suitable temperature for garlic sprouting (Hartman 2002). Sampling was carried out for 2 weeks up to sprouting. Bulbs were observed every 14 days for up to 84 days and were considered sprouting when the bud was developed and greenish (Fig. 1).

Determination of traits

Soluble sugar content

Soluble sugar was determined according to the Omokolo et al. (1996) method by application of 80% ethanol.

Total sugar content

Total sugar was determined according to the Antron Method by spectrophotometry (S 2000 UV/Vis) at 620 nm (McCready et al. 1950).

Glucose content

Glucose content was calculated using dinitrosalicylic acid by spectrophotometry at 575 nm (Miller 1959).

Sucrose content

Sucrose content was determined according to the Antron Method by spectrophotometry at 620 nm (Handel 1968).

Fructose content

Fructose content was calculated by resorcinal Method by spectrophotometry at 520 nm (Ashwell 1957).

Starch measurement

Starch was determined according to the Anthrone Method by spectrophotometry at 620 nm (McCready et al. 1950).

Carotenoid and chlorophyll contents

Carotenoid and chlorophyll contents were extracted using acetone, from 1 g of garlic. The amount of these pigments was measured by Arnon (1956) method pectrophotometry (S 2000 UV/Vis) at 480, 510, 645, 652, and 663 nm, and expressed as mg/g fresh weight.

Anthocyanin content

Anthocyanin contents of garlic cloves were measured according to Wanger (1979). One gram of clove tissue was extracted via 10 mL methanol and incubated overnight at 4°C in the dark. The slurry was centrifuged (SIGMA-3K30) at 4000 g for 10 min. The supernatant, which contained anthocyanin, was determined by pectrophotometry at 520 nm.

α-Amylase activities

The amount of α-amylase activities was measured by 3,5-dinitro salicylic acid color indicator and starch substrate of 1%, spectrophotometry at 540 nm (Bernfeld 1955).

Lipase activities

Lipase activities was estimated according to Sadeghipour and Bhatla (2002). A suspension of urea-washed garlic bodies treated with trypsin was taken in 0.1 mol/L Tris

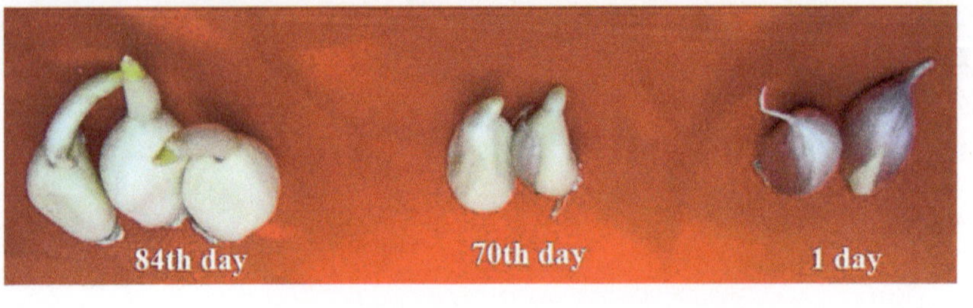

Figure 1. Sprouting of garlic bulbs from 1 day up to 84 days. Developed and greenish bud was considered as sprouting.

Table 1. ANOVA of garlic storage at 21 and 4°C during different times.

Source of variance	df	Starch	Total sugar	Sucrose	Glucose	Fructose	Anthocyanin	Chlorophyll *a*
Temperature (*a*)	1	32.31**	3.44 ns	952.5 ns	675.2**	20.11*	0.0003ns	0.0009ns
Time (*b*)	6	124.29**	1555.2**	27,385.5**	7084.6**	27.42**	0.015**	0.18**
a × *b*	6	17.83**	166.2 ns	288.15 ns	187.9**	29.48**	0.003*	0.02**
Error	154	2.80	252.6	479.5	60.57	3.18	0.001	0.002
CV%		21.32	31.72	25.41	14.56	32.06	29.35	22.97

Source of variance	df	Chlorophyll *b*	Chlorophyll *ab*	Carotenoid	α-Amylase	Lipase	Protease
Temperature (*a*)	1	0.033**	0.027*	0.78 ns	29.25 ns	36.90**	0.05**
Time (*b*)	6	0.329**	0.54**	22.57**	3017.3**	48.20**	0.52**
a × *b*	6	0.042**	0.048**	0.73**	28.5ns	26.86**	0.003ns
Error	154	0.004	0.006	0.23	26.73	0.46	0.004
CV%		26.12	24.19	34.43	24.27	18.40	20.09

$^{**}P < 0.01$, $^{*}P < 0.05$, $^{ns}P > 0.05$.

buffer (pH 7.5). Lipolysis was started by the addition of 20 μL of a garlic membrane preparation containing lipase. To 1 mL of benzene extract, 0.5 mL Rhodamine 6G reagent was added and the fatty acids released were quantified by reading the absorbance at 535 nm. A standard curve was made using palmitic acid. Lipase activity was expressed as μmol fatty acids released per minute/g FW.

Protease activities

Protease assay was determined by the Anson (1938) method. Anson unit is the amount of enzyme which, under the specified test conditions (2% casein as substrate, pH 7.0; for 15 min, at different temperatures analyzed) hydrolyzes casein at a speed that facilitates release, in 1 min, of hydrolysis products soluble in trichloroacetic acid; this provides coloration equivalent, measured at OD_{670nm}, to 1 μmol of tyrosine, in the presence of the Folin-Ciocalteu reagent by using a tyrosine standard curve over the range 0.02–0.24 μmol/mL.

Statistical analysis

The experiment was established in a factorial (two levels of temperature and seven levels of storage time) layout based on completely randomized design with 12 replications. Data were analyzed statistically using analysis of variance in SAS 9.1 software (SAS Institute Inc., Cary, NC). The data of anthocyanin, carotenoid, chlorophyll *a*, *b*, and *ab* were normalized by root square ($\sqrt{X}$). Differences among the means were determined for significance at $P < 0.05$ using Duncan test.

Results and Discussions

The results of ANOVA (Table 1) demonstrated that starch was affected by temperature and time of storage ($P < 0.01$). Results revealed that garlic cloves stored at 4 and 21°C showed a similar pattern of changes in carbohydrates and similar time for sprouting. Cantwell et al. (2003) suggested that storage of garlic at temperatures of 5–18°C had promoted garlic sprouting. In accordance with this result, in this study, starch decomposed gradually at 84 days of storage (Fig. 2). Lee (2007) demonstrated that the hydrolysis of starch at different temperatures is associated with physiological processes. Onion bud dormancy is broken by chilling treatment which causes changes in soluble sugars and oligosaccharides (Benkeblia and Selselet-Attou 1999).

In the present study, starch content strongly declined 14 days after harvesting in both the 4 and 21°C storage periods (Fig. 2). Previous research indicated that the content of starch was the highest in the beginning of storage and reached its lowest value after chilling treatment at 4°C (Atashi et al. 2011).

ANOVA (Table 1) showed that total soluble sugar (TSS) was statistically affected by time of storage ($P < 0.01$). The TSS content decreased 14 days after storage and then increased at temperatures of 4 and 21°C (Fig. 3),

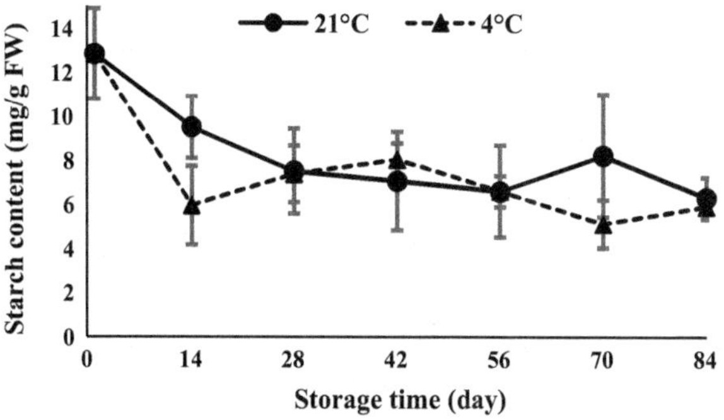

Figure 2. Starch content changes during storage period at 4 and 21°C.

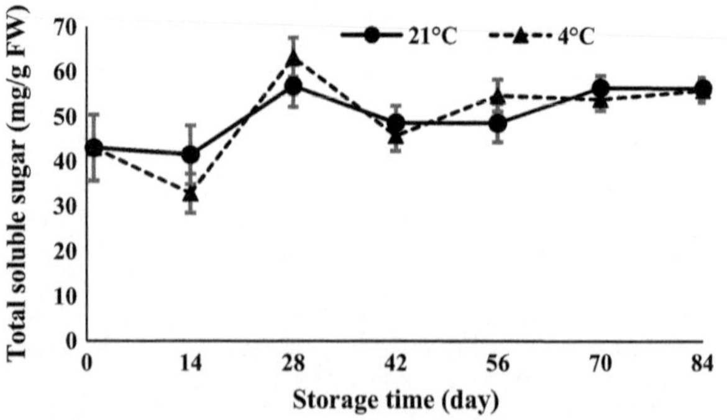

Figure 3. Total soluble sugar content changes during storage period at 4 and 21°C.

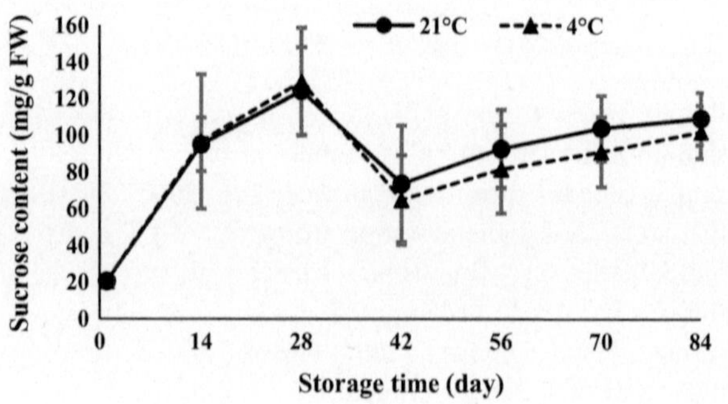

Figure 4. Sucrose content changes during storage period at 4 and 21°C.

indicating reduced sugar consumption in the metabolic pathway of the central bud of the clove. Vazquez-Barrios et al. (2006) observed that storage of garlic at 5°C resulted in a 33% reduction in TSS.

The results of ANOVA (Table 1) revealed that sucrose was affected by time of storage ($P < 0.01$). The results suggested that sucrose content strongly increased 28 days after storage at both 4 and 21°C (Fig. 4). Sucrose is the most important plant disaccharide and is the most common form of carbohydrate transported in plants (Hapkins 1999). Changes in the form of simple non-structural carbohydrates (sucrose, glucose, and fructose) at the time of onion bulb formation demonstrated that glucose and sucrose had the highest and lowest increase, respectively (Kahane et al. 2001). Rosa et al. (2009) showed that starch content of *Chenopodium quinoa* exposed to low temperature (2.5°C) followed a decreasing trend on the second day, whereas sucrose content increased until Day 4 and then decreased until Day 9 of the experiment.

The results of ANOVA (Table 1) demonstrated that glucose and fructose were affected by temperature and time of storage ($P < 0.01$). Glucose showed a decreasing trend in the first 14 days after harvesting and then increased toward the end of storage time at both 4 and

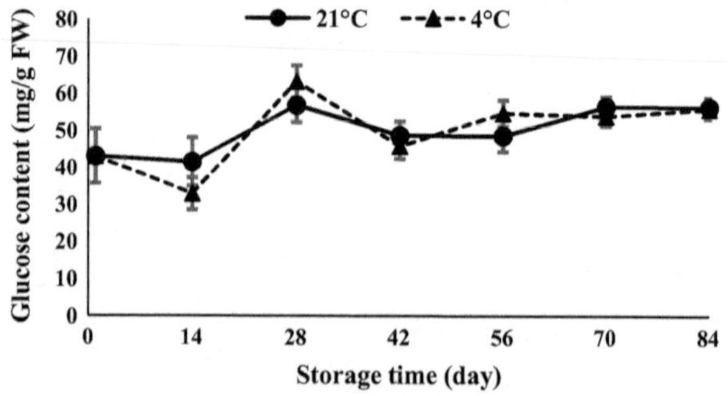

Figure 5. Glucose content changes during storage period at 4 and 21°C.

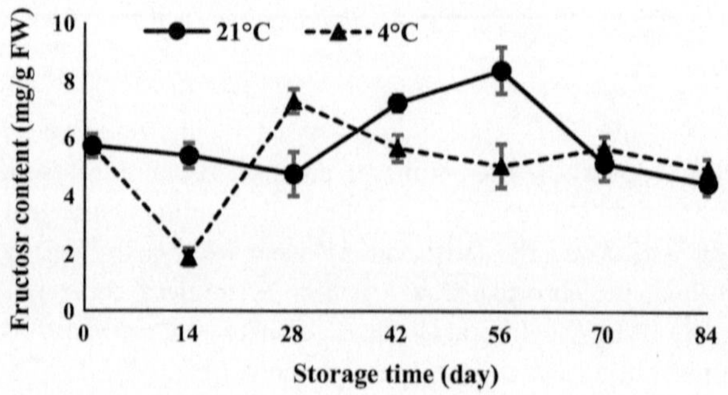

Figure 6. Fructose content changes during storage period at 4 and 21°C.

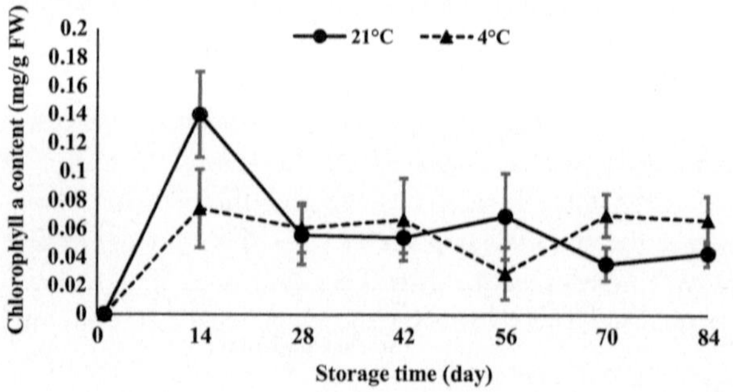

Figure 7. Chlorophyll *a* content changes during storage period at 4 and 21°C.

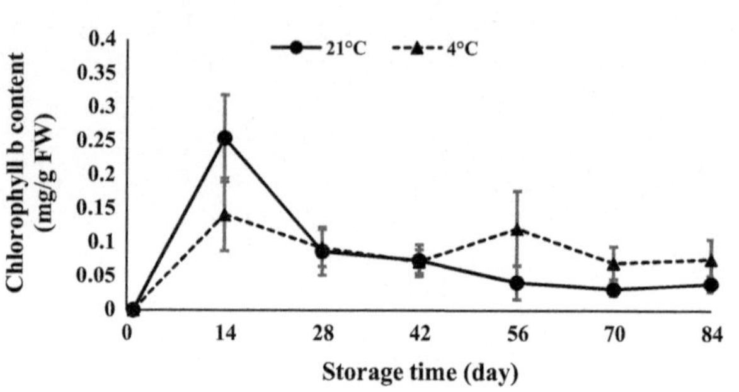

Figure 8. Chlorophyll *b* content changes during storage period at 4 and 21°C.

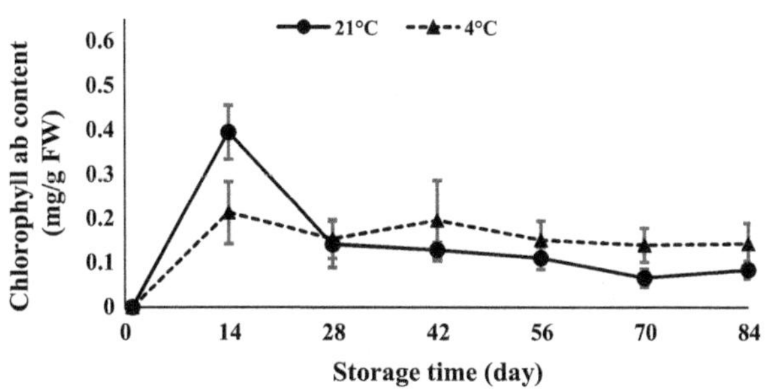

Figure 9. Chlorophyll *ab* content changes during storage period at 4 and 21°C.

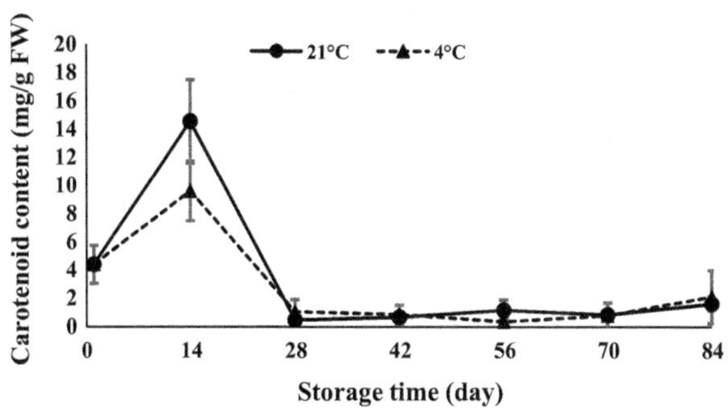

Figure 10. Carotenoid content changes during storage period at 4 and 21°C.

21°C (Fig. 5). On the other hand, the results demonstrated that fructose declined 28 and 14 days after the storage period at both 21 and 4°C, respectively (Fig. 6). Glucose content in thc first 14 days (Fig. 5) and sucrose content at 42 days (Fig. 4) showed a decreasing trend due to growing of buds. The levels of fructose (Fig. 6) oscillated during germination. Each of the sugars plays a role in bud growth. Due to the increase or decrease in each of the sugars during storage, the amount of total soluble sugars (Fig. 4) also increases or decreases. During processes such as seed germination, relatively large amounts of simple sugars are produced (Hapkins 1999). Garlic microbulblets physiologically mature and are able to sprout after 90 days of storage (Arguello et al. 2001). Cloves exposed to 5°C for 15–30 days before sowing accelerate the maturity of bulbs compared with cloves at room temperature or 20°C (Rahim and Fordham 2001). Cold storage at 5°C for 5 weeks before planting enhanced the purple color of the garlic bulb (Dufoo-Hurtado et al. 2013).

ANOVA (Table 1) demonstrated that anthocyanin, carotenoid, chlorophyll *a*, *b*, *ab*, and lipase were statistically affected by interaction of temperature and time of storage. The results revealed that chlorophyll *a*, *b*, *ab*, and carotenoid content strongly increased in the first 14 days after storage and then decreased at both 4 and 21°C (Figs. 7–10). The results showed that the content of chlorophyll *a*, *b*,

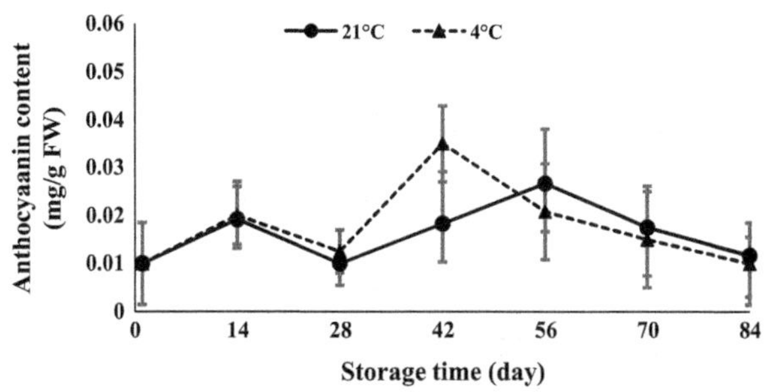

Figure 11. Anthocyanin content changes during storage period at 4 and 21°C.

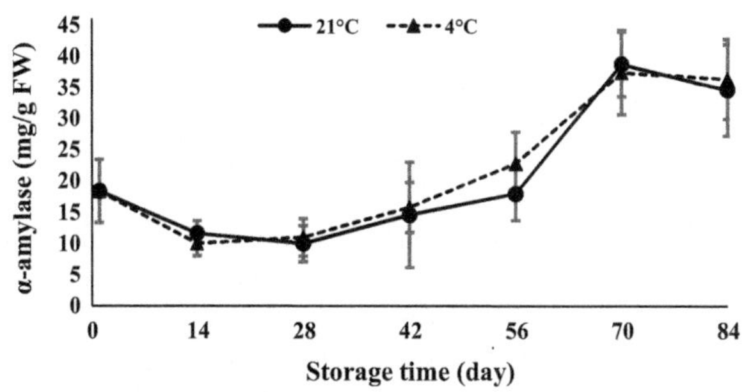

Figure 12. α-Amylase content changes during storage period at 4 and 21°C.

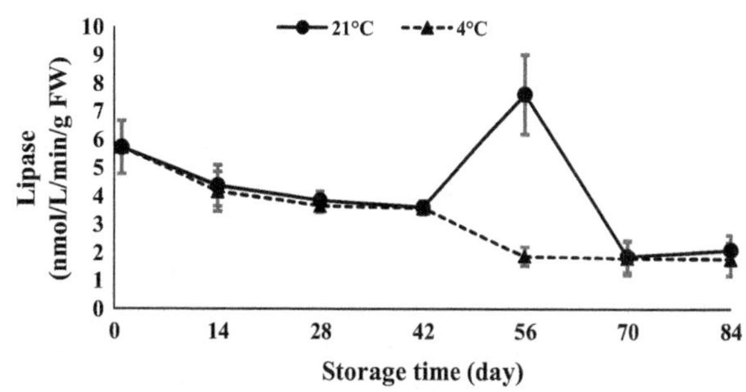

Figure 13. Lipase content changes during storage period at 4 and 21°C.

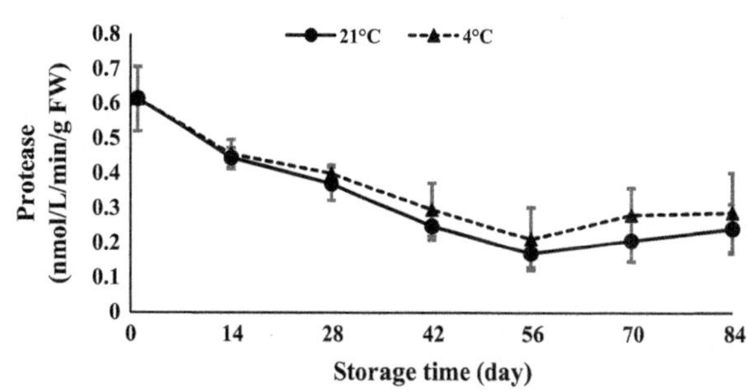

Figure 14. Protease content changes during storage period at 4 and 21°C.

and *ab* increased when glucose was decreased at day 14, which indicated that the glucose was used to produce chlorophyll. Atashi et al. (2011) reported that chlorophyll *a*, *b*, *ab*, and carotenoids exhibited the highest values after the 30-day chilling period at 4°C. Anthocyanin showed an increasing trend 14 and 42 days after harvesting and then decreased toward the end of storage (when sprouting began) at both 4 and 21°C (Fig. 11).

α-Amylase and protease were statistically affected by time of storage ($P < 0.01$). α-Amylase showed a decreasing trend in the first 14 days after storage and then increased toward the end of storage at both 4 and 21°C (Fig. 12). The activity of α-amylase was increased in response to an increase in chilling period at 4°C (Atashi et al. 2011). Amylase activity in Ruditapes variegatus has been reported during storage temperature of 4–35°C by Lin et al. (2009). Lipase enzyme slowly decreased at 84 days of storage (Fig. 13). A sudden jump was observed 56 days after storage for 21°C storage. Levels of protease declined at the end of storage when clove sprouting started at both 4 and 21°C (Fig. 14). Arguello et al. (2001) stated that at the end of garlic dormancy, peaks of peroxidase activity were observed. During both cold stratification and warm incubation of walnut kernels, storage protein mobilization occurred in the cotyledon (Einali and Sadeghipour 2007).

Conclusion

Some physiological changes occurred in garlic during storage time. The results of this experiment indicated that storage at both 4 and 21°C caused starch and sugar changes in garlic leading to sprouting. Some part of starch decomposed, leading to an increase in the content of glucose and sucrose in garlic tissue. When glucose increases, lipase and protease activity are reduced. However, starch, glucose, and sucrose are useful indices to predict sprouting time of garlic.

Conflict of Interest

None declared.

References

Anson, M. L. 1938. The estimation of pepsin, trypsin, papain and cathepsin with hemoglobin. J. Gen. Physiol. 22:79–89.

Arguello, J. A., L. R. Falcon, L. Seisdedos, S. Milrad, and R. Bottini. 2001. Morphological changes in garlic (*Allium sativum* L.) microbulblets during dormancy and sprouting as related to peroxidase activity and gibberellin GA3 content. Biocell 25:1–9.

Arnon, D. I. 1956. Photosynthesis by isolated chloroplast. Biochem. Biphys. 20:440–461.

Ashwell, G. 1957. Methods in Enzymology. p. 75. In: S. J. Colowick and N. O. Kaplan, eds. Methods in enzymol, Vol. 3 Academic Press, New York.

Atashi, S., V. Akbarpour, K. Mashayekhi, and S. J. Mousavizadeh. 2011. Garlic physiological characteristics from harvest in response to low temperature. J. Stored Prod. Postharvest. Res. 15:285–291.

Benkeblia, N., and G. Selselet-Attou. 1999. Effects of low temperatures on changes in oligosaccharids, phenolics and peroxidase in inner bud of onion (*Allium cepa* L.) during break of dormancy. Acta Agric. Scand. 49:98–102.

Bernfeld, P. 1955. Amylases: alpha and beta methods. Enzymol. 1:149–158.

Cantwell, M. I., J. Kang, and G. Hong. 2003. Heat treatments control sprouting and rooting of garlic cloves. Postharvest Biol. Technol. 30:57–65.

Dufoo-Hurtado, M. D., K. G. Zavala-Gutierrez, C. M. Cao, L. Cisneros-Zevallos, R. G. Guevara-Gonzalez, I. Torres-Pacheco, et al. 2013. Low-temperature conditioning of "seed" cloves enhances the expression of phenolic metabolism related genes and anthocyanin content in 'Coreano' garlic (*Allium sativum*) during plant development. J. Agric. Food Chem. 61:10439–10446.

Einali, A. R., and H. R. Sadeghipour. 2007. Alleviation of dormancy in walnut kernels by moist chilling is independent from storage protein mobilization. Tree Physiol. 27:519–525.

Fulton, T. A., A. J. Hall, and J. L. Catley. 2001. Chilling requirements of Paeonia cultivars. Sci. Hort. 89:237–248.

Gupta, A. K., and N. Kaur. 2005. Sugar signalling and gene expression in relation to carbohydrate metabolism under abiotic stresses in plants. J. Biosci. 30:761–776.

Handel, E. V. 1968. Direct microdetermination of sucrose. Anal. Biochem. 22:280–283.

Hapkins, W. G. 1999. Introduction to plant physiology. Vol. 1 and 2. John Wiley and Sons, New York.

Hartman, H. T. 2002. Plant propagation, principles and practices. 880 pp, Prentice hall, Upper Saddle River, NJ.

Iraqi, D., V. QuyLe, M. S. Lamhamedi, and F. M. Tremblay. 2005. Sucrose utilization during somatic embryo development in black spruce: involvement of apoplastic invertase in the tissue and of extracellular invertase in the medium. J. Plant Physiol. 162:115–124.

Kahane, R., E. Vialle, B. Ietje, and T. Dimitris. 2001. Changes in non-structural carbohydrate composition during bulbing in sweet and high-solid onions in field experiments. Environ. Exp. Bot. 45:73–83.

Langens-Grrits, M. M., W. B. Miller, A. F. Croes, and G. J. DeKlerk. 2003. Effects of low temperature on dormancy breaking and growth after planting in lily bulblets regenerated *in vitro*. Plant Growth Regul. 40:267–275.

Lee, H. C. 2007. Study on the expression of b-amylase genes in *Oryza sativa* cv. Nipponbare. Taipei, Taiwan. [Master Thesis] of National Taiwan Univ., Taipei, Taiwan. 125 p.

Lin, J., Y. Lin, Sh. Ku, C. M. Jiang, and M. Ch. Wu. 2009. Purification of soybean amylase by superparamagnetic particles. Food Chem. 117:94–98.

McCready, R. M., J. Guggolz, V. Silviera, and H. S. Owens. 1950. Determination of starch and amylase in vegetables. Anal. Chem. 22:1156–1158.

Miller, G. N. 1959. Use of dinitrosalicylic acid reagent for determination of reducing sugars. Anal. Chem. 31:426–428.

Omokolo, N., D. Tsalam, and F. P. Djogoue. 1996. Change in carbohydrate, amino acid and phenol content in cocoa pods from three clones after infection with *Phytophtora megakarya* Bra and Grif. Ann. Bot. 77:153–158.

Rahim, M. A., and R. Fordham. 2001. Environmental manipulation for controlling bulbing in garlic. Acta Hortic. 555:180–188.

Rosa, M., M. Hilal, J. A. Gonzalez, and F. E. Prado. 2009. Low-temperature effect on enzyme activities involved in sucrose–starch partitioning in salt-stressed and salt-acclimated cotyledons of quinoa (*Chenopodium quinoa* Willd.) seedlings. Plant Physiol. Biochem. 47:300–307.

Rubatzky, E. V., and M. Yamaguchi. 1997. World vegetables, principles, production and nutritive values, 2nd edn. 843 pp. Chapman and Hall, International Thompson Publishing, New York

Sadeghipour, H. R., and S. C. Bhatla. 2002. Differential sensitivity of oleosins to proteolysis during oil body mobilization in sunflower seedlings. Plant Cell Physiol. 43:1117–1126.

Vazquez-Barrios, M. E., G. Lopez-Echevarria, E. Mercado-Silva, E. Castano-Tostado, and F. Leon-Gonzalez. 2006. Study and prediction of quality changes in garlic cv. Perla (*Allium sativum* L.) stored at different temperatures. Sci. Hortic. 108:127–132.

Wanger, G. J. 1979. Content and vacuole extra vacuole distribution of neutral sugars, free amino acids and anthocyanins in protoplasts. Plant Physiol. 64:88–93.

8

Mathematical modeling of drying of potato slices in a forced convective dryer based on important parameters

Samira Naderinezhad, Nasrin Etesami, Arefe Poormalek Najafabady & Majid Ghasemi Falavarjani

Department of Chemical Engineering, Isfahan University of Technology, Isfahan, 84156-8311, Iran

Keywords
Air temperature, forced air convective dryer, mathematical kinetics model, potato slices, sample shape

Correspondence
Nasrin Etesami, Department of Chemical Engineering, Isfahan University of Technology, Isfahan, 84156-8311, Iran.

E-mail: netesami@cc.iut.ac.ir

Funding Information
The authors acknowledge the Isfahan Science & Technology Town for providing financial support.

Abstract

The effect of air temperature, air velocity, and sample shapes (circle and square with the same cross- sectional area) on kinetic drying of potato slices in a tunnel dryer was investigated experimentally and a suitable drying model was developed. The experiments of drying of potato slices were conducted at an air temperature of 45–70°C with an air velocity 1.60 and 1.81 m sec^{-1}. Results showed that drying temperature was the most effective parameter in the drying rate. The influence of air velocity was more profound in low temperature. The time for drying square slices was lower compared to the circle ones. Furthermore, drying data were fitted to different empirical models. Among the models, Midilli–Kucuk was the best to explain the single layer drying of potato slices. The parameters of this model were determined as functions of air velocity and temperature by multiple regression analysis for circle and square slices. Various statistical parameters were examined for evaluating the model.

Introduction

Drying of agricultural products is one of the main goals of preservation, transportation, and commerce. Drying process reduces the content of moisture and then chemical alterations help minimizing microbiological activity in the product during the storage. Therefore, the persistence of product and its stability will increase.

The traditional method which is used in drying of fruits and vegetables through sunlight is not common nowadays, it takes more time leading to a low-quality product with microbial growth and low process capability. Some effective and rapid methods are required to solve these problems in the process of industrial drying. The most common method in drying foodstuffs is the hot air drying which causes rapidity, produces high capacity, reduces its weight and volume, and also minimizes the cost of packing, storage, and transportation. Dried products are affected by drying conditions such as temperature, relative humidity, air velocity, and physical and chemical parameters of raw materials.

An important source of carbohydrate which is rich in β-carotene, fiber, and potassium ion is sweet potato. Potatoes are also the fourth most important vegetable crop for human nutrition in the world. The starch of sweet potato can be used as an ingredient in bread, biscuits, cake, etc.

Dried potato is used to produce potato flakes, powder, animal feed, and chips. Prepared potato's powder is useful for sore salve, concentrate conserves, cake flour, flavor improver, bread paste improver, pizza paste, etc.

One of the important aspects of drying technology is the modeling of drying process. It has been (study of

Table 1. Single layer mathematical drying model.

No.	Model name	Model	References
1	Page	$MR = \exp(-kt^n)$	Guarte (1996), Zhang and Litchfield (1991)
2	Modified page	$MR = \exp[-(kt)^n]$	White et al. (1981)
3	Two term	$MR = a\exp(-k_0t) + b\exp(-k_1t)$	Rahman et al. (1997)
4	Diffusion approach	$MR = a\exp(-kt) + (1 - a)\exp(-kbt)$	Kassem (1998)
5	Verma et al.	$MR = a\exp(-kt) + (1-a)\exp(-gt)$	Verma et al. (1985)
6	Midilli–Kucuk	$MR = a\exp(-kt^n) + bt$	Midilli et al. (2002)
7	Weibull	$MR = \exp(-((t/b)^a))$	Marabi et al. (2003)
8	Modified page equation 2	$MR = \exp(-c^* ((t/(b^2))^n))$	Diamante and Munro (1991)

drying behavior of different materials) an interesting subject for many researchers, in both theoretical and application way. Drying kinetics of food is a complex process. To predict the rate of drying and optimization of drying parameters need suitable kinetic models. Many models have been proposed by researchers for kinetics drying of biological materials. Models of the thin layer drying are very common (see Table 1). The process of drying which includes a thin layer of sample particles or slices is called thin-layer drying.

Hatamipour et al. (2007) analyzed changes in the structure and color of potato samples/slices in different dryers and in different conditions.

Aghbashlo et al. (2009) developed the kinetic model by investigating the thin layer drying kinetics of potato slices in continuous dryer under different air temperatures and air velocity.

Akpinar (2006) examined drying of potato, apple, and pumpkin in the cyclone dryer under forced airflow and estimated kinetic models as a function of sample area, temperature, air velocity, and time for prediction of moisture ratio on trays of dryer. Hassini et al. (2007) measured water loss and volume variation curves for potato samples during drying. They evaluated potato moisture diffusivity from convective drying kinetics with correction for shrinkage and presented correlations for prediction of moisture diffusivity as a function of moisture content and air temperature.

Senadeera et al. (2003) investigated the effect of temperature and samples aspect ratio on drying behavior of parallelepiped shaped potato, cylinder shaped green bean, and sphere shaped pea in fluidized bed dryer and established kinetic models for drying them.

Tripathy and Kumar (2008) investigated the drying process of potato in slice and cylinder shapes in natural convection mixed mode solar dryer. They provided models for each sample and represented temperature which was dependent on drying parameters for cylinders and slices of potato.

Drying of potato with different air temperature, air velocity, and size of the samples was studied experimentally in the cyclone dryer by Akpinar et al. (2003). They developed models as a function of mentioned parameters for trays of dryer.

Reyes et al. (2007) studied the effects of drying conditions such as type of dryer, drying temperature, and air velocity on drying time and the quality of dehydrated potato slices. They also established a model to explain drying curves of potato slices.

Although some of the previous researchers provided general models as a function of parameter that affect drying process (Akpinar et al. 2003; Akpinar 2006; Tripathy and Kumar 2008). While there is not any study about the effect of sample shape on drying rate of potato. In this study, the effects of some important parameters such as air temperature, air velocity, and sample shape on drying behavior of potato in a force convective dryer are experimentally investigated. There is also a general mathematical kinetic model as a function of air temperature and air velocity for two sample shapes with the same surface area which is developed and compared with experimental data.

Materials and Methods

Experimental setup

A schematic diagram of the designed experimental setup has been shown in Figure 1. It includes a blower with 90 $m^3\ h^{-1}$ of nominal flow rate, heater elements with variable power (100–3600 W), and air channel with dimensions $0.15 \times 0.15 \times 2.43\ m^3$ that contains a polymer mesh tray. As a uniform airflow forms near the tray, it has been located 2 m from the entrance of the channel. Air temperature and air velocity are adjusted for the samples on the tray by changing the power of the heater and valve of the blower, respectively. Hot airflows parallel to the tray over and under the samples and the samples are dried in two directions, top and bottom. Before the tray, the air temperature is measured by thermometer with readability of ±1°C. A digital balance (Shimadzo Co., Nakagyo-ku, Kyoto, Japan) was used to measure the sample weight on line. Its readability is 0.01 g.

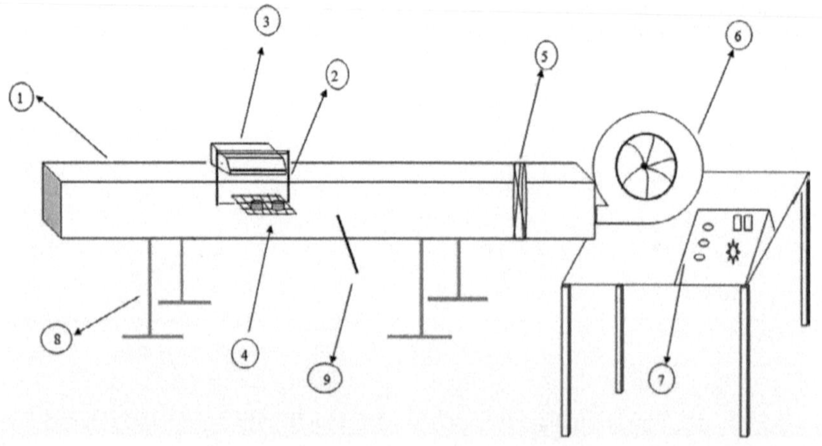

Figure 1. Experimental setup: 1, duct; 2, digital balance; 3, lever; 4, tray and samples; 5, mesh elements of heater; 6, fan; 7, control panel; 8, stand; 9, thermometer.

All experiments were carried out in the same environmental conditions (ambient pressure is 610 mmHg and ambient temperature is 26°C). Multifunction measuring instrument (Testo-400, Lenzkirch, Germany) was used to measure the velocity of airflow. The range of velocity measurement is 0 to10 m sec^{-1} with this instrument and an accuracy of ±0.03 m sec^{-1}. Some experiments were repeated three times in the same conditions to check the repeatability of results and the average of standard deviation was 0.0346.

The samples were placed on the tray after reaching to a steady-state condition for airflow velocity and temperature. The loss of weight is measured by gravimetric method during that time. In order to measure the dry solid of samples, samples were dried in a vacuum oven at 70°C for 24 h.

Sample preparation

Potatoes used for sample preparation were from the same race, fresh, and uniform. They were kept in dark and cold place (4°C) before the experiments were conducted. The average initial moisture content of the samples was approximately 449.1% (dry weight basis).

Potato samples/slices were cut into circle and square shapes with the same cross-sectional area (about 20 cm^2) and thickness (7 mm).

In order to maintain the quality of products, such as color of the sample while drying, pretreatment procedure was done (Akpinar et al. 2003; Agarry et al. 2005; Aghbashlo et al. 2009).

For this purpose, samples were blanched for 5 min in boiling water at 90°C before drying and exactly after the cutting. The time of heating should not be so much that the samples get on the verge of being cooked. Samples were then immediately immerged in 500 mL of cold water at 10°C for 2 min, the water on the surface of the samples was removed by a tissue or filter paper, and finally the samples are ready for drying test.

In order to investigate the effect of various parameters on the drying of potato samples, three series of experiments were designed which are as follows:

1. Experiments with different average velocities (1.6 and 1.81 m sec^{-1}).
2. Experiments with different temperatures (45, 50, 55, 60, 65, and 70°C).
3. Experiments with different shape of samples (square and circle with the same cross-sectional area).

In each series of experiments, other parameters had been fixed.

Drying data processing

Moisture content (g water/g dry solid) of the sample (M) is calculated by the following equation (1):

$$M = \frac{m_t - m_s}{m_s} \tag{1}$$

where m_t is the mass of sample at time t and m_s is mass of dry solid.

The moisture content is essential to be the same for all samples in the base measure because of natural and inherent differences in initial moisture content of the samples. Therefore, the moisture ratio (MR) expression is calculated using the following equation:

$$\mathrm{MR} = \frac{M_t - M_e}{M_o - M_e} \tag{2}$$

where M_t, M_e, and M_0 are moisture content at any time, equilibrium moisture content, and initial moisture content, respectively. In this method, samples were placed in an environment maintaining relative humidity and temperature constant. When the change in the weight of samples was insignificant, the moisture of the samples was measured and adopted as the equilibrium moisture content (M_e). In order to low humidity in ambient (dry and hot weather), equilibrium moisture content is negligible and MR = M_t/M_0.

Drying curves were constructed by MR versus time. Numerical differentiation of drying curves is proportional with drying rate. This concept is used as dimensionless drying rate (DR) through the paper.

Mathematical drying model

Various mathematical and semi-empirical models have been reported in order to study the mathematical modeling of thin layer drying kinetics. In this study, 21 different expressions were examined. Between those expressions, the best eight were selected that can be seen in Table 1.

Nonlinear regression analysis was performed using MATLAB software (version 7.8).

Root mean square error (RMSE) (Procopio (2007)), chi-square (χ^2) (Peck and Devore (2011)), R-square (R^2) (Vidakovic (2011)), and mean absolute error (MAE) (Frees (2010)) were used to determine the quality of the fit. Higher values of R^2 and lower values of χ^2, MAE, and RMSE indicate better goodness of fit (Doymaz 2008; Usub et al. 2010). These can be calculated as:

$$\chi^2 = \frac{\sum_{i=1}^{N}(\text{MRexp}, i - \text{MRpre}, i)^2}{N - Z} \quad (3)$$

$$\text{RMSE} = \left[\frac{1}{N}\sum_{i=1}^{N}(\text{MRpre}, i - \text{MRexp}, i)^2\right]^{1/2} \quad (4)$$

$$R^2 = 1 - \frac{\sum_{i=1}^{N}(\text{MRexp}, i - \text{MRpre}, i)^2}{\sum_{i=1}^{N}(\overline{\text{MRexp}} - \text{MRexp}, i)^2} \quad (5)$$

$$\text{MAE} = \frac{1}{N}\sum_{i=1}^{N}\left|\text{MR}_{\text{pre}, i} - MR_{\text{exp}, i}\right| \quad (6)$$

where $\text{MR}_{\text{exp},i}$ is the experimental moisture ratio found in any measurement, $\text{MR}_{\text{pre},i}$ is predicted moisture ratio for this measurement, N is the number of observations, Z is the number of model constants, $\overline{\text{MR}_{\text{exp}}}$ is the total average data, and i is ith data.

Results and Discussion

The operating conditions for different sets of the experiments are presented in Table 2. In this section the effect of various parameters on the potato drying process is investigated.

Table 2. Operating conditions in different sets of experiments.

Parameter	Unit	Value
Velocity	m sec^{-1}	1.60, 1.81
Shape	–	Circle, Square
Temperature	°C	45, 55, 60, 65, 70 (circle) 50, 60, 70 (square)

Plotted drying curves for all experiments showed that there is no constant rate period in drying of potato slices and falling rate period occurs in drying process of potato due to diffusion controlled mechanism inside the potato. In the early stage of drying process, heat and mass transfer rate is high in thin layer drying. The drying process decreases exponentially and becomes slower and eventually stops by decreasing the gradient of water concentration in the sample. The lack of a constant rate period of drying can be due to changes in the internal moisture and surface changes owing to the shrinkage of the samples during the drying process.

Effect of air temperature

Figures 2 and 3 indicate the effect of air temperature on dimensionless moisture content and dimensionless drying rate in high and low velocity of airflow for circle sample during drying. Figures 2A and 3A illustrate that total drying time decreases and drying rate increases with temperature. For example, the time of drying reaching MR = 0.11 was reduced from about 335 to 256 min by changing temperature from 45°C to 55°C for circular sample at 1.60 m sec^{-1} air velocity.

As shown in these figures, the effect of temperature on drying process at first stage is great. This behavior is attributed to the fact that driving force for evaporation of water from the samples increases by heating the sample.

It is also found that the effect of temperature on dimensionless drying rate is more profound in lower air velocity by comparing Figures 2B and 3B. Similar trend was seen for square shape samples for variation dimensionless moisture and dimensionless drying rate as shown in Figure 4.

Similar results can be found from drying curve that have been presented by Aghbashlo et al. (2009) in the length of continuous band dryer. The results show that the increment in drying rate of potato with air temperature in low air velocity is more than that in high air velocity.

The effect of temperature on drying behavior of potato has been investigated by several researchers at various air velocities; in a cyclone dryer at 50, 60, 70°C (Akpinar

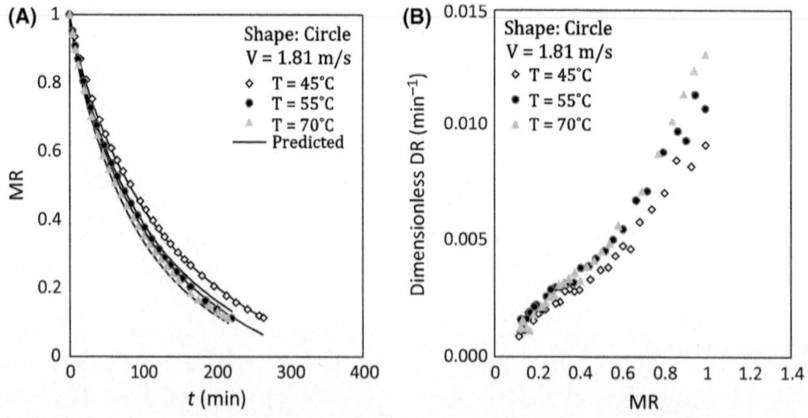

Figure 2. (A) Moisture ratio versus time and (B) dimensionless drying rate versus moisture ratio at different temperatures, 1.81 m sec^{-1} of air velocity, and circle sample.

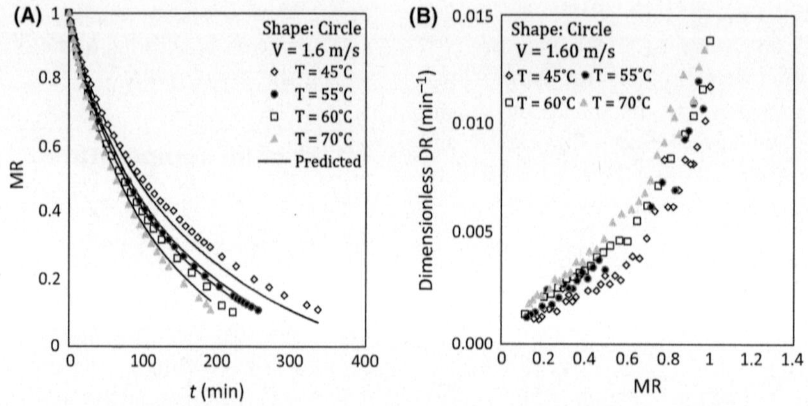

Figure 3. (A) Moisture ratio versus time and (B) dimensionless drying rate versus moisture ratio at different temperatures, 1.60 m sec^{-1} of air velocity, and circle sample.

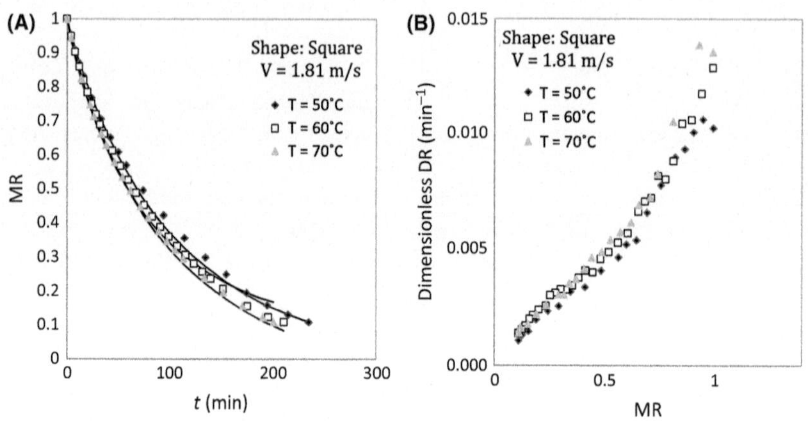

Figure 4. (A) Moisture ratio versus time and (B) dimensionless drying rate versus moisture ratio at different temperatures, 1.81 m sec^{-1} of air velocity, and square sample.

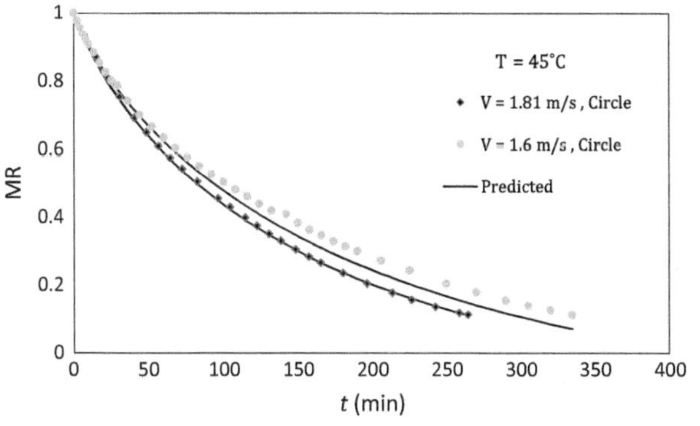

Figure 5. Moisture ratio versus time at different air velocities, 45°C air temperature, and circle sample.

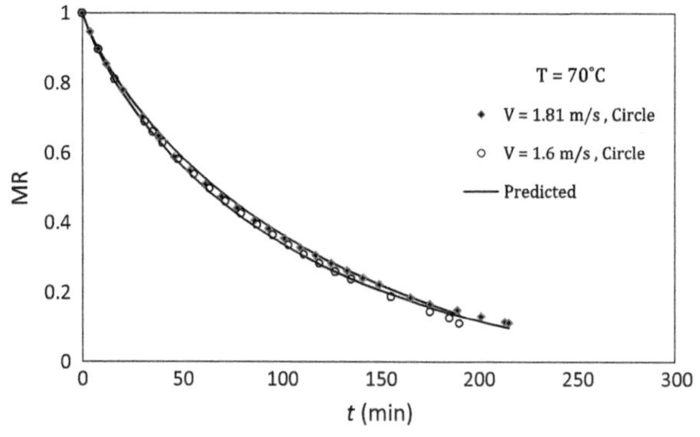

Figure 6. Variation in moisture ratio versus time at different air velocities, 70°C air temperature, and circle sample.

et al. 2003), in a laboratory scale, convective vertical downward flow dryer at 40, 55, 70, 85°C (Hassini et al. 2007), in fluidized bed dryers at 30, 40, 50°C (Senadeera et al. 2003). Similar findings are reported by them.

Effect of air velocity

The variation in dimensionless moisture content with time in low and high temperature has been shown in Figures 5 and 6, respectively. It is found that drying rate is increased with air velocity.

The resistance to mass transfer is mixed in the potato samples and in the external layer. Thickness of the boundary layer and thus the mass transfer resistance in the gas phase decreases with blowing airflow on the sample and increases drying rate consequently. Toward the end of the drying, the effect of air velocity would become negligible because of the greater internal resistance to moisture transfer caused in part by structure changes. Similar results can be found in the previous works (Akpinar et al. 2003).

Comparing Figures 5 and 6 show that the influence of air velocity on drying rate accretion in low temperature is more than that in high temperature (square samples showed similar trends). This effect has not been directly discussed in the previous studies, but similar results can be understood from drying curves that are reported in some of the previous works (Hassini et al. 2007; Aghbashlo et al. 2009).

Effect of sample shape

Figure 7 illustrates the variations in dimensionless moisture during drying and dimensionless drying rate against dimensionless moisture for two samples, respectively. The effect of shape parameter (circle and square section area) with the same surface area (=20 cm^2) has not been examined in the previous studies. According to the Figure 7A, sample in square shape dried faster than the circle shaped sample. Figure 7B shows that the shape parameter has much influence on drying rate.

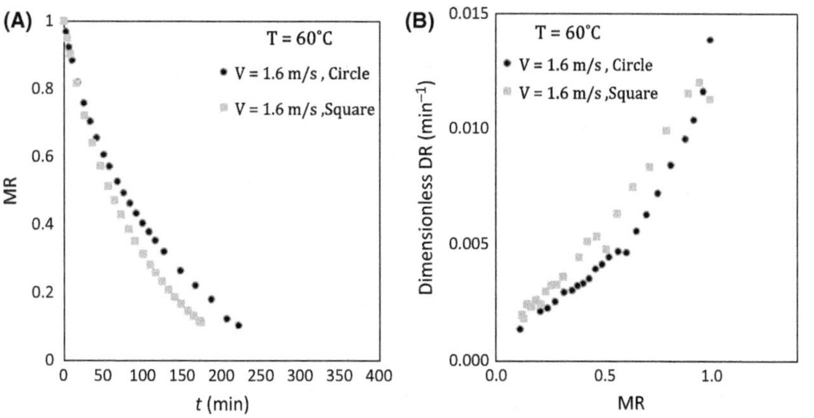

Figure 7. (A) Moisture ratio versus time and (B) dimensionless drying rate versus moisture ratio at different shapes, 60°C air temperature, and 1.60 m sec^{-1} air velocity.

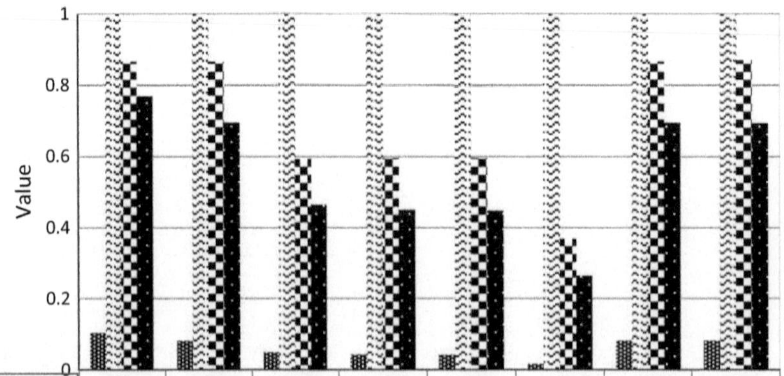

Model number	1	2	3	4	5	6	7	8
X2*1000	0.104	0.0813	0.0488	0.0425	0.0413	0.015	0.0813	0.0813
R2	0.99894	0.99894	0.99946	0.99945	0.99945	0.99981	0.99894	0.99894
RMSE*100	0.8661	0.8661	0.5934	0.5962	0.5962	0.3678	0.8661	0.8704
MAE*100	0.7694	0.6948	0.4641	0.4496	0.447	0.263	0.695	0.6946

Figure 8. Average of various statistical parameters in comparison with eight of the best model for circle shape tests.

Although the cross-sectional area is considered equal in both samples, lateral surface area of the square sample is more than that in circle sample. This would increase the surface exposed with airflow and increase the evaporation rate consequently. In addition the ratio of perimeter to cross-sectional area for square shapes is more than circle. This increases the heat transfer and since the temperature in the drying was most effective parameter, mass transfer increases.

Mathematical modeling

Averages of various statistical parameters were calculated determining the quality of the fit for the best eight models in Table 1 (Fig. 8). As seen in this figure, Midilli–Kucuk model (with the number 6 in Table 1) is the best (parameters calculation were repeated for square samples and similar results obtained).

Several researchers have investigated kinetic drying model of potato. But only some of them (Akpinar et al. 2003; Akpinar 2006) have developed a general model with significant statistical parameters. Nonlinear regression analysis is performed to develop a comprehensive model with goodness of fit in this study.

It is assumed that there is no resistance in airflow to transfer moisture in proposed model. Selected model (Midilli–Kucuk model) is:

$$MR = a\exp(-k(t^n)) + bt \quad (7)$$

Table 3. Midilli–Kucuk coefficient (eq. 7).

Test no.	*V* m sec^{-1}	*T* °C	Shape	*a*	*b*	*n*	*K*	R^2	χ^2	RMSE	MAE
1	1.81	45	Circle	1.00900	0.00019-	0.87280	0.01404	0.99986	0.00001	0.00299	0.00249
2	1.81	55	Circle	1.00700	−0.00031	0.85460	0.01722	0.99990	0.00001	0.00268	0.00222
3	1.81	60	Circle	1.00800	−0.00019	0.82340	0.01873	0.99991	0.00001	0.00245	0.00182
4	1.81	70	Circle	1.00800	−0.00019	0.84520	0.02004	0.99986	0.00001	0.00323	0.00247
5	1.6	45	Circle	1.00600	−0.00020	0.79850	0.01658	0.99979	0.00002	0.00385	0.00268
6	1.6	55	Circle	1.00800	−0.00018	0.84670	0.01680	0.99988	0.00001	0.00345	0.00288
7	1.6	60	Circle	1.00100	−0.00024	0.86600	0.01596	0.99937	0.00005	0.00694	0.0042
8	1.6	65	Circle	1.00700	−0.00036	0.84050	0.01806	0.99988	0.00001	0.00285	0.00231
9	1.6	70	Circle	1.00800	−0.00038	0.83610	0.02042	0.99982	0.00001	0.00383	0.00228
10	1.81	50	Square	0.99020	−0.00003	0.94170	0.01207	0.99927	0.00008	0.00892	0.00759
11	1.81	60	Square	1.00400	−0.00025	0.86840	0.01775	0.99983	0.00001	0.00350	0.00248
12	1.81	70	Square	1.00200	−0.00017	0.86070	0.01981	0.99974	0.00002	0.00447	0.00376
13	1.6	50	Square	0.99520	−0.00005	0.93500	0.01173	0.99928	0.00008	0.00869	0.00729
14	1.6	60	Square	1.00100	−0.00019	0.94360	0.01451	0.99972	0.00002	0.00475	0.00397
15	1.34	50	Square	0.99720	−0.00008	0.99900	0.00911	0.99983	0.00002	0.00393	0.00322
Extra run											

Table 4. Constant parameter of presented models (Midilli–Kucuk kinetic model).

Shape	α	β	γ	ϕ	τ	ω	Θ	ρ	σ
Circle	−1.80211	2.24510E+4	−3.04645E+2	−0.00021	0.7859	0.00019	0.11191	0.00137	0.55637
Square	0.00859	−3.23366E+10	6.46733E+8	−0.00020	1.29904	−0.00339	−0.29405	0.00005	1.25228

where a and n are dimensionless, dimension k is (time^{-n}), and dimension b is (time^{-1}).

Coefficients of the selected model have been calculated in Table 3 for all tests. Statistical parameters have been calculated to compare the goodness of fit by equations 3 to 6 and they have been listed in this table. According to Table 3, high value of average R^2 (0.99973) and low value of average χ^2 (0.000025) indicate that fit is good.

In order to generalize the drying kinetic model, coefficients of Midilli–Kucuk expression were modeled with various parameters such as temperature, air velocity, and sample shape by multiple regression technique. Some researchers have done this for potato, in the past (Akpinar et al. 2003; Akpinar 2006; Aghbashlo et al. 2009; Tripathy and Kumar 2008).

In addition to air temperature and air velocity, the shape of samples is considered in the model too. Coefficients of Midilli–Kucuk model as the best fitting model involves the drying variable such as temperature, air velocity for two shapes of potato sample were determined as follows:

$$a = 1.00389$$

$$b = \frac{\alpha + V}{\beta + \gamma T} + \varphi$$

$$n = \tau \exp(\omega T) \times V^{\theta}$$

$$k = \rho (\mathrm{TV})^{\sigma}$$

where α, β, γ, ϕ, τ, ω, θ, ρ, σ are constants and they are determined in Table 4.

Validation of these three functions is evaluated with %E (Mean of relative error percent), RMSE, and χ^2. Low values of %E, RMSE, and χ^2 show good fit of Midilli coefficients model with presented model. These values are reported in Table 5.

Table 5. Validation of Midilli–Kucuk coefficient model with statistical parameters.

Shape	Coefficient	% E	χ^2	RMSE
Circle	b	15.73	4.6E-09	0.00005
	n	1.90	0.00061	0.02022
	k	5.17	1.58E-06	0.00111
Square	b	11.11	3.39E-09	0.00003
	n	1.81	0.00086	0.01858
	k	6.63	2.51E-06	0.00123

Table 6. Slope and R^2 for predicted MR versus experimental MR.

Test no.	R^2	Slope
1	0.9998	0.9835
2	0.9998	0.9697
3	0.9996	1.0522
4	0.9998	1.0114
5	0.9997	1.0565
6	0.9996	0.9899
7	0.9993	0.9762
8	0.9999	0.9775
9	0.9996	0.978
10	0.9989	1.0069
11	0.9993	1.029
12	0.9949	0.9089
13	0.9978	1.0248
14	0.9996	0.9859
15	0.9991	1.0218
Extra run		

By comparing computed dimensionless moisture contents with measured ones, the validation of final established model for drying kinetic of potato with coefficients as the function of process parameters was made in all drying runs (14 runs). R^2 and slopes have been provided for all runs for measured MR versus predicted MR in Table 6. A good agreement between model and experiment data has been shown in Table 6. It also can be seen that the drying model has successfully predicted the drying of potato in Figures 2A, 3A, 4A, 5, and 6.

The derived model (by 14 runs) is examined by test 15 as extra run; air velocity 1.34 m sec^{-1} with 50°C air temperature and square shape sample; that it was not included in the multiple regressions. The results confirm that present model is suitable for tests which are out-of-range for multiple regression tests.

Conclusion

Drying process of potato slices was investigated in hot air convective dryer. No constant drying rate period was observed. The effect of air temperature, air velocity, and sample shape of potato slices were examined on behavior of potato drying. Results showed that air temperature has the most effect on decreasing of drying time. The influence of air velocity on drying rate in low temperature is more than that in high temperature due to the dominant temperature effect. The time of drying for square slices of potato is lower than circle ones under the same test conditions according to greater lateral surface area. A suitable drying model was developed by incorporating the effect of above parameters on potato drying process. The regression coefficients and statistical parameters RMSE, χ^2, and MAE values show that the derived model is a good agreement with data and it would be a useful engineering application such as design and optimization.

Acknowledgment

The authors thank Maryam Hozhabri researcher from Isfahan University of Technology for scientific assistance during the project and the authors acknowledge the Isfahan Science & Technology Town for providing financial support.

Conflict of Interest

None declared.

References

Agarry, S. E., A. O. Durojaiye, and T. J. Afolabi. 2005. Effect of pretreatment on the drying rate and drying time of potato. J. Food Technol. 3:361–364.

Aghbashlo, M., M. H. Kianmehr, and A. Arabhosseini. 2009. Modeling of thin-layer drying of potato slices in length of continuous band dryer. Energy Convers. Manage. 50:1348–1355.

Akpinar, E. K. 2006. Determination of suitable thin layer drying curve model for some vegetables and fruits. J. Food Eng. 73:75–84.

Akpinar, E., A. Midilli, and Y. Bicer. 2003. Single layer drying behavior of potato slices in a convective cyclone dryer and mathematical modeling. Energy Convers. Manage. 44:1689–1705.

Diamante, L. M., and P. A. Munro. 1991. Mathematical modeling of hot air drying of sweet potato slices. Int. J. Food Sci. Technol. 26:99–109.

Doymaz, I. 2008. Convective drying kinetics of strawberry. Chem. Eng. Process. 47:914–919.

Frees, E. W. 2010. Regression modeling with actuarial and financial applications, 1th edn. pp. 656. Cambridge University Press, New York.

Guarte, R. C. 1996. Modeling the drying behavior of copra and development of a natural convection dryer for production of high quality copra in the Philippines. PhD Dissertation. 287, Hohenheim University, Stuttgart, Germany.

Hassini, L., S. Azzouz, R. Peczalski, and A. Belghith. 2007. Estimation of potato moisture diffusivity from convective drying kinetics with correction for shrinkage. J. Food Eng. 79:47–56.

Hatamipour, M. S., H. H. Kazemi, A. Nooralivand, and A. Nozarpoor. 2007. Drying characteristics of six varieties of sweet potatoes in different dryers. Food Bioprod. Process. 85:171–177.

Kassem, A. S. 1998. Comparative studies on thin layer drying models for wheat. *in* 13th International congress on agricultural engineering, Morocco.

Marabi, A. M., S. L. Livings, M. J. Jacobson, and I. S. S. Saguy. 2003. Normalized Weibull distribution for modeling rehydration of food particulates. Eur. Food Res. Technol. 217:311–318.

Midilli, A., H. Kucuk, and Z. Yapar. 2002. A new model for single layer drying. Drying Technol. 20:1503–1513.

Peck, R., and J. L. Devore. 2011. Statistics: The exploration and analysis of data, 7th edn. pp. 6.6. Brooks/Cole, Boston, MA.

Procopio, M. J. 2007. An experimental analysis of classifier ensembles for learning drifting concepts over time in autonomous outdoor robot navigation. pp. 116. University of Colorado at Boulder, Boulder.

Rahman, M. S., C. O. Perera, and C. Theband. 1997. Desorption isotherm and heat pump drying kinetics of peas. Int. Food Res. J. 30:485–491.

Reyes, A., S. Cerón, R. Zúñiga, and P. Moyano. 2007. A comparative study of microwave-assisted air drying of potato slices. Biosyst. Eng. 98:310–318.

Senadeera, W., B. R. Bhandari, G. Young, and B. Wijesinghe. 2003. Influence of shapes of selected vegetable materials on drying kinetics during fluidized bed drying. J. Food Eng. 58:277–283.

Tripathy, P. P., and S. Kumar. 2008. Determination of temperature dependent drying parameters for potato cylinders and slices during solar drying. Energy Convers. Manage. 49:2941–2948.

Usub, T., C. Lertsatitthankorn, N. Poomsa-ad, L. Wiset, S. Siriamornpun, and S. Soponronnarit. 2010. Thin layer solar drying characteristics of silkworm pupae. Food Bioprod. Process. 88:149–160.

Verma, L. R., R. A. Bucklin, J. B. Endan, and F. T. Wratten. 1985. Effects of drying air parameters on rice drying models. Trans. ASAE 28:296–301.

Vidakovic, B. V. 2011. Statistics for bioengineering sciences: with MATLAB and WinBUGS support, 2th edn. pp. 623. Springer, Germany.

White, G. M., I. J. Ross, and R. Ponelert. 1981. Fully exposed drying of popcorn. Trans. ASAE 24:466–468.

Zhang, Q., and J. B. Litchfield. 1991. An optimization of intermittent corn drying in a laboratory scale thin layer dryer. Drying Technol. 9:383–395.

9

Effect of tamarind (*Tamarindus indica* L.) seed on antioxidant activity, phytocompounds, physicochemical characteristics, and sensory acceptability of enriched cookies and mango juice

Sheilla Natukunda, John H. Muyonga & Ivan M. Mukisa

School of Food Technology, Nutrition & Bioengineering, Makerere University, P.O. Box 7062 Kampala, Uganda

Keywords
Antioxidant activity, condensed tannin, flavonoid, phenolics, phytocompounds, tamarind seed

Correspondence
Ivan M. Mukisa, School of Food Technology, Nutrition and Bioengineering, Makerere University, P.O. Box 7062 Kampala, Uganda.

E-mail: ivanmukisa@caes.mak.ac.ug

Funding Information
Swedish International Development Co-operation Agency, Department for Research Cooperation (Sida-Sarec).

Abstract

Tamarind seeds are not consumed despite their high antioxidative activity. In this study, 0–10% tamarind seed powder (TSP) was incorporated into mango juice and cookies. Total phenolics (Folin–Ciocalteu assay), antioxidant activity (2,2-diphenyl-1 picrylhydrazyl (DPPH) radical scavenging assay), flavonoid (aluminum chloride assay), condensed tannins content (Vanillin-HCl assay), and consumer acceptability (n = 50) of the products were determined. TSP increased the pH and viscosity and reduced titratable acidity of juice. Incorporation of TSP increased the: total phenolic content (6.84 ± 0.21 to 88.44 ± 0.8 mg GAE/100 mL); flavonoid (4.64 ± 0.03–21.7 ± 0.36 mg CE/100 mL); condensed tannins (0.24 ± 0.01–21.81 ± 0.08 mg CE/100 mL) and total antioxidant activity (4.65 ± 0.88–21.70 ± 0.03 mg VCE/100 mL) of juice. A similar trend was observed for cookies. Maximum sensorially acceptable TSP levels were 1.5% and 6%, respectively, for juice and cookies. TSP can thus be utilized as a source of natural antioxidants in food products.

Introduction

Epidemiological studies have consistently demonstrated that consumption of plant-derived foods rich in bioactive phytochemicals has a protective effect against oxidation stress (Librandi et al. 2007; Ovaskainen et al. 2008; Galili and Hovav 2014). Oxidative stress is strongly associated with mutagenesis, carcinogenesis (Abnet et al. 2015), aging (Everitt et al. 2006), and atherosclerosis in humans. The bioactive phytochemical compounds thus decrease the risk of chronic diseases, cardiovascular disease, cancer, and degenerative diseases of the aging (Keservani et al. 2010).

Currently, industries are interested in developing value-added products from the waste-by products generated by both the food and agricultural processing industries (Balasundram et al. 2006). The waste products including seeds, peels, stalks, stems, and leaves of plants contain substantial amount of phenolics and thus can be used as cheap sources of natural antioxidants for pharmaceutical, cosmetic, and food application (Bucić-Kojić et al. 2009). Fruits and vegetable waste products including seeds have been reported to have higher content of bioactive phytochemicals than the edible portions (Soong and Barlow 2004). Fruit seeds contain a variety of biologically active phytochemical compounds, especially phenolic constituents, flavonoids, anthocyaninins, vitamin C, and carotenoids. These phytochemicals positively influence human health and indicate high antioxidant activity (Pérez-Jiménez et al. 2008). Hence, it is considered crucial to increase the antioxidant intake in the human diet and one way of achieving this is can be through enriching food products with seeds which are rich in phytochemicals.

Tamarind (*Tamarindus indica*) seed is a by-product in the tamarind pulp industry. Recently, a large amount of the seed waste is discarded from the tamarind industry (Oluseyi and Temitayo 2015). Tamarind seed is a rich source of phytochemicals (Tsuda et al. 1994; Andabati and Muyonga 2014) which consists of phenolic antioxidants, such as 2-hydroxy-3′,4′-dihydoxyacetophenone, methyl 3, 4-dihydroxybenzoate, 3,4-dihydroxyphenyl acetate and epicatechin (Sudjaroen et al. 2005; El-Siddig et al. 2006). Tamarind seed extracts exhibit antioxidant potential by reducing lipid peroxidation in vitro (Tsuda et al. 1994) and anti-microbial activity. Tamarind seed therefore has the potential of providing low cost nutritional and nutraceutical value.

In this study, tamarind seed powder (TSP was evaluated as a source of antioxidants for inclusion in two commonly consumed products; cookies and mango juice. Cookies and mango juice are regularly consumed by nearly all age groups in developing countries. Cookies are popular compared to other processed foods because of their low cost, diverse taste, myriad shapes, and long shelf life (Davidov-Pardo et al. 2012). Jesionkowska et al. (2009) reported that cookies were selected by consumers as a good vehicle for antioxidants. Cookies also contain fat which possess' sensory characteristics that are ideal to mask the astringent flavor and taste associated with tamarind seed which is undesirable for most consumers.

Mango (*Mangifera indica)* is the most vital and widely cultivated among the tropical and subtropical fruits (Akhter et al. 2012). Thus, mango juice was selected because of the abundance, seasonal availability, popularity, and distinctive flavor and taste. Mangoes also have a strong flavor and substantial levels of pectin which can mask the astringency of the tamarind seed without affecting antioxidant activity (Laaksonen 2011; Soultani et al. 2014).

While tamarind seeds are known to contain substantial levels of bioactive phytocompounds, it was not clear if they could be used to enhance nutraceutical properties of widely consumed processed foods while retaining product acceptability. This study was therefore undertaken to assess the effect of tamarind seed powder on the physicochemical properties, phytonutrient content, antioxidant, and sensory properties of the enriched selected food products.

Material and Methods

Materials

Fresh tamarind fruits were purchased from the local markets in Mbale district, Uganda and transported to the Department of Food Technology and Nutrition, Makerere University. Fresh and fully ripened mangoes were obtained from the local market in Kampala, Uganda and transported to the Department of Food Technology and Nutrition, Makerere University. The fruits were selected for uniformity in shape and color, washed carefully with clean portable water and stored in a refrigerator at 8°C prior to further use.

Commercial wheat flour (Bakhresa Grain Milling (U) Ltd, Uganda), sugar (Kakira Sugar Works, Jinja, Uganda) and sodium bicarbonate (Bidco oil Refineries, Nairobi, Kenya) were purchased from the local supermarkets in Kampala Uganda.

Methods

Preparation of tamarind seed powder

Tamarind fruit pods were manually cracked and from each pod the pulp containing seeds was separated along with the fibers. Tamarind seed with fibers were soaked overnight in clean portable water (1: 3 w/v) to enable removal of the pulp and fiber strands. The seeds were then washed using clean distilled water. The cleaned seeds were sun dried in a shaded for 14 days, milled into fine flour using a Wonder mill (Grain of Truth Bread Company, Arlington, VA). The flour was sieved using a 300 μm screen and stored in an airtight container in a freezer at −18°C prior to further use.

Mango juice enrichment with tamarind seed powder

Preparation of mango juice

The mangoes were rinsed with portable water, peeled, and sliced. Mango juice was then extracted using a blender (Royal Philips, model HR 2167/40, Amsterdam, The Netherlands) and filtered using a sterile cheese cloth. The filtered juice was then blended with clean portable water (1: 3 of mango juice: water) and sugar 3% (w/v) was added to make the desired concentration of 9°Brix. The Mango juice was mixed with TSP powder in different proportions 0%, 0.5%, 1.5%, 1%, 2% and 2.5% (w/v) using a portable hand mixer (sun beam model SHM 100, Nu world industries Ltd, 2000).

Pasteurization treatment of tamarind seed mango juice and storage conditions

The tamarind seed and mango juice blend of 600 mL in a 1 L capacity container was pasteurized at 85°C with a holding time of 25 sec (Moyer and Aitken 1980). The beaker containing the juice was placed in a water bath maintained at 95°C and the juice was heated for 20 min while stirring until it reached 85°C. It was maintained at this temperature for 25 sec before hot filling in amber plastic bottles. The enriched juice was pasteurized to enable extraction of phytochemical compounds as well as to destroy spoilage microorganisms(Andabati and Muyonga 2014). The juice was previously filtered with a clean sterile cheese cloth before hot filling in amber plastic bottles. The amber bottles containing juice were capped and cooled to room temperature in a water bath. The bottles with pasteurized juice were stored in the refrigerator at 8°C subsequent to further analyses.

Cookie enrichment with tamarind seed powder

Preparation of flour mixtures and baking of enriched cookies

Cookies were prepared according to the method number 10–50D AACC (2000) with some modifications in the recipe (Table 1). Control samples were prepared without addition of TSP. TSP-enriched cookies were prepared by substituting wheat flour with of 2%, 4%, 6%, 8% and 10% TSP. Tamarind seed powder was well blended with wheat flour, sugar, and fat. The sugar and fat were creamed manually. The baking flour, baking powder, and TSP were sieved together and added to the cream before mixing it uniformly. The cookie dough was rolled, sheeted to a thickness of 3.5 mm and cut using a circular mould (5 cm diameter). Baking was done at 150°C for 40 min. After baking, cookies were cooled to room temperature and packed into airtight polythene bags until further analysis.

Physicochemical analyses

pH

The pH of TSP-enriched mango juice samples and control was measured with a pH-meter (pH meter, Hanna instrument H12210, Crison Instruments S.A., Barcelona, Spain) at room temperature (~25°C) according to AOAC official method 943.02 (1995). Buffer solutions of pH 4.0 and 7.0 were used for periodical calibration of pH meter. Three readings were performed for each replicate.

Color

The color of the juice was determined using a color tintometer (Lovibond Model E, AF-900; Tintometer Limited, Salisbury. U.K.). The juice was filled in the one inch optical glass cell which was placed into the cell channel. Sample colors were matched by a suitable combination of the three primary colors together with neutral filters using a viewing tube and adjusting the color filter knobs. The resulting set of Lovibond red, blue, yellow, and neutral (RYBN) units were used to define the color of the mango juice and TSP-enriched mango.

Viscosity measurements and analysis

Viscosity of the tamarind seed-enriched mango juice and control juice was measured using a Brookfield Viscometer (Brookfield LVDV-II+P, Brookfield Engineering Laboratories, Inc., Middleboro, MA). TSP-enriched mango juice of 500 mL was loaded into a glass beaker reservoir (cylindrical shape) of 600 mL capacity and was allowed to equilibrate at room temperature. Spindle LV- 1 was used to measure viscosity of juice, using rotational speeds ranging between 0.3 and 1.5 revolutions per minute (RPM). The recording of the viscometer output commenced 3 min after the onset of the experiment.

Total soluble solids

Total soluble solids content of the tamarind seed-enriched mango juice and control was determined with a handheld refractometer (Westover Model RHB-32; Southwest United Industries, Tulsa, OK) using AOAC (1999) method 981.12. The results were reported as °Brix at 20°C.

Titratable acidity

The total titratable acidity of the juices was determined according to AOAC (1999) by titration, using 0.1N sodium

Table 1. Formulation for tamarind seed-enriched cookies.

Formulation description	Wheat flour (g)	Sugar (g)	Fat (g)	TSP (g)	Egg	Baking powder (g)
Control	250	80	100	0	1	3
2% TSP	245	80	100	5	1	3
4% TSP	240	80	100	10	1	3
6% TSP	235	80	100	15	1	3
8% TSP	230	80	100	20	1	3
10% TSP	225	80	100	25	1	3

hydroxide with phenolphthalein. The results were expressed as % tartaric acid, using the weight of the molar mass of tartaric acid as the equivalent weight of acid (Banigo and Muller 1972).

Quantification of total carotenoids

Total carotenoids in tamarind seed powder-enriched mango and control juice was determined according to the method of Rodriguez-Amaya and Kimura (2004). Briefly, 2 mL of TSP-enriched mango juice was extracted by mixing with 50 mL cold acetone in the dark. The acetone was removed through the slow addition of 250 mL double distilled water to prevent the formation of emulsions. The aqueous phase was discarded and this procedure was repeated four times until there was no residual no residual acetone. The extract was then transferred through a funnel into a 50 mL volumetric flask containing glass wool with 15 g of anhydrous sodium sulfate. The final volume was adjusted with petroleum ether. Absorbance was measured at 450 nm (Genesys 10-UV spectrophotometer, Thermo Electron Corporation, Madison, WI) against petroleum ether as a blank. The total carotenoid content was calculated using the following formula:

$$\text{Total carotenoid content } (\mu g/mL) = \frac{\text{Absorbance} \times \text{Total volume of extract} \times 10^4}{\text{Absorption coefficient of beta carotene (2592)} \times \text{sample volume (mL)}}$$

Phytochemical analysis

Tamarind seed-enriched mango juices and cookies including controls (without TSP) were analyzed for total phenolic content, total condensed tannins, total flavonoid content and total antioxidant activity.

Extraction of phenolics

The extraction method described by (Makkar 2000) was used with slight modifications. Briefly, 100 mg of TSP-enriched cookies and control was extracted, using 5 mL of 50% methanol: 50% water solution (v/v). The falcon tube containing the mixture was suspended in ultrasonic water (Bransonic series, M 2800-E; Branson Ultrasonics Co, Danbury, CT) and subjected to ultrasonic treatment for 20 min at room temperature. The extract was immediately cooled at 4°C in a freezer for 10 min and then centrifuged at 3000 g for 10 min using a centrifuge (Fischer scientific 225, Fisher Scientific Co. St. Louis, MO). The supernatant was collected into a separate tube and stored at 4°C. The pellet was then further re-extracted under the conditions previously described to ensure efficient extraction. The two supernatants were pooled in an air tight container and stored in a freezer at 4°C to be used in the determination of total phenolics content (TPC), total antioxidant activity (TAA), total flavonoid contents (TFC) and total condensed tannins (TCT).

Determination of total phenolic content of TSP-enriched products

The total phenolic content of the juices and cookies were determined, using the Folin-Ciocalteu colorimetric method (Makkar 2000) with some modifications. In brief, 100 μL of the diluted juice (1: 10 of juice to water v/v) or cookie extract was pipetted into a test tube covered with aluminum foil and topped up to 0.5 mL with double distilled water. Subsequently 0.25 mL of Folin–Ciocalteu reagent (1 N) was added followed by 1.25 mL of sodium carbonate (20% w/v) and the mixture homogenized using a vortex. The mixture was then incubated at room temperature for 40 min to allow for color development. Absorbance was measured at 725 nm (Genesys 10-UV spectrophotometer, Thermo Electron Corporation) against methanol as the blank. The total phenolic content was determined using the standard gallic acid calibration curve with varying concentrations (0.02– 0.125) mg/mL). The total phenolic content was expressed as milligram gallic acid equivalent (GAE)/100 mL of the enriched mango juice and mg GAE/100 mg of the enriched cookies.

Determination of total condensed tannins of TSP-enriched products

Total condensed tannins were determined using the method described by (Sun et al. 1998) with slight modifications. Briefly, 1.5 mL of vanillin solution (4%) w/v was added to 50 μL of diluted juice (1:10 of juice to water v/v) or cookie extract in a test tube. Immediately, 0.75 mL of concentrated HCl was added and the mixture vortexed. The mixture was incubated at room temperature for 10 min to allow for color development. Absorbance was read at 500 nm (Genesys 10-UV spectrophotometer, Thermo Electron Corporation) with water as a blank. A standard curve was developed using catechin standards of varying concentrations (0.02 to 0.06 mg/mL). Total condensed tannins values were expressed as mg catechin equivalent/100 mL of the juice and mg catechin equivalent/100 g of cookies.

Determination of total flavonoids content of TSP-enriched products

Total flavonoid content was determined using the method of Muanda et al. (2011). In brief, 0.5 mL of catechin standard solution or juice sample or cookie extract was mixed with 2 mL of deionized water and 0.15 mL of sodium nitrite (5% w/v). After 5 min, 0.15 mL of 10% aluminum chloride was added followed by the addition of 1 mL of molar sodium hydroxide after another 6 min. Finally distilled water was used to adjust the total volume to 5 mL and absorbance was read at 510 nm (Genesys 10-UV spectrophotometer, Thermo Electron Corporation). A standard calibration curve was plotted using different concentrations of catechin (0.002 to 0.125 mg/mL). Total flavonoid content values were expressed in milligram catechin equivalents per 100 mL of juice (mg CE/100 mL) and cookies in mg CE/100 g of enriched cookies.

Total antioxidant activity of TSP-enriched products

The total antioxidant capacity (TAA) of the tamarind seed and products was determined, using the free-radical scavenging capacity by use of 1, 1-diphenyl-2-picrylhydrazyl (DPPH) (Brand-Williams et al. 1995) with minimal modification (Stratil et al. 2006). Briefly, 50 μL of the tamarind seed-enriched mango juice or cookie extract was added to 2.9 mL of freshly prepared 80% ethanol solution of 100 μM DPPH. The mixture was vortexed and allowed to stand for 30 min in the dark at room temperature. Absorbance of the resulting mixture was measured at 515 nm, using Genesys 10-UV spectrophotometer (Thermo Electron Corporation) against a blank (80% ethanol). The free-radical scavenging activity of the juice and cookies was calculated as follows

$$\text{Scavenging activity (\%)} = \left[1-\left(\frac{\text{absorbance of sample}}{\text{absorbance of control}}\right)\right]\times 100 \qquad (1)$$

The antioxidant content was determined using a standard curve of ascorbic acid (0.1–8 μg/mL). The results were expressed as milligram vitamin C equivalents per 100 mL of tamarind seed mango juice (mg VCE/100 mL) and cookies as mg VCE/100 g of the cookie.

Sensory evaluation of tamarind seed-enriched products

Sensory analysis of tamarind seed-enriched mango juice involved the participation of 50 untrained panelists who comprised of students from the Department of Food Technology and Nutrition. The recommended minimum number of panelists for assessing sensory acceptability of a product is 50 since a big number best represents the population (Hough et al. 2006). Each individual evaluated eight sensory characteristics (appearance, taste, color, flavor, consistency, mouth feel, sweetness and thickness) of the enriched juices and control. Each sensory attribute was rated on a 9-point Hedonic scale. The ratings on the 9-point hedonic scale used were (9 = "like extremely";8 = "like very much"; 7 = "like moderately"; 6 = "like slightly"; 5 = "neither like nor dislike"; 4 = "dislike slightly"; 3 = "dislike moderately"; 2 = "dislike very much"; 1 = "dislike extremely") (Carr et al. 1999). Each subject received six samples (unidentified, with randomly assigned three-digit codes) of each juice (mango juice with tamarind seed and a control). A control juice sample (without tamarind seed) and five samples with different tamarind seed powder formulations (0.5, 1.0, 1.5, 2.0 and 2.5%). The panelists were presented with 50 mL of each juice sample at room temperature under normal lighting conditions. The tamarind seed-enriched juice and control samples were prepared the day before and stored in a refrigerator. Bottled water was provided to rinse the mouth between tasting samples.

Sensory analysis of tamarind seed-enriched cookies was done as described above for the juices. However, cookies were evaluated for color, appearance, texture, taste, flavor, and overall quality. The samples comprised a control cookie sample (without tamarind seed) and five samples with different tamarind seed powder formulations (2%, 4%, 6%, 8% and 10%). Cookies were formulated according to the experimental design and prepared the day before the evaluation day and stored at room temperature.

Data analysis

All experiments were conducted in triplicate. Statistical analysis of the data was performed by analysis of variance (ANOVA), using Student Edition of Statistix 9.0 software (Analytical Software, Tallahassee, FL). A probability value of difference $P \leq 0.05$ was considered to denote statistical significance. All data are presented as mean values ± standard deviation (SD). Regression analysis was performed to indicate the relationship between total phenolic and/or flavonoid contents and antioxidant activity.

Results

Effect of tamarind seed powder on physicochemical properties of mango juice

The addition of tamarind seed powder (TSP) to mango juice significantly ($P < 0.05$) affected the total soluble

Table 2. Effect of tamarind seed powder (TSP) on total soluble solids, pH, titratable acidity and beta carotene of mango juice.

TSP concentration (%)	TSS (^{O}Brix)	pH	%TTA	β-carotene (μg/100 mL)
Control	9.03 ± 0.04^{a}	4.7 ± 0.01^{a}	0.17 ± 0.01^{a}	892.49 ± 11.79^{a}
0.5%	9.00 ± 0.00^{a}	4.9 ± 0.01^{b}	0.16 ± 0.00^{a}	563.27 ± 26.73^{b}
1.0%	9.00 ± 00^{a}	5.36 ± 0.01^{c}	0.15 ± 0.00^{b}	468.11 ± 8.90^{c}
1.5%	9.00 ± 00^{a}	5.51 ± 0.20^{d}	0.14 ± 0.01^{b}	416.67 ± 20.45^{d}
2.0%	10.00 ± 00^{b}	5.56 ± 0.01^{e}	0.12 ± 0.00^{c}	272.63 ± 17.81^{e}
2.5%	10 ± 00^{b}	5.7 ± 0.00^{f}	0.09 ± 0.00^{d}	195.47 ± 4.45^{f}

TTA, titratable acidity. Data are means of triplicate determination ± standard deviation. Mean values in the same column with different superscript letters are significantly different ($P < 0.05$).

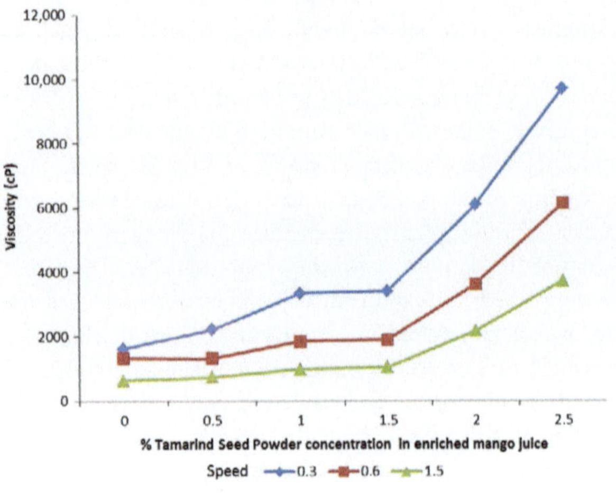

Figure 1. Effect of TSP on viscosity of mango juice.

solids, pH, titratable acidity, and beta carotene of mango juice (Table 2).

The pH ranged from 4.7 to 5.7 and increased with increase in tamarind seed concentration in the order of control <0.5% <1% <1.5% <2.0% <2.5. Total acidity of TSP-enriched mango juices decreased with increase in TSP. The total carotenoids decreased in the order of control >0.5% >1% >2% >2.5%. Total soluble solids only significantly increased at 2.0% tamarind seed powder concentration.

Color

The color of mango juice varied at different concentration of tamarind seed powder. The color of mango juices was generally pale yellow to dull orange color on adding TSP. The highest orange color (2.4 and 2.6 units) of the mango juice was observed at 2% and 2.5% concentration, respectively. The juice appeared as yellow/orange with a shade of yellow (2.3 and 1.9) at 2% and 2.5%, respectively. The color of the juice at 0%, 0.5%, 1%, and 1.5% concentration was 1.5, 1.8, 1.8, and 0.9 orange values, respectively, while the shade of yellow was 5.8, 6.0, 5.0, and 2.3 respectively. Tamarind seed-enriched mango juice of 0.5% and 1% appeared paler than the rest due to a higher yellow shade.

Effect of TSP on viscosity of mango juice

The viscosity of enriched mango juice increased with increase in tamarind seed powder concentration for all viscometer speeds (Fig. 1). It is clear from Figure 1 that addition of TSP to juices increases the viscosity of enriched juices compared to the control.

Effect of tamarind seed powder on phytochemical composition of mango juice

Incorporation of tamarind seed powder in mango juice formulation significantly increased the total phenolic, total flavonoids, and total condensed tannin content as well as the total antioxidant activity as compared to the control (Table 3).

Addition of tamarind seed powder resulted in an increase in the content of total phenolic from 6.54 ± 0.8 to 88.44 ± 0.21 mg GAE/100 mL of the juice. There was a more than 13 fold increase in total phenolic content of enriched juices that received higher TSP (2.5%) as compared to the control.

Mango juice enriched with TSP also showed a similar pattern, with respect to total flavonoid content (TFC), with the value for the 2.5% TSP – enriched juice increased by 20-fold compared to the control. The total antioxidant activity of the enriched juice increased from 4.64 ± 0.58 for control to 21.70 ± 0.04 mg VCE/100 mL for mango juice containing 3% TSP, while total condensed tannins increased from 3.59 to 21.81 ± 0.08 mg CE/100 mL of the juice.

Effect of tamarind seed powder on phytochemical composition of cookies

Cookies with tamarind seed powder had significantly higher antioxidant activity and content of the different

Table 3. Effect of tamarind seed powder (TSP) on phytochemical composition of mango juice.

TSP concentration	TPC (mg GAE 100 mL^{-1})	TFC (Mg CE 100 mL^{-1})	TAA (Mg VCE 100 mL^{-1})	TCT (Mg CE 100 mL^{-1})
Control	6.54 ± 0.21^{a}	1.04 ± 0.03^{a}	4.64 ± 0.58^{a}	0.24 ± 0.01^{a}
0.5% TSP	19.50 ± 0.29^{b}	8.36 ± 0.06^{b}	8.84 ± 0.15^{b}	3.59 ± 0.24^{b}
1.0% TSP	29.60 ± 0.36^{c}	11.87 ± 0.14^{c}	13.96 ± 0.28^{c}	8.62 ± 0.84^{c}
1.5% TSP	43.90 ± 0.14^{d}	13.06 ± 0.15^{d}	17.91 ± 0.95^{d}	11.33 ± 0.29^{d}
2.0% TSP	56.06 ± 0.67^{e}	17.75 ± 0.28^{e}	20.33 ± 0.08^{e}	15.99 ± 0.40^{e}
2.5% TSP	88.44 ± 0.8^{f}	22.48 ± 0.36^{f}	21.70 ± 0.04^{f}	21.81 ± 0.08^{f}

TPC, total phenolic content; TFC, total flavonoid content; TAA, total antioxidant activity; TCT, total condensed tannins. Data are means ± standard deviation from three independent experiments (n = 3). Mean values in the same column with different superscript letters are significantly different ($P < 0.05$).

Table 4. Effect of tamarind seed powder (TSP) on phytochemical composition of cookies.

TSP concentration	TPC (mg GAE 100 mg^{-1})	TFC (mg CE 100 mg^{-1})	TAA (mg VCE 100 mg^{-1})	TTC (mg CE 100 mg^{-1})
Control	20.43 ± 0.29^{a}	4.06 ± 0.06^{a}	5.6 ± 0.01^{a}	8.3 ± 0.73^{a}
2.0% TSP	23.41 ± 0.31^{b}	5.35 ± 0.07^{b}	8.9 ± 0.07^{b}	11.70 ± 1.06^{b}
4.0% TSP	25.37 ± 0.20^{c}	5.71 ± 0.05^{c}	12.7 ± 0.08^{c}	12.35 ± 0.5^{c}
6% TSP	26.1 ± 0.05^{d}	6.67 ± 0.29^{d}	17.2 ± 0.06^{d}	13.54 ± 0.27^{d}
8% TSP	27.41 ± 0.09^{e}	8.2 ± 0.08^{e}	19.2 ± 0.03^{e}	15.48 ± 0.43^{e}
10% TSP	29.08 ± 0.23^{f}	10.29 ± 0.07^{f}	25.5 ± 0.04^{f}	19.24 ± 0.40^{f}

TPC, total phenolic content; TFC, total flavonoid content; TAA, total antioxidant activity; TCT, total condensed tannins. Data are means ± standard deviation from three independent experiments (n = 3). Mean values in the same column with different superscript letters are significantly different ($P < 0.05$).

bioactive compounds (Table 4). Total phenolics ranged from 20.43 ± 0.29 for control to 29.08 ± 0.23 mg GAE/100 g for cookies containing 10% TSP. Tannins content ranged from 8.3 ± 0.73 to 19.24 ± 0.40 mg CE/100 g (Table 4). Enriched cookies that received higher TSP concentration (10%) showed an increase of fivefold and 2.5 fold in both total antioxidant activity and flavonoid content, respectively, as compared to the control juice (without TSP).

There was a significant positive correlation between total phenolic content (TPC) and total antioxidant activity (TAC) ($R^2 = 0.922$, $P < 0.05$) as shown in Figure 2.

There was a significant positive correlation ($R^2 = 0.923$, $P < 0.05$) between TAC and TFC as shown in Figure 3.

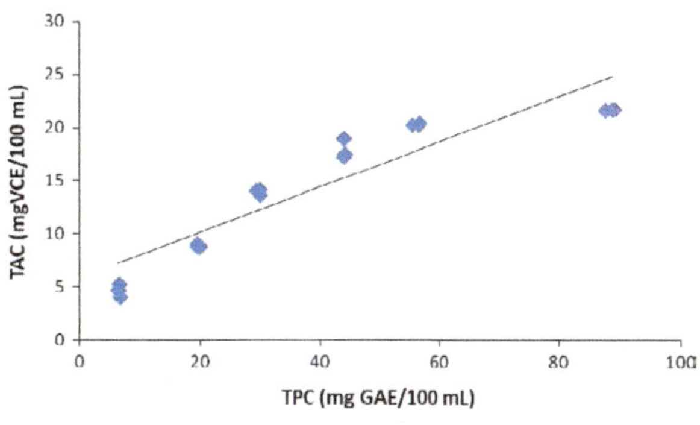

Figure 2. Relationship between antioxidant activity and total phenolic content mango juice enriched with TSP ($R^2 = 0.922$).

Effect of tamarind seed powder on sensory acceptability of enriched mango juice

The acceptability scores of all sensory attributes lowered with increase in concentration of tamarind seed powder in enriched mango juice (Table 5). Mango juice enriched with 2.5% TSP received the lowest perceived scores in all sensory attributes (Table 5). The general acceptability of the enriched juice ranged from 4.9 to 8.1. Overall Sensory attributes of 0.5%, 1%, and 1.5% mango–tamarind seed juices were well accepted with a score between 6.6 and 7 (like moderately). Addition of TSP up to 0.5% negatively affected all sensory attributes apart from thickness. Majority the of panelists mentioned that 2.5% TSP-enriched mango juices was more viscous/thicker than 0%, 0.5%, 1.0%, 1.5% and 2%. Some panelists also noted that 2.5% TSP-enriched mango juice was more astringent in flavor compared to the other juices. There was no significant difference ($P < 0.05$) between 0.5%, 1.0% and 1.5% TSP-enriched mango juice in terms of flavor, taste, consistency, sweetness, and overall acceptability.

Correlation of overall acceptability with taste ($r = 0.744$), mouth feel ($r = 0.738$), sweetness ($r = 0.783$) and flavor ($r = 0.682$) showed that each of the properties

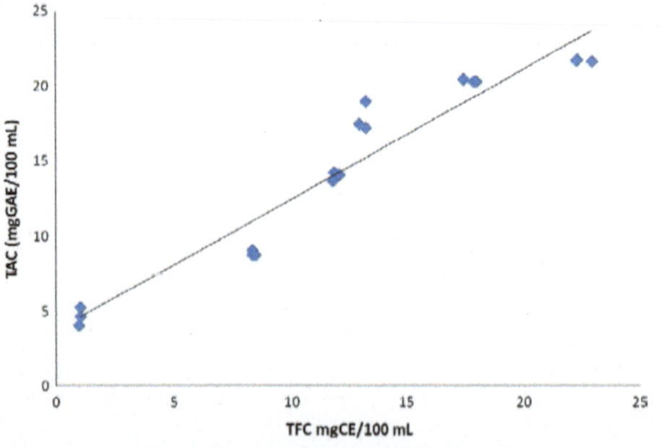

Figure 3. Relationship between antioxidant activity and total flavonoid content of mango juice enriched with TSP ($R^2 = 0.923$).

is of high significance ($P < 0.01$) in determining the acceptability of the TSP-enriched mango juice (Table 6).

Effect of tamarind seed powder on sensory acceptability of enriched cookies

The scores of all sensory attributes lowered with increase in concentration of tamarind seed powder in enriched cookies (Table 7).

The results show that the addition TSP in cookie formulation resulted in lower scores in all sensory attributes at high concentrations with an overall acceptability ranging from 6.6 ± 1.47 to 7.8.1 ± 1.83. Addition of TSP up to 2.0% did not affect acceptability for appearance, color, flavor, crunchiness and taste of the enriched cookies (Table 7). Addition of tamarind seed powder above 8% significantly ($P < 0.05$) reduces the acceptability for color of the enriched cookies. Incorporation of tamarind seed powder significantly affected texture in relation to the control. In terms of overall acceptability tamarind seed powder-enriched cookies were acceptable up to 10% tamarind seed powder (6.6 = like slightly). Although, 6% tamarind seed powder-enriched cookie was not significantly different from 8% tamarind seed-enriched cookie in terms of overall acceptability, it differed in terms of flavor.

Discussion

Effect of tamarind seed on physicochemical properties of mango juice and cookies

Addition of tamarind seed powder led to a significant increase ($P < 0.05$) in pH of mango juice. Tamarind seed powder has a pH 5.2 ± 0.01 (Oluseyi and Temitayo 2015) and therefore may be responsible for the increase of the pH of the enriched mango juice that was observed. The reduction of total titratable acidity is consistent with the increase in pH of the enriched mango juices. The reduction in titratable

Table 5. Effect of tamarind seed powder (TSP) on sensory acceptability of enriched mango juice.

	Inclusion level of TSP (%)					
Attribute	0 (Control)	0.5	1.0	1.5	2.0	2.5
Appearance	7.9 ± 1.88^{a}	6.9 ± 1.37^{bc}	6.8 ± 1.27^{b}	6.5 ± 1.24^{c}	6.1 ± 1.48^{cd}	5.9 ± 1.93^{d}
Color	8.0 ± 1.71^{a}	7.0 ± 1.07^{b}	6.7 ± 1.27^{b}	6.5 ± 1.29^{cb}	6.0 ± 1.51^{c}	6.1 ± 1.82^{c}
Flavor	7.9 ± 1.09^{a}	6.5 ± 1.50^{b}	6.0 ± 1.93^{b}	5.9 ± 1.87^{b}	5.2 ± 1.97^{c}	4.9 ± 2.14^{c}
Taste	7.7 ± 1.41^{a}	6.4 ± 1.41^{b}	6.2 ± 1.81^{b}	5.8 ± 1.93^{b}	4.9 ± 2.07^{c}	4.8 ± 2.12^{c}
Thickness	6.7 ± 2.03^{ab}	6.7 ± 1.76^{ab}	6.9 ± 1.57^{a}	6.0 ± 1.85^{b}	6.3 ± 1.82^{ab}	5.9 ± 2.42^{b}
Consistency	7.2 ± 1.67^{a}	6.4 ± 1.33^{b}	6.4 ± 1.86^{b}	6.4 ± 1.50^{b}	5.8 ± 1.85^{bc}	5.4 ± 1.89^{c}
Mouth feel	7.4 ± 1.59^{a}	6.3 ± 1.88^{bc}	6.3 ± 1.77^{c}	6.0 ± 1.95^{b}	5.3 ± 2.24^{db}	5.2 ± 2.20^{d}
Sweetness	7.7 ± 1.49^{a}	6.3 ± 1.69^{b}	6.1 ± 1.93^{b}	5.9 ± 2.27^{bc}	5.2 ± 2.16^{c}	4.9 ± 2.26^{c}
Overall acceptability	8.1 ± 1.03^{a}	7.0 ± 1.46^{b}	6.7 ± 1.61^{b}	6.6 ± 1.99^{b}	5.3 ± 2.02^{c}	4.9 ± 1.98^{c}

Values are means ± standard deviation ($n = 50$). Mean values in the same row with different superscripts (a–d) are significantly different ($P < 0.05$). Anchors for the hedonic scale used were: 9 = like extremely, 8 = like very much, 7 = like moderately, 6 = like slightly, 5 = neither like nor dislike, 4 = dislike slightly, 3 = dislike moderately, 2 = dislike very much, 1 = dislike extremely.

Table 6. Correlation coefficient of the acceptability selected sensory attributes and general acceptability.

Attribute	Flavor	Taste	Consistency	Mouthful	Sweetness	Overall acceptability
Flavor	1	0.758**	0.464**	0.552**	0.603**	0.682**
Taste	0.758**	1	0.528**	0.624**	0.707**	0.744**
Mouth feel	0.552**	0.624**	0.579**	1	0.710**	0.738**
Sweetness	0.603**	0.707**	0.485**	0.710**	1	0.783**

**$P < 0.01$.

Table 7. Effect of tamarind seed powder (TSP) on sensory acceptability of enriched cookies.

	Inclusion level of TSP (%)					
Attribute	0 (Control)	2.0	4.0	6.0	8.0	10
Appearance	7.7 ± 1.33^{a}	7.6 ± 0.90^{a}	6.8 ± 1.61^{b}	6.6 ± 1.31^{bc}	6.8 ± 1.37^{b}	6.2 ± 1.50^{c}
Color	7.4 ± 1.5^{a}	7.4 ± 1.06^{a}	6.8 ± 1.53^{b}	6.6 ± 1.45^{b}	6.8 ± 1.36^{b}	6.0 ± 1.51^{c}
Flavor	7.6 ± 1.19^{a}	7.5 ± 1.20^{a}	7.1 ± 1.52^{ab}	6.7 ± 1.29^{b}	6.4 ± 1.58^{c}	6.1 ± 1.14^{c}
Taste	7.5 ± 1.40^{a}	7.4 ± 1.19^{a}	7.0 ± 1.33^{ab}	6.6 ± 1.40^{bc}	6.6 ± 1.38^{bc}	6.3 ± 1.70^{c}
Texture	8.4 ± 6.03^{a}	7.2 ± 1.20^{b}	7.3 ± 1.30^{b}	6.7 ± 1.11^{b}	7.1 ± 1.30^{b}	6.6 ± 1.50^{b}
Mouth feel	7.3 ± 1.51^{a}	7.2 ± 1.26^{ab}	7.1 ± 1.16^{ab}	6.8 ± 1.49^{ab}	6.9 ± 1.35^{ab}	6.6 ± 1.89^{b}
After taste	7.3 ± 1.45^{a}	7.0 ± 1.59^{ab}	6.8 ± 1.42^{abc}	6.5 ± 1.50^{bc}	6.8 ± 1.34^{abc}	6.4 ± 1.48^{c}
Crunchiness	7.7 ± 1.37^{a}	7.6 ± 1.39^{a}	7.7 ± 0.92^{a}	7.5 ± 1.06^{ab}	7.02 ± 1.41^{b}	7.1 ± 1.45^{b}
Overall acceptability	7.8.1 ± 1.83^{a}	7.7 ± 0.90^{ab}	7.3 ± 1.15^{bc}	7.0 ± 1.07^{cd}	6.9 ± 1.03^{cd}	6.6 ± 1.47^{d}

Data are means ± standard deviation (n = 50). Mean values in the same row with different superscript letters are significantly different ($P < 0.05$). Anchors for the hedonic scale used were: 9 = like extremely, 8 = like very much, 7 = like moderately, 6 = like slightly, 5 = neither like nor dislike, 4 = dislike slightly, 3 = dislike moderately, 2 = dislike very much, 1 = dislike extremely.

acidity may be attributed to tamarind seed powder since there was increase in pH with increase in tamarind seed powder concentration. The low titratable acidity and high pH are associated with reduction in shelf life. Acidulants like citric acid should be added to tamarind seed powder-enriched mango juice to increase its shelf life (Pundhir and Murtaza 2015).

Results of this study revealed that addition of tamarind seed powder led to a concentration-dependent increase in mango juice viscosity. These results are consistent with observations by Kumar and Bhattacharya (2008) who studied the rheological behavior of Tamarind Kernel Powder (TKP) of varying concentration (2, 4, 6, 8, and 10%) and observed an increase in apparent viscosity with increase in TKP concentration. The increment in viscosity of the enriched mango juices may be attributed to large proportions (65.1–72.2%) of galactoxyloglucan found in tamarind seed (Bhattacharya et al. 1994). Galactoxyloglucan is composed of a β- (1–4) linked D- glucan backbone that is substituted with side-chains of α-d-xylopyranose and β-d-galactopyranosyl (1-2)-α-d-xylopyranose linked to (1–6) glucose residue (Yamanaka et al. 2000). Galactoxyloglucan exhibits high water-holding capacity with good stability to heat, acids, and shear and thus its wide application in the food industry as a thickener, stabilizer, or starch modifier. It is used to improve rheological and thermal properties of many products including, salad dressing, mayonnaise, and stew (Nishinari et al. 2000). This therefore implies that tamarind seed powder can potentially be utilized as a food stabilizer.

The coloration of the enriched juices became more orange and dull with increased concentration of tamarind seed powder. A similar observation was made by Andabati and Muyonga (2014) where addition of tamarind seed powder to the tamarind pulp juice led to discoloration of the enriched juices. This may be attributed to the activity of polyphenol oxidase. TSP is rich in polyphenols which are substrates for the polyphenol oxidases. In presence of oxygen, the enzymes catalyze the hydroxylation of monophenols to diphenols and then subsequently to corresponding quinine intermediates. It is the intermediates that are responsible for discoloration. More so, TSP has a dark brownish color (Kumar and Bhattacharya 2008), and therefore incorporation of TSP in mango juice decreases its brightness. Color is very important when consumers are making choices on food products (Tril et al. 2014). It is therefore important to use low concentration of TSP in juices to avoid discoloration/darkening of juices which potentially has an effect on consumer preference. High concentrations of TSP can be tried in other products such as sausages whose color may not be affected (Tril et al. 2014).

Effect of TSP on phytochemical composition of enriched mango juices and cookies

The effect of TSP on phytochemical content of enriched mango juice and cookies was concentration dependent. In their studies Andabati and Muyonga (2014) found that addition of tamarind seed powder in tamarind pulp juice led to a significant enrichment in total phenolic compounds, total flavonoids and total antioxidant activity. The observed increase in TFC, TPC and TAA in enriched juices is attributed to the high phenolic content, flavonoid content, and antioxidant activity in *Tamarindus indica* L. seeds (Tsuda et al. 1994; Soong and Barlow 2004; Siddhuraju 2007). A similar observation was reported by Salgado et al. (2012) where addition of antioxidant-rich pomegranate peel (*Punica granatum*) extract to orange and tomato juice led to increase in antioxidant activity. The total phenolic content of TSP-enriched mango juices was in the range 6.54 ± 0.21 to 88.44 ± 0.8 mg GAE/100 mL. This is higher than the phenolic content in tomato juice (5.97 mg GAE/100 mL) (Owusu et al. 2015), passion fruit (27.1–38.1 mg GAE/100 g) (Ramaiya et al. 2013), mango (6.25 mg GAE/100 g) (Gorinstein et al. 1999), jackfruit 0.36 mg GAE/100 g (Swami et al. 2012) and fruit juices enriched with roselle fruit (53.7-10.8 GAE mg/100 g) (Mgaya et al. 2014). There was a 13-fold increase in the total phenolic content at 2.5% of tamarind seed powder-enriched juice compared to the control. This suggests that addition of tamarind seed powder highly enhances the content of bioactive compounds, thus increasing the nutraceutical properties of the enriched mango juices. It is therefore important to further utilize the seeds rather than just discarding them as waste as it is a common practice currently. Flavonoid intake of about 14.33 mg/day has been reported to reduce memory loss in elderly people (Letenneur et al. 2007). Daily consumption of 110 mL of 1.5% TSP-enriched mango juice is adequate to meet flavonoid content of 14.33 mg/day. Therefore, the findings from the current study show the potential of tamarind seed-enriched mango juices in mitigating memory loss in elderly people.

Antioxidant activity is very important in human health mainly because of its free-radical scavenging activity and protection against oxidative stress (Haghju and Almasi 2015; Valdes et al. 2015) and thus prevents development of diseases such as heart disease and cancer (González-Vallinas et al. 2013; Farias et al. 2014). Numerous studies have demonstrated that polyphenol and flavonoid compounds are the most effective antioxidative constituents in fruits, vegetables and grains (Choi et al. 2007; Dykes and Rooney 2007). This is consistent with significant positive correlation between total antioxidant activity and the concentrations of total phenolics and total flavonoid in tamarind seed-enriched juices observed in this study. Similar relations have been reported for other foods such as Chilean blackberries, barley, mushrooms, mulberries, flaxseed, wheat, oats, ginseng rice, and bread enriched with ginger (Choi et al. 2007; Céspedes et al. 2008; Jayaprakasha et al. 2008; Shen et al. 2009; Balestra et al. 2011).

The addition of tamarind seed powder to mango juices increased the content of total phenolics, flavonoid, antioxidant activity, and tannin in the enriched cookies in a concentration-dependent manner. In a related study Ajila et al. (2008) observed that incorporation of mango peel powder (0, 5, 10, 15, 20%) increased total phenolics and antioxidant activity in a concentration-dependent manner. The assay of DPPH-scavenging activity showed that TSP was a good source of active compounds, and adding it significantly enhanced the antioxidant properties of the cookies. A similar study Mildner-Szkudlarz et al. (2013) reported that incorporation of white grape pomace (residue) significantly increased the content of phenolics and antioxidants in biscuits.

The beta carotene levels decreased with increase in tamarind seed powder concentration in enriched juices. Addition of TSP may have contributed to dilution of beta carotene content. However, it was added in quite small quantities up to 2.5% to account for all the change. Another reason is probably formation of the complexes between the proteins in the seed powder with carotenoids in the enriched mango juices. This reduces carotenoid concentration in juice with increase in tamarind seed (Sweeney and Marsh 1971).

Effect of tamarind seed powder on sensory properties of enriched products

Addition of tamarind seed powder in mango juice resulted in reduced scores in all the sensory attributes including color, flavor, consistency, thickness, and general acceptability. In a related study, Salgado et al. (2012) observed low scores when pomegranate peel powder was added to orange and tomato juice. Both powders have high phenolics and tannins which elicit undesired astringent taste (Kumar and Bhattacharya 2008; McRae and Kennedy 2011). Phenolic compounds highly correlate inherently with sensory characteristics of food, such as color, astringency, bitterness, and flavor (Mousavinejad et al. 2009). High levels of phenolics and tannins can elicit negative consumer reactions (Drewnowski and Gomez-Carneros 2000). Astringency is the drying, roughing, and puckering of the epithelium of the oral cavity. The perception of astringency results from binding and subsequent precipitation of tannins with salivary proteins and glycoproteins. This interaction acts as a water barrier resulting in a tactile sensational loss of lubrication in the oral cavity (Kielhorn and Thorngate III 1999). This therefore explains the reduction in scores in sensory acceptability with increase in concentration of TSP in the current study. The lowest score on the sensory attributes was recorded at the highest concentration of 2.5% of the TSP in mango juice. According to Lawless et al. (2012), addition of high level of polyphenol compounds in food formulations negatively affects the sensory attributes and acceptability of finished foods, resulting in changes such as increased bitterness and astringency. The sensory acceptability results of this study confirm the association of astringency to poor acceptability. The low consumer acceptance ratings for the thickness and flavor of the enriched juices scores were substantiated by the findings on viscosity and phytochemical analysis findings in the current study. There was no significant difference in acceptance for flavor, taste, thickness, and overall acceptability between 0.5%, 1.0%, 1.5%, respectively, while at 2.0% and 2.5% there was a significant difference of the enriched juices. The results of this study show that juice with 2% and 2.5% TSP had significantly lower acceptability compared to the control and those with lower TSP concentrations. This therefore suggests that 1.5% is the maximum concentration possible that can be added to enrich mango juice that can have commercial appeal because it was the acceptance limit of sensory evaluation by the tasters.

While consumers may be interested in products with high levels of bioactive products, palatability and taste are key determinants of acceptability. This, therefore, suggests that a concentration of 1.5% of TSP would be an appropriate level to cater for consumer acceptability as well as providing health benefits of phenolics.

Incorporation of tamarind seed powder into cookies resulted in reduced scores in all the sensory attributes. Sensory evaluation studies showed flavor, color, taste, crunchiness, and overall general acceptability of cookies containing tamarind seed were as acceptable as those of control cookies up to 2% level of tamarind seed incorporation and any further increase led to lower scores. The enriched cookies also became relatively harder compared to the control. Tamarind seed powder contains galactoxylose which has high water-binding capacity (Bhattacharya et al. 1994) and this may explain the hardness of the enriched cookies. The addition of TSP influenced the color of each of the cookies. In the cookies made with 10% TSP panelists commented on the unappealing dark color. This may be due to the brown of the tamarind seed (Kumar and Bhattacharya 2008). These comments were reflected in the significantly lower acceptance scores for enriched cookies color compared with the control.

At higher TSP concentration, the acceptability for mouth feel and after taste scores was also low. It is known that the polyphenolic compounds contribute to the astringency of enriched cookies because of the interaction between phenolics, mainly procyanidins and the glycoproteins in saliva (McRae and Kennedy 2011). The tamarind seed has high phenolics and tannins which elicit undesired astringent taste (Kumar and Bhattacharya 2008) which makes products with tamarind seed powder have lower consumer appeal. Based on all these sensory attributes, participants preferred a control cookie, rather than enriched cookies. This is consistent with the study by Bakke and Vickers (2011), in which, the bitterness from added wheat germ extract decreased bread liking. In terms of overall acceptability, cookies enriched with (6%, 8%, 10%) TSP were not significantly different. However, 8% and 10% TSP-enriched cookies had significantly lower scores for flavor (6.4) and color (6.0), respectively. On that basis, the 6% TSP-enriched cookie was selected as the maximum acceptable TSP concentration for TSP-enriched cookies.

Other efforts have been made to add bioactive-rich components to processed foods. (Ajila et al. (2008); Hooda and Jood (2005); Mildner-Szkudlarz et al. (2013)) added mango peel powder, fenugreek, and white grape pomace powder to biscuits and reported no negative effect with levels of up to 10% (Sudha et al. 2007) added apple pomace to biscuits and found that up to 20% could be incorporated without compromising acceptability.

Conclusion

Incorporation of the tamarind seed powder into mango juice and cookies significantly increases their content of bioactive phytochemicals with an associated increase in the antioxidant activity. Based on sensory analysis, it may be concluded that the amount of TSP that can be added to mango juice and cookies need to be limited to 1.5% and 6%, respectively, to ensure consumer acceptability. The findings confirm the potential to utilize tamarind seed powder as a source of natural antioxidants and stabilizer in our search for good human health.

Acknowledgments

This study was funded through a grant from the Swedish International Development Co-operation Agency, Department for Research Cooperation (Sida-Sarec) Program of Makerere University.

Conflict of Interest

The authors did not declare any conflict of interest.

References

AACC. (2000). Approved methods of the AACC. 10th ed. Method 10-50D. American Assoc. Cereal Chemists. St. Paul, MN.

Abnet, C. C., D. A. Corley, N. D. Freedman, and F. Kamangar. 2015. Diet and upper gastrointestinal malignancies. Gastroenterology 148: 1234–1243. e1234.

Ajila, C. M., K. Leelavathi, and U. J. S. Prasada Rao. 2008. Improvement of dietary fiber content and antioxidant properties in soft dough biscuits with the incorporation of mango peel powder. J. Cereal Sci. 48:319–326.

Akhter, S., S. Masood, S. Jadoon, I. Ahmad, and S. Ullah. 2012. Quality evaluation of different brands of Tetra Pak mango juices available in market. Pakistan J. Food Sci. 22:96–100.

Andabati, B., and J. H. Muyonga. 2014. Phenolic content and antioxidant activity of selected Ugandan traditional medicinal foods. Afri. J. Food Sci. 8:427–434.

AOAC. 1995. Official methods of analysis, 16th ed. Association of Official Analytical Chemists, Washington, DC.

AOAC. 1999. Official methods of analysis. AOAC (Association of Offi cial Analytical Chemists) International, 16th ed. AOAC International, Gaithersburg.

Bakke, A., and Z. Vickers. 2011. Effects of bitterness, roughness, PROP taster status, and fungiform papillae density on bread acceptance. Food Qual. Prefer. 22:317–325.

Balasundram, N., K. Sundram, and S. Samman. 2006. Phenolic compounds in plants and agri-industrial by-products: antioxidant activity, occurrence, and potential uses. Food Chem. 99:191–203.

Balestra, F., E. Cocci, G. Pinnavaia, and S. Romani. 2011. Evaluation of antioxidant, rheological and sensorial properties of wheat flour dough and bread containing ginger powder. Food Sci. Technol. – LEB 44:700–705.

Banigo, E., and H. Muller. 1972. Manufacture of ogi (a Nigerian fermented cereal porridge): comparative evaluation of corn, sorghum and millet. Can. I Food Sci. Tech. J. 5:217–221.

Bhattacharya, S., S. Bal, R. K. Mukherjee, and S. Bhattacharya. 1994. Functional and nutritional properties of tamarind (*Tamarindus indica*) kernel protein. Food Chem. 49:1–9.

Brand-Williams, W., M. E. Cuvelier, and C. Berset. 1995. Use of a free radical method to evaluate antioxidant activity. Food Sci. Technol. – LEB 28:25–30.

Bucić-Kojić, A., M. Planinić, S. Tomas, L. Jakobek, and M. Šeruga. 2009. Influence of solvent and temperature on extraction of phenolic compounds from grape seed, antioxidant activity and colour of extract. Int. J. Food Sci. Tech. 44:2394–2401.

Carr, B. T., M. Meilgaard, and G. Civille. 1999. Sensory evaluation techniques. CRC Press, Washington, DC.

Céspedes, C. L., M. El-Hafidi, N. Pavon, and J. Alarcon. 2008. Antioxidant and cardioprotective activities of phenolic extracts from fruits of Chilean blackberry *Aristotelia chilensis* (Elaeocarpaceae). Maqui. Food Chem. 107:820–829.

Choi, Y., H. S. Jeong, and J. Lee. 2007. Antioxidant activity of methanolic extracts from some grains consumed in Korea. Food Chem. 103:130–138.

Davidov-Pardo, G., M. Moreno, I. Arozarena, M. Marín-Arroyo, R. Bleibaum, and C. Bruhn. 2012. Sensory and consumer perception of the addition of grape seed extracts in cookies. J. Food Sci. 77:S430–S438.

Drewnowski, A., and C. Gomez-Carneros. 2000. Bitter taste, phytonutrients, and the consumer: a review. Am. J. Clin. Nutr. 72:1424–1435.

Dykes, L., and L. Rooney. 2007. Phenolic compounds in cereal grains and their health benefits. Cereal Food World 52:105–111.

El-Siddig, K., H. Gunasena, B. Prasad, D. Pushpakumara, K. Ramana, P. Vijayanand, et al. 2006. Tamarind: Tamarindus Indica L (Vol. 1): Crops for the Future.

Everitt, A. V., S. N. Hilmer, J. C. Brand-Miller, H. A. Jamieson, A. S. Truswell, A. P. Sharma, et al. 2006. Dietary approaches that delay age-related diseases. Clin. Interv. Aging 1:11.

Farias, G. A., L. Guzmán-Martínez, C. Delgado, and R. B. Maccioni. 2014. Nutraceuticals: A novel concept in prevention and treatment of Alzheimer's disease and related disorders. J. Alzheimer's Dis. 42:357–367.

Galili, S., and R. Hovav. 2014. Chapter 16 – Determination of polyphenols, flavonoids, and antioxidant capacity in dry seeds. Pp. 305–323 *in* R. R. Watson, ed. Polyphenols in plants. Academic Press, San Diego.

González-Vallinas, M., M. González-Castejón, A. Rodríguez-Casado, and A. R. de Molina. 2013. Dietary phytochemicals in cancer prevention and therapy: a complementary approach with promising perspectives. Nutr. Rev. 71:85–599.

Gorinstein, S., M. Zemser, R. Haruenkit, R. Chuthakorn, F. Grauer, O. Martin-Belloso, et al. 1999. Comparative content of total polyphenols and dietary fiber in tropical fruits and persimmon. J. Nutr. Biochem. 10:367–371.

Haghju, S., and H. Almasi. 2015. Antioxidant, antibacterial and therapeutic properties of some endemic medicinal plants of Iran: a review. Adv. Plants Agric. Res. 2:00053.

Hooda, S., and S. Jood. 2005. Organoleptic and nutritional evaluation of wheat biscuits supplemented with untreated and treated fenugreek flour. Food Chem. 90:427–435.

Hough, G., I. Wakeling, A. Mucci, E. Chambers, I. M. Gallardo, and L. R. Alves. 2006. Number of consumers necessary for sensory acceptability tests. Food Qual. Pref. 17:522–526.

Jayaprakasha, G., B. Girennavar, and B. S. Patil. 2008. Radical scavenging activities of Rio Red grapefruits and Sour orange fruit extracts in different in vitro model systems. Bioresource Technolo. 99:4484–4494.

Jesionkowska, K., S. Sijtsema, D. Konopacka, and R. Symoneaux. 2009. Dried fruit and its functional properties from a consumer's point of view. J. Hortic. Sci. Biotech. 1:85.

Keservani, R. K., R. K. Kesharwani, N. Vyas, S. Jain, R. Raghuvanshi, and A. K. Sharma. 2010. Nutraceutical and functional food as future food: a review. Der. Pharmacia Lettre. 2:106–116.

Kielhorn, S., and I. J. Thorngate III. 1999. Oral sensations associated with the flavan-3-ols (+)-catechin and (−)-epicatechin. Food Qual. Pref. 10:109–116.

Kumar, C. S., and S. Bhattacharya. 2008. Tamarind seed: properties, processing and utilization. Crit. Rev. Food Sci. 48:1–20.

Laaksonen, O. 2011. Astringent food compounds and their interactions with taste properties. PhD thesis. Department of Biochemistry and Food Chemistry. Functional foods forum. University of Turku, Finland.

Lawless, L. J., R. T. Threlfall, L. R. Howard, and J. F. Meullenet. 2012. Sensory, compositional, and color properties of nutraceutical-rich juice blends. Am. J. Enol. Vitic. 63:529–537.

Letenneur, L., C. Proust-Lima, A. Le Gouge, J. F. Dartigues, and P. Barberger-Gateau. 2007. Flavonoid intake and cognitive decline over a 10-year period. Am. J. Epidemiol. 165:1364–1371.

Librandi, L. A. P., T. N. Chrysóstomo, A. E. Azzolini, C. G. V. Recchia, S. A. Uyemura, and A. Assis-Pandochi. 2007. Effect of the extract of the tamarind (*Tamarindus indica*) fruit on the complement system: studies *in vitro and* in hamsters submitted to a cholesterol-enriched diet. Food Chem. Toxicol. 45:1487–1495.

Makkar, H. P. S. 2000. A laboratory manual for the FAO/IAEA co-ordinated research project on 'Use of Nuclear and Related Techniques to Develop Simple Tannin Assays for Predicting and Improving the Safety and Efficiency of Feeding Ruminants on Tanniniferous Tree Foliage'. Animal Production and Health Sub-Progrmme, FAO/IAEA Working Document, IAEA, Vienna, Austria.

McRae, J. M., and J. A. Kennedy. 2011. Wine and grape tannin interactions with salivary proteins and their impact on astringency: a review of current research. Molecules 16:2348–2364.

Mgaya, K., S. Remberg, B. Chove, and T. Wicklund. 2014. Physio-chemical, mineral composition and antioxidant properties of Roselle (*Hibiscus sabdariffa* L.) extract blended with tropical fruit juices. AJFAND 14:8963–9878.

Mildner-Szkudlarz, S., J. Bajerska, R. Zawirska-Wojtasiak, and D. Górecka. 2013. White grape pomace as a source of dietary fibre and polyphenols and its effect on physical and nutraceutical characteristics of wheat biscuits. J. Sci. Food Agri. 93:389–395.

Mousavinejad, G., Z. Emam-Djomeh, K. Rezaei, and M. H. H. Khodaparast. 2009. Identification and quantification of phenolic compounds and their effects on antioxidant activity in pomegranate juices of eight Iranian cultivars. Food Chem. 115:1274–1278.

Moyer, J. C., and H. C. Aitken. 1980. Apple juice in fruit and vegetable juice processing technology. Pp. 212–267 *in* P. E. Nelson and D. K. Tressler, eds. AVI Publishing Company, Westport, CT.

Muanda, F., D. Koné, A. Dicko, R. Soulimani, and C. Younos. 2011. Phytochemical composition and antioxidant capacity of three Malian medicinal plant parts. J. Evid. Based Complement. Altern. 2011:1–8.

Nishinari, K., K. Yamatoya, M. Shirakawa, G. O. Phillips, and P. A. Williams. 2000. Handbook of hydrocolloids. 2nd ed. Pp. 247–267. Woodhead Publ., Cambridge, UK.

Oluseyi, E. O., and O. M. Temitayo. 2015. Chemical and functional properties of fermented, roasted and germinated tamarind (*Tamarindus indica*) seed flours. J. Nutr. Food Sci. 45:97–111.

Ovaskainen, M. L., R. Törrönen, J. M. Koponen, H. Sinkko, J. Hellström, H. Reinivuo, et al. 2008. Dietary intake and major food sources of polyphenols in Finnish adults. J. Nutr. 138:562–566.

Owusu, J., H. Ma, Z. Wang, N. A. Afoakwah, C. Zhou, and A. Amissah. 2015. Effect of pH and temperature on antioxidant levels of tomato wine. J. Food Biochem. 39:91–100.

Pérez-Jiménez, J., S. Arranz, M. Tabernero, M. E. Díaz-Rubio, J. Serrano, I. Goñi, et al. 2008. Updated methodology to determine antioxidant capacity in plant foods, oils and beverages: extraction, measurement and expression of results. Food Res. Int. 41:274–285.

Pundhir, A., and N. Murtaza. 2015. Hurdle technology-an approach towards food preservation. Int. J. Curr. Microbiol. App. Sci. 4:802–809.

Ramaiya, S., J. S. Bujang, M. H. Zakaria, W. S. King, S. Sahrir, and M. Arif. 2013. Sugars, ascorbic acid, total phenolic content and total antioxidant activity in passion fruit (Passiflora) cultivars. J. Sci. Food Agr. 93:1198–1205.

Rodriguez-Amaya, D. B., and M. Kimura. 2004. HarvestPlus handbook for carotenoid analysis. International Food Policy Research Institute (IFPRI), Washington, DC.

Salgado, J. M., T. R. B. Ferreira, F. de Oliveira Biazotto, and C. T. dos Santos Dias. 2012. Increased antioxidant content in juice enriched with dried extract of pomegranate (*Punica granatum*) peel. Plant Food Hum. Nutr. 67:39–43.

Shen, Y., L. Jin, P. Xiao, Y. Lu, and J. Bao. 2009. Total phenolics, flavonoids, antioxidant capacity in rice grain and their relations to grain color, size and weight. J. Cereal Sci. 49:106–111.

Siddhuraju, P. 2007. Antioxidant activity of polyphenolic compounds extracted from defatted raw and dry heated *Tamarindus indica* seed coat. Food Sci. Technol. – LEB 40:982–990.

Soong, Y. Y., and P. J. Barlow. 2004. Antioxidant activity and phenolic content of selected fruit seeds. Food Chem. 88:411–417.

Soultani, G., V. Evageliou, A. E. Koutelidakis, M. Kapsokefalou, and M. Komaitis. 2014. The effect of pectin and other constituents on the antioxidant activity of tea. Food Hydrocoll. 35:727–732.

Stratil, P., B. Klejdus, and V. Kuban. 2006. Determination of total content of phenolic compounds and their antioxidant activity in vegetables evaluation of spectrophotometric methods. J. Agr. Food Chem. 54:607–616.

Sudha, M., V. Baskaran, and K. Leelavathi. 2007. Apple pomace as a source of dietary fiber and polyphenols and its effect on the rheological characteristics and cake making. Food Chem. 104:686–692.

Sudjaroen, Y., R. Haubner, G. Würtele, W. E. Hull, G. Erben, B. Spiegelhalder, et al. 2005. Isolation and structure elucidation of phenolic antioxidants from Tamarind (*Tamarindus indica* L.) seeds and pericarp. Food Chem. Toxicol. 43:1673–1682.

Sun, B., J. M. Ricardo-da-Silva, and I. Spranger. 1998. Critical factors of vanillin assay for catechins and proanthocyanidins. J. Agr. Food Chem. 46:4267–4274.

Swami, S. B., N. Thakor, P. Haldankar, and S. Kalse. 2012. Jackfruit and its many functional components as related to human health: a review. Comp. Rev. Food Sci. F 11:565–576.

Sweeney, J., and A. Marsh. 1971. Effect of processing on provitamin A in vegetables. Amer. Diet Ass. J. 59:238–243.

Tril, U., J. Fernández-López, J. Á. P. Álvarez, and M. Viuda-Martos. 2014. Chemical, physicochemical, technological, antibacterial and antioxidant properties of rich-fibre powder extract obtained from tamarind (*Tamarindus indica* L.). Ind. Crop Prod. 55:155–162.

Tsuda, T., M. Watanabe, K. Ohshima, A. Yamamoto, S. Kawakishi, and T. Osawa. 1994. Antioxidative components isolated from the seed of tamarind (*Tamarindus indica* L.). J. Agr. Food. Chem. 42:2671–2674.

Valdes, L., A. Cuervo, N. Salazar, P. Ruas-Madiedo, M. Gueimonde, and S. González. 2015. Relationship between phenolic compounds from diet and microbiota: impact on human health. Food Funct. 6:2424–2439.

Yamanaka, S., Y. Yuguchi, H. Urakawa, K. Kajiwara, M. Shirakawa, and K. Yamatoya. 2000. Gelation of tamarind seed polysaccharide xyloglucan in the presence of ethanol. Food Hydrocoll. 14:125–128.

10

Development and quality characteristics of shelf-stable soy-agushie: a residual by-product of soymilk production

Christina A. Nti[1], Wisdom A. Plahar[2] & Nana T. Annan[2]

[1]Department of Family and Consumer Sciences, University of Ghana, Legon, Ghana
[2]CSIR-Food Research Institute, Box M.20, Accra, Ghana

Keywords
Product development, quality characteristics, soy-agushie, soymilk by-product

Correspondence
Christina A. Nti, Department of Family and Consumer Sciences, University of Ghana, Legon, Ghana.
E-mail: cnti@ug.edu.gh

Funding Information
No funding information provided.

Abstract

A process was developed for the production of a high-protein food ingredient, soy-agushie, from the residual by-product of soymilk production. The product, with a moisture content of about 6%, was evaluated for its quality characteristics and performance in traditional dishes. The protein content was about 26% with similar amino acids content as that of the whole soybean. Lysine remained high in the dehydrated product (6.57 g/16 g N). While over 60% of the original B vitamins content in the beans was extracted with the milk, high proportions of the minerals were found to be retained in the residual by-product. The process adequately reduced the trypsin inhibitor levels in the beans from 25 to 1.5 mg/g. High sensory scores were obtained for recipes developed with soy-agushie in traditional dishes. The scope of utilization of the soy-agushie could be widened to include several traditional foods and bakery products for maximum nutritional benefits.

Introduction

In many parts of Africa, soybean has been identified as a suitable protein-rich crop that could help improve the economic and nutritional status of the general population through increased production and utilization. It is for this reason that several projects were initiated in the early 2000s with the objective to promote the production and utilization of soybeans in the West African sub-region through the development of home-level and small-scale processing technologies for soy-based foods for rural and urban populations (IDRC Soybean Utilization Project document, 1994). The processing technologies are aimed at developing new food products and improve the quality of local foods by fortifying them with soybeans, taking into account country-specific and within country preferences. Promotion of the production and consumption of soymilk in Ghana is one of the main activities of the soybean utilization research groups in Ghana, Nigeria, and Cote D'Ivoire in one such collaborative project.

Technologies have been developed and extended in past research work for the preparation of soymilk both at the household level and the small-scale enterprise level (Plahar and Annan 1994). One major by-product of soymilk production is the residue after extraction of the milk. Food uses of the wet residue have not been developed. As a result, producers end up giving it to free range domestic animals. The apparent similarities in the physical characteristics of the soy residue and ground melon seed (*agushie*) used extensively for various food preparations in West Africa formed the basis for the present investigation aimed at developing an acceptable substitute for agushie. Agushie is used in countries in the West African sub-region for the preparation of diverse soups and stews which form a major part of the diets of the people. It is, however, relatively expensive and not always readily available. The method of preparation of the mashed agushie is also tedious as it has to be dehulled manually and ground on a stone or mill. It is envisaged that the development of a stable and ready-to-use product from the residual by-product of soymilk production will not only be nutritionally advantageous, but will also add economic value to the utilization of soybean for milk production.

The purpose of the study was therefore to develop an acceptable agushie substitute from the residual by-product of soymilk production and to characterize the product in terms of its nutritional, sensory, and physicochemical properties. Acceptability of the soy-agushie as a substitute for the melon seed was also assessed in a few traditional stews and sauces.

Materials and Methods

Materials

Samples of soybeans used in this study were the *Salintuya* variety obtained from the CSIR-Crops Research Institute, Ghana. All chemicals used were of reagent grade obtained from the Sigma Chemical Co. (St. Louis, MI).

Product development

The standard procedure reported by Plahar and Annan (1994) was followed in the preparation of soymilk samples. For each batch production, cleaned soybeans were soaked in potable water (1:5 w/v) for 30 min. The water was drained and the soaked beans dropped into boiling water (1:10 dry bean weight to water ratio) and allowed to boil for 10 min with 0.2% salt added. A slurry was prepared by grinding the blanched beans for 3 min in a blender using all of the blanch water. The slurry was stirred well and filtered hot through muslin cloth, squeezing to remove as much filtrate as possible. The extract obtained was boiled for 20 min to obtain the milk. The wet residual by-product was dried for about 6 h in a mechanical dryer (Apex, Royce Ross Ltd., Construction Ltd. Chemical Eng., Soho Sq. London) maintained at 70–80°C to obtain the relatively shelf-stable dehydrated meal with a moisture content of 3.6%. The dehydrated meal was milled using a hammer mill (Jacobson Machine Works Inc., Minneapolis, MN) into grits and sealed in double-laminated sealable polyethylene bags as the shelf-stable soy-agushie. Color of the final product was one main physical characteristic used to determine the optimal dehydration parameters. The color of the samples was measured in triplicate using the L*, a*, and b* color space (CIE LAB space) with Colorimeter CR-200 (Minolta, Model CR310, Minolta Camera Company Ltd., Osaka, Japan). The L* value indicates lightness, where L* = 0 is completely black and L* = 100 is completely white. The a* values represent red to green with positive a* and negative a* depicting red and green, respectively. The b* values on the other hand represent yellow to blue, with positive b* representing yellow and negative b* representing blue. The meter was calibrated with a white tile (L* = 97.63, a* = −0.48, and b* = +2.12). ΔE values were calculated to indicate the extent of deviation of color of samples from the standard tile color used. ΔE is calculated as the square root of the sum of the squared deviations of L*, a*, and b* values, that is, $\Delta E = \sqrt{[\Delta L^2 + \Delta a^2 + \Delta b^2]}$ (Morrison and Laignelet 1983; Oduro-Yeboah et al. 2010).

Recipe formulation and sensory evaluation

Recipes were developed with the soy-agushie as a replacement for the melon seed in common traditional stews, sauces, and soups including gravies, ordinary stews, garden egg stew, palaver sauce, vegetable soup, and groundnut soup. In the recipe development with the soy-agushie, the technical development processes for optimization and prototype refining by sensory techniques were applied to arrive at the final ingredient composition and preparation of each recipe. Sensory characteristics of the products were evaluated by a 10-member trained panel of the CSIR-Food Research Institute, Ghana. The quantitative descriptive sensory analysis as described by Johnson et al. (1988) was used to assess the color of the products. To determine the relative intensity of the beany flavor in the samples, the category scaling method of Larmond (1977) was used. Samples were served at room temperature in porcelain plates and judges were asked to evaluate the beany flavor by checking the appropriate terms on a graduated scale with anchor words. The triangle difference test (Larmond 1977) was used to compare traditional agushie (lemon seed) products and the soy substitutes.

Analytical procedures

The following analytical procedures were used for a comprehensive quality assessment of the wet and the dehydrated meal products as well as the milk extract. Product quality factors determined include the proximate composition, minerals (sodium, potassium, calcium, magnesium, phosphorus, iron, manganese, zinc, and copper), vitamins (total pyridoxamine, riboflavin, and biotin), selected disaccharides (fructose, sucrose, and maltose), amino acids, and TIA (trypsin inhibitor activity).

Moisture (AOAC 925.10), protein (AOAC 984.13), fat (AOAC 920.39), and ash (AOAC 923.03) were determined by the AOAC (2000) standard methods, while carbohydrates were calculated by difference, and energy values were obtained using the Atwater factors 3.47, 8.37 and 4.00 for protein, fat, and carbohydrates, respectively (Eyeson and Ankrah 1975). Iron, calcium, and phosphorous were determined by AACC (2000) bipyridyl colorimetric, permanganate titration, and molybdenum methods, respectively, while sodium, potassium, calcium, magnesium, manganese, zinc, and copper were determined using Atomic Absorption Spectrophotometric method with the PerkinElmer atomic absorption spectrophotometer No.3030, (AACC, 1999). The ground samples were ashed and dissolved in a mixture of 0.5 mL nitric acid and 1 mL hydrochloric acid, heated, and diluted after cooling. Measurements were taken against standards.

A modification of the HPLC (high-performance liquid chromatography) method described by Aslam et al. (2008) and Ekinci and Kadakal (2005) was used for the determination of riboflavin (vitamin B_2), pyridoxine (vitamin B_6), and biotin (vitamin B_7), with simultaneous UV and fluorescence detection. Two to seven gram samples were weighed into a 100 mL volumetric flask and hydrolyzed for 30–60 min with 50 mL water + 1 mL 25% HCl at 70°C in a water bath. After cooling to 40°C the sample solution was buffered with 5 mL 2.5 N sodium acetate solution and incubated overnight with 1 mL freshly prepared enzyme solution (4 mg/mL phosphatase and 15 mg/mL Taka-Diastase) at 37°C. The solution was cooled, made up to the mark with deionized water, and filtered. The filtrate was further washed over a C18-SPE ion exchange column and the eluent was measured by HPLC.

The HPLC technique of Müller and Siepe (1980) was used for the determination of fructose, glucose, galactose, sucrose, maltose, and lactose contents of the samples. The watery solution of each sample was clarified with Carrez solution ($K_4(Fe(CN)_6).3H_2O$ and $ZnSO_4.7H_2O$) and cleaned on an SPE column (Waters Sep-Pak No. 51910). Methyl-α-D-glucopyranoside was used as internal standard. The components were then separated on an HPLC (column Nucleosil NH_2, 5 mm, 250 × 4 mm with a 30 × 4 mm fore column), using a refractive index detector. HPLC conditions were flow rate = 1 mL/min, sample volume = 20 mL, column temperature = 30°C, refractive index temperature = 35°C, eluent = acetonitrile:water ratio of 70:20 w/w.

Amino acid composition of samples was determined in triplicate by digestion under vacuum with 6 N HCl in sealed ampoules at 110°C for 22 h. The hydrolysates were derivatized and analyzed for amino acids on a Waters HPLC system controlled by Millenium 2010 software (Waters Div., Millipore Corp., Milford, MA). Cystine was determined as cysteic acid by performic acid oxidation (Hirs 1967) as described by Albert et al. (2008). The colorimetric technique of Opienska-Blauth et al. (1963) was used for the determination of tryptophan in extracts prepared by the method of Subramanian et al. (1970).

Trypsin inhibitor activity was determined by the method of Hammerstrand et al. (1981). One gram portions of the samples were extracted by soaking overnight at 4°C in 50 mL 0.01 NaOH (pH was adjusted to 8.4–10.0). The suspensions were diluted so that 2 mL of the sample extract inhibited 40–60% of standard trypsin used in the analysis. For the analysis on inhibition of trypsin, synthetic BAPNA (benzoyl DL arginine-*p*-nitro anilide) was used as substrate. Residual enzyme activities were determined in systems containing 2 mL aliquots of the sample extracts by measuring the absorbance at 410 nm. TIA in terms of milligrams pure trypsin per gram sample was calculated as

$$TIA = \frac{2.632 \times D \times A_1}{S}$$

where A_1 = change in absorbance due to trypsin inhibition per mL diluted sample extract, D = dilution factor, and S = weight of sample (g).

Statistical analysis

Statistical significance of observed differences among means of experimental results were evaluated by ANOVA (analysis of variance) followed by pairwise comparison of means (Steel and Torie 1981). Significance was accepted at $P < 0.05$.

Results and Discussion

Dehydration of soy-agushie samples

Using the commercial Apex dryer (Apex, Royce Ross Ltd., Construction Ltd. Chemical Eng., Soho Sq. London) the optimal dehydration temperature range for the soy-residue samples was found to be between 70°C and 80°C. The desired physical and sensory characteristics were obtained at this temperature while higher temperatures presented problems of burnt flavor and lower temperatures prolonged the drying rate unduly. There was no detectable beany flavor in the dried meal, and the color of the product was creamy off-white with L*, a*, and b* values of 82.64 ± 0.35, −1.62 ± 0.08, and 12.51 ± 0.39, respectively, and a ΔE value of 18.27. The ΔE value indicates the extent of deviation of color of the product from the standard tile color used (L* = 97.63, a* = −0.48, and b* = +2.12). In other studies ΔE values obtained using the same standard tile for similar products were 15.61 for yam bean flour obtained by drying at 55°C for 5½ h (Buckman et al. 2015), and 29.98 for orange flesh sweet potato flour obtained by drying in a solar tent dryer at 40–50°C for 6 days (Bonsi et al. 2014). Plahar et al. (1983) recommended a dehydration temperature of 62°C for unfortified fermented maize dough to produce dehydrated maize meal with the desired color characteristics.

Chemical characteristics of soy-agushie samples

The proximate composition and trypsin inhibitor activities of soymilk extract and the residual by-product, soy-agushie samples are given in Table 1. On dry weight basis, the protein and fat contents of the soy-residue were significantly ($P < 0.05$) higher than in the soymilk. A large proportion of the protein and fat contents of the original grain were not extracted into the milk, but remained in the residue making the latter highly nutritious. The milk extraction procedure could extract only a small proportion of the protein and fat from the raw grains, with the dried residue containing over 70% and 56%, respectively, of the original content of these nutrients. A similar situation was observed in the ash content of the extract and the residual by-product. The soy-agushie prepared from the residue therefore had nutritional quality quite close to that of the original grains used. The composition of the undehydrated fresh wet residue, when converted to dry weight basis is quite similar to that of the dehydrated meal.

In terms of antinutritional factors, the heat treatment was found adequate in drastically reducing the trypsin inhibitor levels in soy-agushie from an original value of 25 mg CE/g sample to minimal levels of <2 mg CE/g soy-agushie sample, and <0.5 mg CE/g soymilk sample. This situation is quite desirable to guarantee no adverse trypsin inhibitory effects in cases where minimal heat treatments will be applied in culinary preparations of dishes containing soy-agushie. The TIA in the dehydrated soy-agushie meal was found to be lower than that in the wet meal when considered on dry weight basis (Table 1). The dehydration process helped to further destroy the residual activity in the dried product. In other studies, Plahar and Annan (1994) observed a reduction in TIA from 25 to 0.3 mg/g sample after boiling soaked soybeans for 20 min. Such final levels of TIA are considered safe for maximum nutritional benefits.

Table 1. Proximate composition and trypsin inhibitor activity of soymilk and the residual by-product, soy-agushie samples[1].

Component	Whole raw soybean	Soymilk sample	Fresh (wet) soy-agushie	Dehydrated soy-agushie
Moisture (%)	9.54 ± 0.24	88.62 ± 0.72	59.12 ± 0.51	5.73 ± 0.70
Protein (%)	37.41 ± 0.64	2.53 ± 0.91	10.91 ± 1.71	26.40 ± 1.13
Fat (%)	18.72 ± 1.14	1.58 ± 0.66	4.73 ± 0.44	10.50 ± 0.62
Ash (%)	6.12 ± 0.32	0.60 ± 0.15	1.01 ± 0.34	3.72 ± 0.53
Carbohydrates (%)	28.21 ± 1.33	6.67 ± 1.34	24.23 ± 1.87	53.66 ± 1.56
Energy (kcal)	399.34 ± 4.32	48.68 ± 2.90	174.37 ± 5.07	394.13 ± 4.17
TIA (mg/g sample)[2]	25.36 ± 1.72	0.31 ± 0.06	1.82 ± 0.30	1.53 ± 0.44

[1]Values are mean ± standard deviation of triplicate determinations expressed on as-is basis.
[2]Trypsin inhibitor activity.

Table 2. Minerals, vitamins, and sugar content of raw soybean, soymilk, and soy-agushie samples[1].

Component	Whole raw soybean	Soymilk sample	Dehydrated soy-agushie
Minerals (mg/100 g)			
Sodium	1.6 ± 0.28^{c}	2.5 ± 0.34^{b}	12.2 ± 0.68^{a}
Potassium	1,269 ± 8.10^{a}	206.0 ± 5.02^{c}	945.0 ± 6.75^{b}
Calcium	268.0 ± 2.60^{b}	18.5 ± 1.25^{c}	347.0 ± 3.24^{a}
Magnesium	182.0 ± 4.30^{a}	22.0 ± 0.94^{c}	151.0 ± 1.77^{b}
Phosphorus	617.7 ± 3.60^{a}	60.3 ± 1.81^{b}	641.1 ± 2.89^{a}
Iron	9.1 ± 0.81^{a}	0.5 ± 0.08^{b}	9.5 ± 1.23^{a}
Manganese	1.6 ± 0.31^{a}	0.1 ± 0.02^{b}	2.4 ± 0.22^{a}
Zinc	4.0 ± 0.58^{a}	0.3 ± 0.04^{b}	4.5 ± 0.38^{a}
Copper	1.4 ± 0.19^{a}	0.2 ± 0.06^{b}	1.5 ± 0.42^{a}
Vitamins (mg/100 g)			
Pyridoxin—HCl	0.36 ± 0.07^{b}	0.53 ± 0.08^{a}	0.17 ± 0.08^{c}
Pyridoxamine	0.19 ± 0.04^{a}	0.13 ± 0.03^{a}	0.04 ± 0.01^{b}
Total B_6	0.55 ± 0.08^{a}	0.66 ± 0.17^{a}	0.21 ± 0.08^{b}
Riboflavin	0.14 ± 0.02^{a}	0.02 ± 0.01^{c}	0.06 ± 0.01^{b}
Biotin	0.03 ± 0.01^{a}	–	0.02 ± 0.00^{a}
Sugars (g/100 g)			
Fructose	–	0.12 ± 0.09^{a}	–
Sucrose	3.61 ± 0.21^{a}	1.07 ± 0.18^{b}	1.50 ± 0.17^{b}
Maltose	0.44 ± 0.05^{a}	0.15 ± 0.02^{b}	0.03 ± 0.01^{b}

[1]Values are mean ± SD of triplicate determinations expressed on dry weight basis. Means with different superscript letter are significantly different (p<0.05).

Minerals, vitamins, and sugar content of soy-agushie samples

Table 2 gives the concentrations of selected minerals, vitamins, and sugars in soymilk extract and the soy-agushie samples compared to the content in the original raw soybean. It was observed that most of the minerals determined were in greater concentrations in the final dehydrated soy-agushie product than in the raw material. The normal preparation of soymilk involves addition of sodium chloride in the form of crude table salt. The normal crude salt used usually contains small amount of mineral contaminants, and this should account for the greater concentrations of some of the minerals in the product than in the beans. In general, however, large proportions of the mineral content of the raw beans were found to be retained in the residual by-product during soymilk extraction. On dry weight basis, the amount of minerals extracted with the milk was found to be at most 22% of the unextracted portion in the residue. In most cases, the extracted portions were as low as 4% of the unextracted portions. The minerals in the greatest concentrations in the soy-agushie were potassium, calcium, magnesium, and phosphorus. Minor mineral components were sodium, iron, manganese, zinc, and copper (Table 2).

Contrary to the observations made on the minerals, relatively large proportions of the vitamins were extracted with the milk leaving significantly ($P < 0.05$) lower concentrations in the residue. The vitamins determined were water soluble, and were more likely to be concentrated in the aqueous milk phase. In spite of this, the soy-agushie was found to contain significant levels of the B vitamins. Similarly, most of the sugars were extracted into the milk. Although fructose was not determined in the soybean, about 0.12% was observed in the milk extract. This could have been produced during the process. Earlier reports by Hou et al. (2009) mentioned about 4.49 mg/g sucrose, 0.12 mg/g fructose, and 0.18 mg/g glucose in soybeans.

Amino acid composition of soymilk and soy-agushie

Table 3 gives the amino acid composition of raw soybeans, soymilk extract, and the wet and dehydrated residual by-products. The amino acid composition of the soymilk extract was similar to that of the raw soybean. However, the residual by-product was found to have higher concentrations of most of the amino acids than in the original beans. Lysine remained high in both the wet and the dehydrated products, as well as in the milk ranging between 6.47 and 6.57 g/16 g N in the meals and 6.66 g/16 g N in the milk. Tryptophan content was also high in the product. The dehydration temperatures used were also mild enough to prevent loss of available essential amino acids in the process. Considering the fact that traditional cereal-based weaning foods in Ghana are grossly inadequate in these two amino acids, and hence their low nutritive value, the soy-agushie could serve as a fortifying material in these traditional weaning foods for improved amino acids pattern and general protein content and quality.

Previous studies investigated the effects of fortification of traditional cereal-based weaning foods with soy flour. The results showed significant improvements in the protein content and quality of the traditional foods by virtue of

Table 3. Amino acid composition (g/16 g N) of raw soybean, soymilk, and soy-agushie (wet and dried) samples[1].

Component	Whole raw soybean	Soymilk sample	Fresh (wet) soy-agushie	Dehydrated soy-agushie
Aspartic acid	10.80 ± 0.51	11.54 ± 0.42	16.11 ± 0.28	16.09 ± 0.35
Threonine	3.83 ± 0.30	4.11 ± 0.38	5.47 ± 0.39	5.72 ± 0.21
Serine	5.16 ± 0.15	5.24 ± 0.24	7.47 ± 0.40	7.75 ± 0.38
Glutamic acid	17.09 ± 0.13	19.40 ± 0.47	25.47 ± 0.21	25.26 ± 0.32
Proline	5.30 ± 0.20	5.51 ± 0.18	8.21 ± 0.41	8.09 ± 0.44
Glycine	4.02 ± 0.32	4.36 ± 0.19	6.00 ± 0.50	6.09 ± 0.21
Alanine	3.97 ± 0.11	4.14 ± 0.30	6.00 ± 0.22	6.27 ± 0.20
Cystine	1.40 ± 0.10	1.68 ± 0.08	2.00 ± 0.10	1.97 ± 0.12
Valine	4.14 ± 0.20	3.92 ± 0.18	6.63 ± 0.19	6.70 ± 0.23
Methionine	0.98 ± 0.13	1.33 ± 0.22	1.89 ± 0.12	1.38 ± 0.28
Isoleucine	4.09 ± 0.23	3.97 ± 0.27	6.63 ± 0.51	6.55 ± 0.48
Leucine	6.99 ± 0.57	6.75 ± 0.45	10.84 ± 0.55	10.92 ± 0.54
Tyrosine	3.05 ± 0.17	3.53 ± 0.22	5.16 ± 0.36	4.55 ± 0.16
Phenylalanine	4.79 ± 0.27	4.57 ± 0.23	7.68 ± 0.26	7.51 ± 0.18
Lysine	6.34 ± 0.41	6.66 ± 0.12	6.47 ± 0.21	6.57 ± 0.20
Histidine	2.62 ± 0.08	2.82 ± 0.11	3.79 ± 0.17	3.94 ± 0.10
Arginine	6.78 ± 0.27	7.63 ± 0.18	10.63 ± 0.30	10.06 ± 0.26
Tryptophan	1.43 ± 0.60	1.30 ± 0.08	2.00 ± 0.41	2.06 ± 0.13

[1]Values are mean ± SD of triplicate determinations expressed on dry weight basis.

Table 4. Mean sensory scores for recipes developed with soy-agushie in selected traditional dishes[1].

Product	Sensory attributes			
	Taste	Aroma	Texture/consistency	Overall acceptability
Gravy				
Traditional	7.1 ± 0.73	7.4 ± 1.24	8.3 ± 1.02	7.8 ± 0.74
Soy-agushie	6.8 ± 1.10	7.5 ± 0.95	8.4 ± 1.23	7.5 ± 0.68
Tomato stew				
Traditional	7.0 ± 0.75	7.2 ± 0.92	8.1 ± 1.30	7.6 ± 1.03
Soy-agushie	6.7 ± 0.46	7.3 ± 1.19	7.8 ± 1.21	7.4 ± 1.24
Garden egg stew				
Traditional	7.6 ± 1.03	7.8 ± 0.64	7.9 ± 0.92	7.7 ± 0.92
Soy-agushie	7.7 ± 1.18	7.4 ± 0.74	8.1 ± 1.24	7.6 ± 0.64
Palaver sauce				
Traditional	8.2 ± 1.12	8.0 ± 1.19	7.9 ± 0.99	8.0 ± 1.24
Soy-agushie	7.8 ± 1.06	8.1 ± 1.20	7.6 ± 0.75	7.9 ± 1.17
Vegetable soup				
Traditional	6.6 ± 0.75	6.8 ± 0.46	7.5 ± 1.04	7.2 ± 0.74
Soy-agushie	6.8 ± 0.70	6.9 ± 0.64	7.3 ± 1.21	7.0 ± 0.63
Groundnut soup				
Traditional	6.2 ± 0.48	7.5 ± 1.19	8.0 ± 1.03	7.3 ± 0.87
Soy-agushie	6.4 ± 0.74	7.8 ± 1.23	7.5 ± 0.98	7.1 ± 1.06

[1]Interpretation of scores: 9 = like extremely; 8 = like very much; 7 = like moderately; 6 = like slightly; 5 = neither like nor dislike; 4 = dislike slightly; 3 = dislike moderately; 2 = dislike very much; 1 = dislike extremely.

the high-protein content of the soy flour and by the mutual complementation of the limiting amino acids (Plahar et al. 1983, 1997). The protein content of the soy-agushie developed in the present study was comparable to that of the soy flour, with a better amino acids pattern in terms of high concentrations of lysine, tryptophan, and the sulfur amino acids. These qualities would make the soy-agushie an equally good, if not a better material for the development of high-protein weaning foods based on traditional cereal-based weaning foods. Other quality characteristics of blends with respect to their biochemical, hematological, histopathological, and nutritional implications would, however, have to be established through animal studies.

Soy-agushie recipes

Six recipes were developed with soy-agushie as a substitute for the melon seed, based on traditional dishes. The ingredient composition and preparation methods were arrived at after several tests for minimal detectable differences between test samples and traditional controls, as well as maximum consumer acceptability of sensory attributes. The mean sensory scores for the final recipes are shown in Table 4. For all the sensory attributes, mean scores were similar for both traditional agushie products and products with soy-agushie as substitute. Consumer overall acceptability ranged between 7.0 and 7.9 which indicates moderate to very much liking of the products. Mean scores for taste ranged from 6.4 (like slightly) for the groundnut soup to 7.8 (like very much) for the palaver sauce. Aroma scores ranged between 6.9 (like moderately) for vegetable soup and 8.1 (like very much) for palaver sauce. Similarly, texture/consistency scores also indicate high acceptability with scores ranging between 7.3 (like moderately) for vegetable soup and 8.4 (like very much) for the soy-agushie gravy. In general, soy-agushie was more acceptable in stews and sauces than in soups for which the traditional agushie also received relatively low scores.

Conclusion

The process developed in the study effectively produced a nutritious shelf-stable soy-agushie product that could be effectively used as a substitute for agushie in West African traditional dishes. The product contains lysine and tryptophan in concentrations that can contribute significantly to improving the amino acid pattern of cereal–legume blends. The milk extraction procedure was able to extract only small proportions of the protein and fat from the raw seeds, leaving the dried residue soy-agushie with about 26.4% protein and 10.5% fat content. About 50% of the B vitamins in the original content of the beans were extracted with the milk, while very high proportions of the minerals determined were found to be retained in the residue. The heat treatment adequately reduced the trypsin inhibitor levels in the soy-agushie from 25 mg/g to minimal levels of 1.5 mg/g. Recipes developed with the soy-agushie as replacement for melon seed in traditional dishes had sensory scores in the same category of degree of likeness as the traditional dishes. The scope of utilization of the soy-agushie developed could be widened to include several traditional foods, bakery products, and weaning foods. There is however the need to develop appropriate recipes and large-scale consumer acceptability tests.

Acknowledgment

This publication is an output of IDRC/IITA/FRI Soybean Utilization Project.

Conflict of Interest

None declared.

References

AACC. 1999. Approved methods of analysis. 11th ed. American Association of Cereal Chemists, AACC International, St. Paul, MN.

AACC. 2000. Approved methods of analysis. 10th ed. American Association of Cereal Chemists, AACC International, St. Paul, MN.

Albert, C. S., K. L'oki, G. Pohn, E. Varga-Visi, and J. Csap'o. 2008. Investigation of performic acid oxidation in case of thiol-containing amino acid enantiomers. Acta Univ. Sapientiae Alimentaria 1:73–80.

AOAC. 2000. Official methods of analysis, 17th ed. Association of Official Analytical Chemists, Washington, DC.

Aslam, J., M. S. Mohajir, S. A. Khan, and A. Q. Khan. 2008. HPLC analysis of water-soluble vitamins (B_1, B_2, B_3, B_5, B_6,) in *in-vitro* and *ex-vitro* germinated chickpea (*Cicer arietinum* L.). Afr. J. Biotechnol. 7:2310–2314.

Bonsi, E. A., W. A. Plahar, E. C. Chibuzo, and C. K. Bonsi. 2014. Varietal and solar-drying effects on the yield and quality of flours produced from sweetpotato. Eur. J. Sci. Res. 127:432–441.

Buckman, E. S., W. A. Plahar, I. N. Oduro, and E. E. Carey. 2015. Effects of sodium metabisulphite and blanching pretreatments on the quality characteristics of yam bean (*Pachyrhizus erosus*) flour. Br. J. Appl. Sci. Technol. 6:138–144.

Ekinci, R., and C. Kadakal. 2005. Determination of seven water-soluble vitamins in Tarhana, a traditional Turkish cereal food, by High Performance Liquid Chromatography. Acta Chromatographica. 15:289–297.

Eyeson, K. K., and E. K. Ankrah. 1975. Composition of foods commonly used in Ghana. UNDP/FAO Publication, Food Research Institute, Ghana.

Hammerstrand, G. E., L. T. Black, and J. D. Glover. 1981. Trypsin inhibitors in soy products: modification of the standard analytical procedure. Cereal Chem. 58:42–45.

Hirs, C. H. 1967. Determination of cystine as cysteic acid. Methods Enzymol. 11:59–62.

Hou, A., P. Chen, A. Shi, B. Zhang, and Y.-J. Wang. 2009. Sugar variation in soybean seed assessed with a rapid extraction and quantification method. Int. J. Agron. 2009. Article ID 484571, 8 pages. http://dx.doi.org/10.1155/2009/484571.

IDRC Soybean Utilization Project document. 1994. Project Summary submitted to IDRC. International Institute for Tropical Agriculture (IITA), Ibadan, Nigeria.

Johnson, J. M., G. J. Flick, K. A. Long, and J. A. Phillips. 1988. Menhaden (*Brevoortia tyrannus*): thermally processed for a potential food resource. J. Food Sci. 53:323–324.

Larmond, E. 1977. Laboratory methods for sensory evaluation of food. Canada Dept. of Agricultural Publication, Ottawa, Canada.

Morrison, W. R., and B. Laignelet. 1983. An improved colorimetric procedure for determining apparent and total amylose in cereal and other starches. J. Cereal Sci. 1:9–20.

Müller, H., and V. Siepe. 1980. Quantitative determination of several mono- and oligosaccharides in food products by means of high pressure liquid chromatography replacement of the toxic eluent 'acetonitrile/water' by a mixture of harmless solvents. Chromatographia 13:447.

Oduro-Yeboah, C., P.-N. T. Johnson, E. Sakyi-Dawson, and A. Budu. 2010. Effect of processing procedures on the colorimetry and viscoelastic properties of cassava starch, flour and cassava-plantain fufu flour. Int. Food Res. J. 17:699–709.

Opienska-Blauth, J., M. Charrzinski, and H. Merbec. 1963. A new rapid method of determining tryptophan. Anal. Biochem. 6:69–76.

Plahar, W. A., and N. T. Annan. 1994. *Development of balanced protein-energy weaning foods based on local legumes and cereals.* Report submitted to the Association of African Universities. Food Research Institute, Accra, Ghana.

Plahar, W. A., H. K. Leung, and C. N. Coon. 1983. Effects of dehydration and soy fortification on the physicochemical, nutritional and sensory properties of Ghanaian fermented maize meal. J. Food Sci. 48:1255–1259.

Plahar, W. A., C. A. Nti, and N. T. Annan. 1997. Effect of soy-fortification method on the fermentation characteristics and nutritional quality of fermented maize meal. Plant Foods Hum. Nutr. 51:365–380.

Steel, R. G. D., and J. H. Torie. 1981. Principles and procedures of statistics. A biometrical approach, 2nd ed. McGraw-Hill Kogakusha, Tokyo, Japan.

Subramanian, S. S., R. Jambunathan, J. M. Concon, and E. T. Mertz. 1970. Simple methods for determining lysine and tryptophan in high lysine and normal maize. Fed. Proc. 29:761.

11

Phytochemical, antimicrobial, and antioxidant activities of different citrus juice concentrates

Ehigbai I. Oikeh[1], Ehimwenma S. Omoregie[1], Faith E. Oviasogie[2] & Kelly Oriakhi[3]

[1]Department of Biochemistry, Faculty of Life Sciences, University of Benin, PMB 1154 Benin City, Nigeria
[2]Department of Microbiology, Faculty of Life Sciences, University of Benin, PMB 1154 Benin City, Nigeria
[3]Department of Medical Biochemistry, Faculty of Basic Medical Sciences, University of Benin, PMB 1154 Benin City, Nigeria

Keywords
Antimiocrobial, antioxidant, citrus, juice concentrate

Correspondence
Ehigbai I. Oikeh, Department of Biochemistry, Faculty of Life Sciences, University of Benin, PMB 1154, Benin City, Nigeria.

E-mail: ehigbai.oikeh@uniben.edu

Funding Information
No funding information provided.

Abstract

The search for new antimicrobial compounds is ongoing. Its importance cannot be overemphasized in an era of emerging resistant pathogenic organisms. This study therefore investigated the phytochemical composition and antioxidant and antimicrobial activities of different citrus juice concentrates. Fruit juices of *Citrus tangerine* (tangerine), *Citrus paradisi* (grape), *Citrus limon* (lemon), and *Citrus aurantifolia* (lime) were evaluated. Antimicrobial activities against five bacterial and three fungal strains were evaluated. The results revealed the presence of alkaloids, flavonoids, steroids, terpenoids, saponins, cardiac glycosides, and reducing sugars in all the juice concentrates. DPPH (1,1-diphenyl-2-picrylhydrazyl) radical scavenging capacities varied with tangerine and grape juices having better scavenging capacities than lemon and lime juices. Grape juice was observed to have a significantly higher ($P < 0.05$) ferric-reducing antioxidant potential (FRAP) value (364.2 ± 10.25 μmol/L Fe(II)/g of the extract) than the reference antioxidant, ascorbic acid (312.88 ± 5.61 μmol/L). Antimicrobial studies revealed differential antimicrobial activities against different microbial strains. Zones of inhibition ranging from 4 to 26 mm were observed for the antibacterial tests with 0–24 mm for antifungal test. Minimum inhibitory concentrations (MIC) and minimum bacteriostatic concentrations (MBC) for concentrates against bacterial strains ranged from 12.5 to 200 μg/mL. Lemon and lime juice concentrates had lower MIC and MBC values with orange and tangerine having the highest values. Minimum fungicidal concentrations ranged from 50 to 200 μg/mL. The results of this study suggest that these juice concentrates may have beneficial antimicrobial roles that can be exploited in controlling unwanted microbial growth.

Introduction

Normal physiological processes in vivo result in the production of free radicals. Oxidative stress results when there is an insufficient capacity of the biological system to neutralize excess free radicals that have been produced. This may result in aging and disease conditions (Sahreen et al. 2014). Food and fruits are known to contain antioxidants that are linked to in vivo protection from oxidative stress (Jensen et al. 2008).

An estimated 100 million tons of citrus fruits are produced annually; thereby making the citrus family the largest contributor to the world's fruit production (Jwanny et al. 2012). Citrus is one of the largest plant species known, consisting of 40 species that are distributed around the world (Karimi et al. 2012). Among the most commonly consumed citrus fruits in Nigeria are tangerine, lime, lemon, and grape.

Citrus juices are consumed majorly because of their nutritional value and special flavor. Fruit juice consumption is beneficial for the maintenance of good health and prevention of diseases. The positive health benefits of juices have been ascribed in part to vitamin C (ascorbic acid), the major vitamin found in fruits and vegetables (Boudries et al. 2012; Rekha et al. 2012). Citrus fruits are also known to contain bioactive compounds such as phenolics, flavonoids, vitamins, and essential oils which are believed to be responsible for a range of protective health benefits including antioxidative, anti-inflammatory, antitumor, and antimicrobial activities (Aruoma et al. 2012; Karimi et al. 2012).

The problem of resistance of microorganisms to antimicrobial drugs is one of the world's current challenges. On the other hand, plant-based antimicrobials are attractive as they are often devoid of the many side effects associated with synthetic antimicrobials. The search for new antimicrobial compounds from natural sources is, thus, an ongoing one (Parekh et al. 2005).

This study was therefore aimed at evaluating the phytochemical composition and antioxidant and antimicrobial activities of different commonly available citrus juice concentrates in Nigeria.

Materials and Methods

Collection and identification of plant materials

Fresh fruits (tangerine, lemon, lime, and grape) were purchased from New Benin Market, Benin City in Edo State, Nigeria. The fruits were identified by a Botanist in the Department of Plant Biology and Biotechnology of the University of Benin, Benin City, Nigeria.

Preparation of fruit juice concentrates

The fruits were rinsed thoroughly with distilled water and were cut into halves. The juice was extracted from the fruits using a juice extractor. The fruit juices were then lyophilized and the concentrates obtained were preserved at 4°C in airtight containers until subsequent use.

Phytochemical screening

Phytochemical screening was carried out on the juice concentrates using established protocols as described by Trease and Evans (1989), Sofowora (1993), and Harborne (1998).

Stock solutions of each extract with a concentration of 10 mg extract/mL distilled water was prepared and used for the phytochemical screening.

Estimation of antioxidant activity

Determination of DPPH radical scavenging activity

Radical scavenging activity of each concentrate against the 1, 1-diphenyl-1-picryl-hydrazyl radical (DPPH) was done by a slightly modified method by Brand-Williams et al. (1995). Concentrations of each sample was prepared in methanol and used for the assay. Ascorbic acid was used as standard, and the same concentrations, as the test solution in methanol were prepared. Two milliliters of the prepared concentration was placed into test tubes and 0.5 mL of 1 mmol/L DPPH solution in methanol was added. The experiment was carried out in triplicates. The test tubes were incubated for 15 min at room temperature, and the absorbance was read at 517 nm. A blank solution containing the same amount of methanol and DPPH was prepared and the was absorbance read. Lower absorbance of the reaction mixture indicates higher free radical scavenging activity. The radical scavenging activity was calculated using the following formula:

$$\text{DPPH radical scavenging activity}(\%) = [(A_0 - A_1)/(A_0)] \times 100,$$

where A_0 was the absorbance of DPPH radical + methanol; A_1 was the absorbance of DPPH radical + sample or standard. The 50% inhibitory concentration value (IC_{50}) is indicated as the effective concentration of the sample that is required to scavenge 50% of the DPPH free radical.

Ferric-reducing antioxidant power assay

The Benzie and Strain (1996) protocol with slight modification was employed for this assay. Different concentrations (100–500 mg/mL) of the concentrates and the standard were serially diluted with distilled water. One milliliter of FRAP reagent (200 mL of 300 mmol/L sodium acetate buffer at pH 3.6, 20 mL of 10.0 mmol/L 2,4,6-tripyridyl -s- triazine (TPTZ) solution, 20 mL of 20.0 mmol/L $FeCl_3.6H_2O$ solution, and 24 mL of distilled water) was then added to each test tube. The resulting mixture was vigorously shaken and then incubated at 37°C for 4 min and the increase in absorbance at 593 nm was measured and compared with the standard ascorbic acid.

Antimicrobial assay

Test microorganisms

Eight microorganisms were used in this study, consisting of five bacterial strains and three fungal strains. Two were gram positive (*Staphylococcus aureus* and *Enterococcus faecalis*), while the other three were gram negative (*Pseudomonas aeruginosa, Escherichia coli*, and *Salmonella* spp.). The three fungal strains used are *Candida albicans, Aspergillus niger*, and *Penicillum* spp. All microorganisms were obtained from Lahor Research and Diagnostic Laboratories, Benin City, Nigeria.

Antimicrobial susceptibility assay

This was carried out using the protocol described by Owoseni and Ajayi (2010). Test organisms were subcultured onto fresh suitable broth medium. Broth cultures were then incubated at 37°C till the turbidity of 0.5 McFarland's standard was obtained. Mueller–Hinton agar was used as bacterial medium and Sabouraud agar as fungal medium.

All were incubated appropriately as specified for each test organism. The turbidity of the actively growing broth culture was then adjusted with sterile saline to obtain 0.5 McFarland's standard turbidity. This was used to flood the surface of solid Mueller–Hinton agar plates and then drained dry. Wells of 5 mm in diameter and about 2 cm apart were punched in the culture media with sterile cork borer. The extracts were thereafter used to fill the boreholes. Each plate was kept in the refrigerator at 4°C for 1 h before incubating at 37°C for 24 h (bacteria) and 72 h (fungi). Zones of inhibition around the wells, measured in millimeters, were used as positive bioactivity.

Minimum inhibitory concentration

The organisms that showed susceptibility to different solvent extracts were introduced into the broths containing different concentrations of each extract (serial dilutions of the extracts corresponding to 200, 100, 50, 25, and 12.5 μg/mL). The tubes were then incubated for 24 h at 37°C. The minimum inhibitory concentrations (MIC) was taken as the lowest concentration of the extracts that did not permit any visible growth (Owoseni and Ajayi 2010).

Minimum bactericidal concentration and minimum fungicidal concentration

The tubes that showed no turbidity in the MIC test were taken and a loop-full from each tube was streaked on Mueller–Hinton agar. The plates were incubated for 24 h at 37°C and the absence of growth was observed. The concentration of the extracts that showed no growth was recorded as the minimum bactericidal concentration (MBC)/minimum fungicidal concentration (MFC) (CLSI 2008a,b, 2012).

Statistical analysis

The data were expressed as mean ± SEM of three replicates. The data were subjected to one-way analysis of variance (ANOVA), and differences between means were determined by Duncan's multiple range test using the Statistical Analysis System (SPSS Statistics 17.0, SPSS Inc. Chicago, Illinois, USA) where applicable. $P \leq 0.05$ were regarded as significant.

Results and Discussion

Phytochemicals are non-nutritive plant chemicals possessing varying degrees of disease-preventive properties. They are invaluable sources of raw materials for both traditional and orthodox medicine (Oikeh et al. 2013). In this study, the phytochemical composition of the citrus juice concentrates revealed the presence of alkaloids, flavonoids, steroids, terpenoids, saponins, cardiac glycosides, and reducing sugars

Table 1. Phytochemical composition of some citrus fruit juice concentrates.

	Tangerine	Grape	Lemon	Lime
Alkaloids	++	+	+	+
Phenols	+	+++	+	+
Flavonoids	+	+++	+	+
Steroids	++	+	+	+
Terpenoids	++	+	+	+
Reducing sugar	+	+	+	++
Saponins	++	++	+	+
Cardiac glycosides	+	+	+	++

+, slightly detected; ++, moderate amount; +++, high amounts.

Table 2. Percentage inhibition of the 1,1-diphenyl-2-picrylhydrazyl radical scavenging activity of some citrus fruit juice concentrates.

Sample	% inhibition (mg/mL)	
	0.5	1.0
Ascorbic acid	40.10 ± 0.02	70.20 ± 0.20
Tangerine juice concentrate	17.80 ± 0.60*	26.45 ± 0.15*
Grape juice concentrate	2.60 ± 0.30*	24.0 ± 0.10*
Lemon juice concentrate	2.60 ± 0.20*	5.25 ± 0.40*
Lime juice concentrate	2.85 ± 0.20*	6.25 ± 0.06*

Values are expressed as mean ± SEM. n = 3/group.Values in a column with (*) are significantly different (P < 0.05) from the reference antioxidant.

Table 3. Ferric-reducing antioxidant potential (FRAP) of some citrus fruit juice concentrates.

Plant extract	FRAP value (μmol/L Fe(II)/g) of the extract
Ascorbic acid	312.88 ± 5.61
Tangerine juice concentrate	179.75 ± 4.25*
Grape juice concentrate	364.2 ± 10.25*
Lemon juice concentrate	122.75 ± 3.25*
Lime juice concentrate	173.25 ± 0.25*

Values are expressed as mean ± SEM. n = 3/group. Values with (*) are significantly different (P < 0.05) from the reference antioxidant.

(Table 1). However, the abundance of these phytochemicals varied from juice to juice. These results agree in part with the findings of Rauf et al. (2014) who reported the presence of reducing sugars, phenols, flavonoids, and terpenoids in lemon and lime juice. However, they did not detect the presence of alkaloids, saponins, and glycosides, while steroids was absent in lemon. These differences may be due to differences in species and geographical location.

Generally, phytochemicals are known to confer certain health benefits such as anti-inflammatory, antimicrobial, antihypertensive, and antidiabetic effects (Ayoola et al. 2008; Oikeh et al. 2013).

The presence of flavonoids, alkaloids, steroids, terpenoids, saponins, cardiac glycosides, and reducing sugars

Table 4. Antibacterial activities of some citrus juice concentrates (200 μg/mL) against some bacterial strains tested by disc diffusion assay.

	Zone of inhibition (mm)				
	Gram positive		Gram negative		
	Staphylococcus aureus	*Enterococcus faecalis*	*Pseudomonas aeruginosa*	*Escherichia coli*	*Salmonella* spp.
Tangerine	18	26	25	18	6
Grape	10	8	8	4	6
Lemon	20	10	18	12	10
Lime	20	14	16	8	10

in all the juice concentrates studied corroborates the assertion of Mathew et al. (2012) that citrus fruits are rich sources of phytochemicals.

The DPPH radical scavenging assay is a commonly used tool for accessing the antioxidant capacity of plant materials because of the relative cheap cost and speed of completion.

The results from this study showed increase in the radical scavenging activities of all extracts as the concentration increased from 0.5 to 1.0 mg/mL (Table 2). The standard antioxidant, ascorbic acid had significantly higher ($P < 0.05$) percentage inhibitions of the DPPH radical than all the juice concentrates at both concentrations studied (40.10 ± 0.02% and 70.20 ± 0.20% at concentrations of 0.5 and 1.0 mg/mL of extract). Tangerine had the highest DPPH radical scavenging activity of the four studied juice concentrates (17.08 ± 0.60% and 26.45 ± 0.15% inhibition). A comparison of the DPPH radical scavenging activities of the lemon and lime juices corroborates the finding of Rauf et al. (2014) who observed better percentage inhibition of the DPPH radical in lime compared to lemon at all concentrations studied.

The results also revealed that the juice concentrates are not as effective as DPPH radical scavengers when compared to ascorbic acid. At the concentrations studied, ascorbic acid has a significantly higher inhibition of the DPPH radical compared to the juice concentrates.

The FRAP of the citrus juice concentrates revealed that the tangerine, lemon, and lime juice concentrates had significantly lower FRAP values (179.75 ± 4.25, 122.75 ± 3.25, and 173.25 ± 0.25 μmol/L Fe(II)/g of the extract, respectively) compared to the reference antioxidant (312.88 ± 5.61 μmol/L Fe(II)/g of the extract). Grape juice concentrate had a higher FRAP value (364.2 ± 10.25 μmol/L Fe(II)/g of the extract) than that of ascorbic acid (Table 3). This difference was however not significant ($P > 0.05$). The results suggest that grape juice has a good reductive power and may thus possess significant antioxidant activity.

The antibacterial susceptibility test of the juice concentrates against some gram-positive and -negative bacterial strains are shown in Table 4. The observed zones of inhibition varied from one organism to another and from one citrus juice concentrate to another,

The gram-positive strains showed higher susceptibility values than the gram-negative strains. *Staphylococcus aureus* recorded zones of inhibition ranging from 10 to 20 mm. *Enterococcus faecalis* had zones of inhibition from 8 mm for grape juice concentrate to 26 mm for tangerine juice concentrate. *Salmonella* spp. had the lowest zones of inhibition for the juices studied (6–10 mm). Tangerine produced the higher zones of inhibition for the bacterial strains studied while grape had the lowest zones of inhibition.

The lower zones of inhibition observed in the gram-negative organisms compared to the gram-positive organisms is not all together surprising. This is very likely due to the peptidoglycan-containing periplasmic space and the outer membrane lipopolysaccharide layer of gram-negative bacteria.

The gram-negative outer membrane acts as a barrier, preventing the penetration of numerous environmental substances, including antimicrobial substances into the organism. The periplasmic space is also known to contain enzymes capable of breaking down foreign molecules attempting to gain entry into the microorganism (Holetz et al. 2002; Cheruiyot et al. 2009).

The antifungal activities of citrus juice concentrates revealed that *C. albicans* was most susceptible to the juice concentrates with observed zones of inhibition ranging from 8 mm for grape juice to 24 mm for lemon juice

Table 5. Antifungal activities of some citrus juice concentrates (200 μg/mL) against some fungal strains tested by disc diffusion assay.

	Zone of inhibition (mm)		
	Candida albicans	*Aspergillus niger*	*Penicillum* spp.
Tangerine	14	2	4
Grape	8	6	–
Lemon	24	4	10
Lime	16	4	2

Table 6. Minimum inhibitory and bacteriostatic concentrations of some citrus juice concentrates against some bacterial strains expressed in μg/mL.

	Gram positive				Gram negative					
	Staphylococcus aureus		*Enterococcus faecalis*		*Pseudomonas aeruginosa*		*Escherichia coli*		*Salmonella* spp.	
	MIC	MBC	MIC	MBC	MIC	MBC	MIC	MBC	MIC	MBC
Tangerine	100	200	100	200	12.5	25	100	200	100	200
Grape	25	50	25	50	100	200	100	200	50	100
Lemon	25	50	50	100	12.5	50	50	100	25	50
Lime	12.5	50	50	100	25	50	25	50	12.5	50

MIC, minimum inhibitory concentration; MBC, minimum bacteriocidal concentration.

(Table 5), while *A. niger* and *Penicillum* spp. were less susceptible to the juice concentrates. Zones of inhibition ranging from 2 mm in tangerine juice to 6 mm for grape juice concentrates were observed for *A. niger*. However, *Penicillum* spp. was not susceptible to grape juice. While a 10-mm zone of inhibition of *Penicillum* spp. growth was observed for lemon juice concentrates.

These results suggest that citrus juice concentrates at the concentration studied may not possess very good antifungal activities for controlling *A. niger* and *Penicillum* spp. growth as evidenced by the small zones of inhibition observed for these fungal strains. *Candida albicans* growth was however significantly inhibited by the juice concentrates.

This is especially important in light of the increasing incidence of candiadiasis infections as well as the emergence of resistant Candida species to existing antifungal drugs (Bardaweel et al. 2014).

Table 6 shows the inhibitory and bacteriocidal concentrations of the citrus juice concentrates against some bacterial strains. MIC values ranged from 12.25 to 100 μg/mL, while MBC values ranged from 50 to 200 μg/mL for all the juices studied. The results obtained showed that the MIC values for the juice concentrates were lower than their MBC values. Thus, suggesting that the concentrates were bacteriostatic at lower concentrations, but bacteriocidal at higher concentrations.

The grape, lemon, and lime juices were more effective in inhibiting the growth of *S. aureus*, *E. faecalis*, and *Salmonella* spp. Tangerine juice was most effective against *P. aeruginosa*.

Infections caused by *P. aeruginosa* are among the most difficult to treat with conventional antibiotics (Abu-Shanab et al. 2004). Our study shows that tangerine and lemon juice concentrates significantly inhibited the growth of *P. aeruginosa* (MIC 12.5 μg/mL). Lime juice concentrate also shows good inhibitory effect on the organism (MIC 25 μg/mL). These juice concentrates may therefore hold promise in the management of *P. aeruginosa* infection.

Staphylococcus aureus is one of the most common bacteria implicated in food poisoning. The grape, lemon, and lime juice concentrates showed good inhibitory and bacteriocidal activities against this pathogen (MIC values of 25, 25, and 12.5 μg/mL, respectively).

Escherichia coli was not as susceptible to the juice concentrates. Higher MIC values of the extracts were observed (25 μg/mL for lime juice, 50 μg/mL for lemon juice, and 100 μg/mL for tangerine and grape juice). *Escherichia coli* is a naturally occurring bacteria in the intestinal tract of man. The acquisition of invasion factors increases their ability to adapt to new niches and their disease-causing abilities (Akinjogunla et al. 2010). Our results show that the lime juice concentrate may be an alternative source of antimicrobial agent for this organism.

The inhibitory and fungicidal concentrations of the citrus juice concentrates against three fungal strains is shown in Table 7. The MFC was observed to be higher than the MIC in all the juices. *Candida albicans* was the most susceptible organism with MIC values of 25 μg/mL for tangerine, grape, and lemon juices. *Penicillum* spp. was least susceptible to the juice concentrates with MIC values of 100 μg/mL for lemon and lime juices and 50 μg/mL for tangerine juice. *Penicillum* spp. was not susceptible to grape juice.

The results of this study showed that grape juice was least effective both as an antibacterial and as an antifungal agent. This is evidenced by the smaller zones of inhibition and larger MIC, MBC, and MFC values obtained for grape juice concentrate. However, grape juice had

Table 7. Minimum inhibitory and fungicidal concentrations of some citrus juice concentrates against some fungal strains expressed in μg/mL.

	Candida albicans		*Aspergillus niger*		*Penicillum* spp.	
	MIC	MFC	MIC	MFC	MIC	MFC
Tangerine	25	50	100	200	50	100
Grape	25	50	100	200	–	–
Lemon	25	50	50	100	100	200
Lime	50	100	50	100	100	200

MIC, minimum inhibitory concentration; MFC, minimum fungicidal concentration.

more promising antioxidant activities than the other juice concentrates as evidenced by its higher FRAP values and high percentage of inhibition of the DPPH radical. This juice may therefore have other health benefits that may not necessarily be antimicrobial.

A lot of data exists on the antimicrobial activities of a wide range of extracts of plant origin. This is especially useful for dwellers in rural communities in developing countries who have limited access to synthetic antimicrobial drugs. This study has therefore provided additional information on the health benefits of consuming fruits.

The results of this study have revealed that these commonly consumed citrus juices may contain promising antimicrobial leads. This study, however, provides in vitro data which may not be exactly replicated in vivo. Further studies directed at isolation of novel antimicrobial compounds and in vivo studies that may validate the in vitro findings are recommended.

Conflict of Interest

None declared.

References

Abu-Shanab, B., G. Adwan, D. Abu-Safiya, N. Jarrar, and K. Adwan. 2004. Antibacterial activities of some plant extracts utilized in popular medicine in Palestine. Turk. J. Biol. 28:99–102.

Akinjogunla, O. J., N. O. Eghafona, I. O. Enabulele, C. I. Mboto, and F. O. Ogbemudia. 2010. Antibacterial activity of ethanolic extracts *of Phyllanthus amarus* against extended spectrum β- lactamase producing *Escherichia coli* isolated from stool samples of HIV sero-positive patients with or without diarrhea. Afr. J. Pharm. Pharmacol. 4:402–407.

Aruoma, O. I., B. Landes, D. Ramful-Baboolall, E. Bourdond, V. Neergheen-Bhujune, K. Wagnerf, et al. 2012. Functional benefits of citrus fruits in the management of diabetes. Prev. Med. 54:S12–S16.

Ayoola, G. A., A. D. Folawewo, S. A. Adesegun, O. O. Abioro, A. A. Adepoju-Bello, and H. A. B. Coker. 2008. Phytochemical and antioxidant screening of some plants of Apocynaceae from South West Nigeria. Afr. J. Plant Sci. 2:124–128.

Bardaweel, S. K., K. A. Tawaha, and M. M. Hudaib. 2014. Antioxidant, antimicrobial and antiproliferative activities of *Anthemis palestina* essential oil. BMC Complement. Altern. Med. 14:297.

Benzie, I. F. F., and J. J. Strain. 1996. The ferric reducing ability of plasma (FRAP) as a measure of "antioxidant power": the FRAP assay. Anal. Biochem. 239:70–76.

Boudries, H., K. Madani, N. Touati, S. Souagui, S. Medouni, and M. Chibane. 2012. Pulp antioxidant activities, mineral contents and juice nutritional properties of Algerian Clementine Cultivars and Mandarin. Afr. J. Biotechnol. 11:4258–4267.

Brand-Williams, W., M. E. Cuvelier, and C. Berset. 1995. Use of free radical method to evaluate antioxidant activity. Lebenson. Wiss. Technol. 28:25–30.

Cheruiyot, K. R., D. Olila, and J. Kateregga. 2009. *In-vitro* antibacterial activity of selected medicinal plants from Longisa region of Bomet district, Kenya. Afr. Health Sci. 9(S1):42–46.

CLSI (Clinical and Laboratory Standards Institute). 2008a. Reference method for broth dilution antifungal susceptibility testing of yeasts; approved standard-third edition; CLSI document M27-A3 . Clinical and Laboratory Standards Institute, Wayne, PA.

CLSI (Clinical and Laboratory Standards Institute). 2008b. Reference method for broth dilution antifungal susceptibility testing of filamentous fungi; approved standard CLSI document M38-A2. Clinical and Laboratory Standards Institute, Wayne, PA.

CLSI (Clinical and Laboratory Standards Institute). 2012. Methods for dilution antimicrobial susceptibility tests for bacteria that grow aerobically; approved standard CLSI document M07-A9. Clinical and Laboratory Standards Institute, Wayne, PA.

Harborne, J. B.. 1998. Phytochemical methods: a guide to modern techniques of plant analysis. 3rd ed. New York, NY: Chapman and Hall. Pp. 49–188.

Holetz, F. B., G. L. Pessini, N. R. Sanches, D. A Cortez, C. V. Nakamura, and B. P. D. Filho. 2002. Screening of some plants used in the Brazilian folk medicine for the treatment of infectious diseases. Mem. Inst. Oswaldo Cruz, 97:1027–1031.

Jensen, G. S., X. Wu, K. M. Patterson, J. Barnes, S. G. Carter, L. Scherwitz, et al. 2008. *In vitro* and *in vivo* antioxidant and anti-inflammatory capacities of an antioxidant-rich fruit and berry juice blend. Results of a pilot and randomized, double-blinded, placebo-controlled, crossover study. J. Agric. Food Chem. 56:8326–8333.

Jwanny, E. W., S. T. El-Sayed, A. M. Salem, N. A. Mabrouk, and A. N. Shehata. 2012. Fractionation, identification and biological activities of Egyptian citrus peel extracts. Aust. J. Basic Appl. Sci. 6:34–40.

Karimi, E., E. Oskoueian, R. Hendra, A. Oskoueian, and H. Z. E. Jaafar. 2012. Phenolic compounds characterization and biological activities of *Citrus aurantium* bloom. Molecules 17:1203–1218.

Mathew, B. B., S. K. Jatawa, and A. Tiwaari. 2012. Phytochemical analysis of Citrus limonum pulp and peel. Int. J. Pharm. Pharm. Sci. 4:269–371.

Oikeh, E. I., K. Oriakhi, and E. S. Omoregie. 2013. Proximate analysis and phytochemical screening of *Citrus sinensis* fruit wastes. Bioscientist 1:164–170.

Owoseni, A. A., and A. Ajayi. 2010. Antimicrobial properties of ethanolic and aqueous extracts of *Cymbopogon citratus* on selected bacteria and fungi. J. Med. Appl. Biosci. 2:64–73.

Parekh, J., D. Jadeja, and S. Chanda. 2005. Efficacy of aqueous and methanol extracts of some medicinal plants for potential antibacterial activity. Turk. J. Biol. 29:203–210.

Rauf, A., G. Uddin, and J. Ali. 2014. Phytochemical analysis and radical scavenging profile of juices of *Citrus sinensis*, *Citrus anrantifolia*, and *Citrus limonum*. Org. Med. Chem. Lett. 4:5.

Rekha, C., G. Poornima, M. Manasa, V. Abhipsa, J. Pavithra Devi, H. T. Vijay Kumar, et al. 2012. Ascorbic acid, total phenol content and antioxidant activity of fresh juices of four ripe and unripe citrus fruits. Chem. Sci. Trans. 1:303–310.

Sahreen, S., M. R. Khan, and R. A. Khan. 2014. Comprehensive assessment of phenolics and antiradical potential of Rumex hastatus D. Don. roots. BMC Complement. Altern. Med. 14:47.

Sofowora, A. 1993. Medicinal plants and traditional medicine in Africa. 2nd ed. Ibadan: Spectrum Books Limited. Pp. 134–156.

Trease, G. E., and W. C. Evans. 1989. A textbook of pharmacognosy. 13th ed. London: Bailliere-Tyndall Ltd. Pp. 345–356.

12

Nutritional composition of raw fresh cashew (*Anacardium occidentale* L.) kernels from different origin

Ricard Rico[1], Mònica Bulló[2] & Jordi Salas-Salvadó[2]

[1]International Nut and Dried Fruit Council, Reus, Spain
[2]Department of Biochemistry and Biotechnology, IISPV, School of Medicine, Rovira i Virgili University, CIBERobn Physiopathology of Obesity and Nutrition, Instituto de Salud Carlos III, Madrid, Spain

Keywords
Anacardium occidentale L., cashew nut, fatty acids, nutritional composition, nuts, sterols

Correspondence
Ricard Rico, International Nut and Dried Fruit Council, C/ de la Fruita Seca, 4 (Polígon Tecnoparc), 43204 Reus, Spain.

E-mail: ricardo.rico@estudiants.urv.cat

Funding Information
This work was supported by the Global Cashew Council and the International Nut and Dried Fruit Council.

Abstract

The total dietary fiber, sugar, protein, lipid profile, sodium, and energy contents of 11 raw cashew kernel (*Anacardium occidentale* L.) samples from India, Brazil, Ivory Coast, Kenya, Mozambique, and Vietnam were determined. Total fat was the major component accounting for 48.3% of the total weight, of which 79.7% were unsaturated FA (fatty acids), 20.1% saturated FA, and 0.2% trans FA. Proteins, with 21.3 g/100 g, were ranked second followed by carbohydrates (20.5 g/100 g). The average sodium content was 144 mg/kg. Fourteen FA were identified among which oleic acid was the most abundant with a contribution of 60.7% to the total fat, followed by linoleic (17.77%), palmitic (10.2%), and stearic (8.93%) acids. The mean energy content was 2525 kJ/100g. Furthermore, the sterol profile and content, amino acids, vitamins, and minerals of four raw cashew kernel samples from Brazil, India, Ivory Coast, and Vietnam were determined. β- Sitosterol with 2380 ± 4 mg/kg fat was the most occurring sterol. Glutamic acid, with 4.60 g/100 g, was the amino acid with highest presence, whereas tryptophan with 0.32 g/100 g was the one with lower presence. Vitamin E with an average contribution of 5.80 mg/100 g was the most abundant vita-min. Potassium with a mean value of 6225 mg/kg was the mineral with highest amount in cashew samples.

Introduction

Nuts played an important role in diets of many cultures and civilizations for centuries due to its high energy and nutritional value as well as its huge variety of flavors and unique taste. Furthermore, consumption of tree nuts had been linked with several health benefits during the last years due to its particular nutritional composition. Tree nuts are known to contain a high content of unsaturated FA (fatty acids), both mono- and polyunsaturated FA, combined with a huge variety of vitamins, minerals, amino acids, phytosterols, and a generous content of fiber. Consumption of nuts incorporated in a healthy diet was associated not only to a reduced risk of cardiovascular disease and mortality (Kris-Etherton et al. 2008; Ros et al. 2010), especially in case of stroke (Estruch et al. 2013), but also to a decreased risk of metabolic syndrome (Fernández-Montero et al. 2013; Mitjavila et al. 2013) and diabetes (Kendall et al. 2011). Furthermore, in some studies nuts had been found to improve mental health (Carey et al. 2012; Herbison et al. 2012), increase bone mineral density (Rivas et al. 2013), and decrease the risk of depression (Sanhueza et al. 2013). Its long-term consumption was also associated with a decreased risk of weight gain and obesity (Bes-Rastrollo et al. 2009). In addition, no association between nut consumption and weight gain was recently demonstrated in a meta-analysis of clinical trials (Flores-Mateo et al. 2013). Furthermore, adding cashew nuts in the diet resulted in an increased antioxidant capacity in subjects with metabolic syndrome (Davis et al. 2007). The benefits of the addition of nuts in a healthy diet in front of a low-fat diet have been recently highlighted by Estruch et al. (2013) confirming that the incidence of major cardiovascular events and mortality is 30% lower for those individuals consuming a Mediterranean diet supplemented with a handful of nuts a day, compared to those that are advised to consume a low-fat diet.

Among tree nuts, cashew nuts ranks third in world-wide production (kernel basis), with a world average production of 547,371 metric tons (kernel basis) in the last 10 years with a continuous raising trend. In 2014, the total production of cashew kernels achieved 629,668 MT (metric tons), led by India with 164,286 MT and followed by Vietnam with 119,048 MT, Ivory Coast with 109,583 MT, Guinea-Bissau with 48,300 MT, and Tanzania with 35,200 MT (unpublished results from the International Nut and Dried Council database).

Cashew nuts, *Anacardium occidentale* L., belongs to the Anacardiaceae family and is an evergreen tree native from northeast region of Brazil which expanded spontaneously in South American countries (Asogwa et al. 2008). During the 16th century, it was introduced into India and Africa by Portuguese (Aiyadurai 1966; Asogwa et al. 2008). From India, cashew trees spread all over southeast Asia. Cashew trees can grow from sea level to an altitude of 1000 m (Davis 1999). The tree produces a soft, shiny, and juicy fruit known as cashew apple which bears a single-seeded nut in its bottom covered with a hard gray shell. Cashew nut plays a massive social aid in many developing countries, where thousands of families live from cashew cultivation. The processing of cashew nuts in shell is difficult and expensive due to the specific characteristics of the shell. African cashew nuts with shell are mostly processed in India and Vietnam. However, year by year, more processing factories are being implemented in Africa helping the local industry and farmers to obtain more benefit and expanding the harvested areas and families living from its cultivation and becoming one of the most important economies in the growing areas.

Although being the third most produced nut worldwide, to date, very little research has been made on cashews. As for its nutritional composition, phenolic lipids (Shobha et al. 1992), saturated and unsaturated FA, tocopherols, squalenes, and phytosterols (Ryan et al. 2006), bioactive compounds such as β-carotene, lutein, zeaxanthin, α-tocopherol, γ-tocopherol, thiamin, stearic acid, oleic acid, and linoleic acid (Trox et al. 2010) were already identified and determined in cashew nuts. Cashew trees are widely spread over tropical areas close to the equator; therefore, the nutritional composition of cashew nuts may vary by origin. The aim of the present study was to determine the nutrient composition of raw fresh cashew (*Anacardium occidentale* L.) kernels and its variability by origin, including cashews from the major world producing areas such as Brazil, India, Vietnam, and East and West Africa.

Materials and Methods

Materials

Raw fresh cashew kernels (*Anacardium occidentale* L.) from 11 different origins were used in this study to determine the total dietary fiber, sugar, protein, lipid profile, salt, and energy contents. Six samples proceed from several parts of India, of which two were from Kerala (south west), one from Goa (central west), one from Panruti (south east), one from Andhra Pradesh (central east), and one from Maharashtra (central India). The rest of the samples originated from Brazil, Ivory Coast, Kenya, Mozambique, and Vietnam. Four samples of raw fresh cashew kernels from Brazil, India, Ivory Coast, and Vietnam were used to determine the sterol profile and content, amino acids, vitamins, and heavy metals. One kilogram sample of each origin was obtained, sent to the central laboratory, was protected from light, and then chilled (<21°C). Composition analysis were conducted within 3 months after harvest, and analysis of dietary fiber, sugar, protein, lipid profile, salt, and energy contents were conducted by duplicate.

Methods

Total dietary fiber was determined by gravimetry. One hundred grams of sample material was digested with different enzymes at 37°C, fat and sugars were removed by solvent extraction and fibers were precipitated and determined gravimetrically with a LOQ (limit of quantification) lower than 0.5 g/100 g (§64 LFGB L 00.00-18). Sugars were extracted with hot water/methanol (90/10), insoluble matter was precipitated by Carrez reagent, the extract was filtered by a 0.45-μm filter and sugars were determined by HPLC (high-performance liquid chromatography) with RID (refractive index detector) (HPLC-RID; Agilent Technologies, Santa Clara, CA) using the column Merck LiChospher 100 NH2 (Merck, Darmstadt, Germany) and acetonitrile/water (74/26) as eluent. Fat composition of samples was measured after the hydrolysis with 4 mol/L hydrochloric acid. After filtering, the solid matter was washed until neutral and free from chloride and dried (60°C, vacuum). The matter was extracted by petroleum spirit (boiling range 40–60°C), the solvent was evaporated, and the residue was dried (60°C, vacuum). To measure ash content, the sample material was given in a muffle furnace and the organic matter was combusted. The residue was determined gravimetrically (§64 LFGB L 06.00-4, mod.). Raw protein content was calculated through titrimetry by multiplying the nitrogen (N2) content by 6.25. The sample material was digested in concentrated sulfuric acid at 400°C. All organic bound nitrogen was converted in ammonium sulfate which was extracted in a water steam distillation as ammonia. Ammonia content was determined by a titration with sulfuric acid and protein was then calculated by multiplying the content of nitrogen with factor 6.25 (§64 LFGB L 06.00-7, mod.). Water content was determined by drying the sample material at 103°C and the residue (dry matter) was determined gravimetrically. Water content was calculated (100 − dry matter) (§64 LFGB L 06.00-3, mod.). Fatty acid profile was determined by GC (gas chromatography) with FID (flame ionization detector) (GC-FID CN10703016) (Agilent, Technologies, Santa Clara, CA). The fat yielded by the fat total method was transesterified with methanol–boron trifluoride reagent. The fatty acid methyl esters were analyzed via GC-FID. The column used was Supelco SP-2560, 100 m, 0.25 mm i.d., 0.2 μm phase, and hydrogen as carrier gas (Sigma-Aldrich, St. Louis, MO). The distribution of the peak areas was calculated as the distribution of the mass fraction of the different FA. Isomers were separated according to their molecular weight, number, and position of double bonds as well as configuration of double bounds (*cis/trans*) (DGF C-VI 10a/11a). To determine sodium content, the sample was incinerated at 550°C and the resulting ash was measured via atomic emission spectroscopy (§64 LFGB L 07.00-56) (Sherwood Scientific, Cambridge, U.K.). The sterol profile and content was determined by saponification, extraction of the unsaponifiable matter and separation of sterols from the unsaponifiable matter by thin-layer chromatography, analysis of the derivated sterols by capillary gas–liquid column chromatography with FID detector (GC-FID US00038388)(Agilent Technologies). Vitamin B6 was extracted from the sample in autoclave using acid hydrolysis followed by enzymatic dephosphorylation, reacted with glyoxylic acid in the presence of Fe^{2+}, and then reduced with sodium borohydride in alkaline medium, and quantified by reverse-phase HPLC with fluorometric detection (EX [excitation wavelengths]: 290 nm [nanometers], EM [emission wavelengths]: 395 nm) (EN 14164:2008). Vitamin D3 was saponified using alcoholic potassium hydroxide solution and extracted with hexane:ethylacetate. The extract is concentrated and cleaned up by solid phase extraction (SPE), followed by normal phase semipreparative, and determined by reverse-phase HPLC with DAD (diode array detection) at 265 nm (Agilent Technologies/Thermo Fisher Scientifics Inc., Waltham, MA) (EN 12821:2009). β-Carotene fat containing samples was released from the sample by hydrolysis using ethanolic potassium hydroxide solution for 16 h at room temperature and extracted one time with ethanol:hexane (4:3 v/v) and two times with hexane. The determination was carried out by reverse-phase HPLC with ultraviolet (UV)/DAD detection at 450 nm (Agilent Technologies/Thermo Fisher Scientifics Inc.) (EN 12823-2:2000). Vitamin A (retinol) was released from the sample by alkaline hydrolysis using ethanolic potassium hydroxide solution, extracted three times with hexane:ethylacetate (85:15 v/v), and determined by RP-HPLC (reverse-phase HPLC) with UV/DAD detection at 325 nm (Agilent Technologies/Thermo Fisher Scientifics Inc.) (EN 12823-1:2000). Vitamin B1 was extracted by acid hydrolysis followed by enzyme dephosphorylation and quantified by RP-HPLC with fluorometric detection (EX:368 nm, EM: 440 nm) after postcolumn oxidation to thiochrome (Agilent Technologies/Thermo Fisher Scientifics Inc.) (EN 14122:2006 mod.). Vitamin B2 (riboflavin) was extracted from the sample using acid hydrolysis and quantified by RP-HPLC with fluorometric detection (EX: 468 nm, EM: 520 nm) (Agilent Technologies/Thermo Fisher Scientifics Inc.) (En 14152:2006, mod.). Vitamin B5 (pantothenic acid) was measured microbiologically comparing *Lactobacillus plantarum* (ATCC 8014) growth response to calibration solutions (AOAC 945.74/45.2.05 [1990]). Vitamin B8 (biotin) was also measured microbiologically with *Lactobacillus plantarum* (ATCC 8014) and compared to calibration solutions (LST AB 266.1, 1995). Vitamin B9 (total folate) was calculated microbiologically with *Lactobacillus rhamnosus* (ATCC 8043) and compared to calibration solutions (AOAC 45.2.09 [2004]). Vitamin B12 was extracted from the sample in autoclave using a buffered solution, measured microbiologically with *Lactobacillus leichmannii* (ATCC 7830) and compared to calibration solutions (AOAC 952.20/45.2.02). Vitamin C (ascorbic acid + dehydroascorbic acid) was measured by extraction in an aqueous solution containing trichloroacetic acid and the antioxidant tris(2-carboxyethyl)phosphine. Vitamin C is degraded in a basic environment. The final extract was analyzed by reverse-phase HPLC with UV detection at 265 nm (Agilent Technologies) (Food Chemistry, 94 626–631). Vitamin K1 was enzymatically treated to remove fat and extracted by *n*-hexane, the determination was carried out using reverse-phase HPLC with postcolumn reduction and fluorometric detection (EX: 243 nm, EM: 430 nm) (Agilent Technologies/Thermo Fisher Scientifics Inc.) (EN 14148:2003). Vitamin D2 was saponified in the sample using alcoholic potassium hydroxide solution and extracted with hexane:ethylacetate, the extract was concentrated and cleaned up by solid-phase extraction followed by normal-phase semipreparative and then determined by RP-HPLC with DAD at 265 nm (Agilent Technologies/Thermo Fisher Scientifics Inc.) (EN 12821:2009). Vitamin E (tocopherol profile) (includes δ-tocopherol, α-tocopherol, β-tocopherol, and γ-tocopherol) was released from the sample by alkaline hydrolysis using ethanolic potassium hydroxide solution and then extracted three times with hexane:ethylacetate (85:15 v/v); the determination was carried out by reverse-phase HPLC with FLD detection (EX/EM: 290/327 nm) (Agilent Technologies/Thermo Fisher Scientifics Inc.) (EN 12822:2000). Vitamin B3 (total niacin) was extracted from the sample in a mild hydrochloric solution at 100°C, adjusted to pH 4.5 with sodium acetate and filtrated; the determination was carried out by RP-HPLC-FLD (EX: 322 nm, EM: 380 nm) after a postcolumn oxidation with hydrogen peroxide and Cu(II) ions activated by UV

Table 1. Water, protein, ash, and sodium contents of the different cashew samples.

	Central West India—Goa origin	South West India—Kerala origin 1	South West India—Kerala origin 2	South East India—Panruti origin	Central East India—Andhra Pradesh origin	Central India—Maharashtra origin	Ivory Coast	Brazil	Viet Nam	Kenya	Mozambique	Mean	SD
Water content (g/100 g)	3.5	4.0	4.4	2.3	3.6	4.0	3.4	5.3	4.4	3.9	3.4	3.8	0.8
Raw Protein (g/100 g)	20.1	21.5	21.3	23.0	21.6	20.5	21.4	20.2	21.0	21.5	22.0	21.3	0.8
Ash (g/100 g)	2.5	2.6	2.5	2.8	2.5	2.4	2.6	2.6	2.4	2.5	2.6	2.5	0.1
Sodium (Na) (mg/kg)	120	165	175	105	150	140	115	140	105	205	165	144	32

radiation at 365 nm (Agilent Technologies/Thermo Fisher Scientifics Inc.) (EN 15652:2009). Amino acid profile was determined with a Biochrom 30 amino acid analyzer (Biochrom Ltd, Cambourne, UK). Heavy metals (Na, K, Mg, P, Ca, Zn, Se, and Fe) were digested with nitric acid using microwave technique at temperatures up to 235°C. For heavy metals, the sample was digested with nitric acid using microwave technique at temperatures up to 235°C and analyzed by atomic absorption spectroscopy (PerkinElmer, Waltham, MA), ICP-OES (inductively coupled plasma optical emission spectroscopy) (Varian Inc./Agilent Technologies) and ICP-MS (inductively coupled plasma mass spectroscopy) (Agilent Technologies) (DIN EN ISO 11885, mod.).

Results and Discussion

Dietary fiber, sugars, protein, lipids profile, salt, and energy contents

The water content of cashew kernels was 3.8 ± 0.8% fresh weight of edible food (Table 1). Total protein content was 21.3 ± 0.8% (Table 1). Content on sodium had an average of 144 ± 32 mg/kg (Table 1).

Fat is the major macronutrient present in cashews accounting for 48.3 ± 1.6% (average) of the total weight, of which 61.8 ± 1.8% were monounsaturated FA, 17.9 ± 0.8% polyunsaturated FA, 20.1 ± 1.7% saturated FA, and 0.19 ± 0.02% trans FA (Table 2).

Fourteen FA were identified among which oleic acid was the most abundant with a contribution of 60.7 ± 1.7% to the total fat content, followed by linoleic (17.8 ± 0.8%), palmitic (10.2 ± 0.8%), stearic (8.9 ± 0.9%), and with lower amount of arachidic (0.63 ± 0.07%), palmitoleic (0.41 ± 0.03%), vaccenic (0.41 ± 0.03%), gadoleic (0.20 ± 0.00%), lignoceric (0.20 ± 0.00%), linolenic (0.13 ± 0.04%), behenic (0.12 ± 0.04%), margaric (0.10 ± 0.00%), elaidic (0.03 ± 0.04%), and lauric (0.02 ± 0.08%) acids (Table 2).

Table 3 shows the total fiber, sugar profile, carbohydrates, and energy contents of the different cashew samples analyzed. Among sugars, sucrose was found with a mean of 6.3 ± 0.5 g/100 g. Total dietary fiber had an average content of 3.6 ± 0.2 g/100 g.

The energy profile showed a mean content of energy of 2525 ± 35.8 kJ/100 g (Table 3).

Sterol profile and content, amino acids, vitamins, and heavy metals

Table 4 describes the sterol profile and content of different cashew samples. Total sterols in fat were 286 ± 24 mg/100 g of fat. β-Sitosterol was the major component accounting for 83.3 ± 1.5% of total sterols

Table 2. Fatty acid profile and content, % weight of total fatty acids of the different cashew samples.

	Central West India—Goa origin	South West India—Kerala origin 1	South West India—Kerala origin 2	South East India—Panruti origin	Central East India—Andhra Pradesh origin	Central India—Maharashtra origin	Ivory Coast	Brazil	Viet Nam	Kenya	Mozambique	Mean	SD
Total fatty acid (g/100 g)	49.05	48.60	48.20	48.05	49.35	49.40	49.25	47.40	45.05	50.40	46.20	48.27	1.55
Fatty acid profile, % weight of total FA													
Saturated fatty acid	20.25	20.55	20.45	21.55	22.30	20.30	16.95	17.30	21.65	19.90	20.00	20.11	1.66
Monounsaturated fatty acid	60.90	61.65	61.50	60.65	60.75	60.20	64.95	65.40	60.85	62.05	60.70	61.78	1.76
Polyunsaturated fatty acid	18.65	17.60	17.85	17.65	16.75	19.30	17.95	17.10	17.25	17.90	19.10	17.92	0.81
Trans fatty acid	0.20	0.20	0.15	0.20	0.20	0.20	0.15	0.20	0.20	0.20	0.20	0.19	0.02
C12:0 Dodecanoic acid (lauric acid)	n/d	n/d	n/d	n/d	0.25	n/d	n/d	n/d	n/d	n/d	n/d	0.02	0.08
C16:0 Hexadecanoic acid (palmitic acid)	9.90	10.65	10.35	10.40	10.65	10.00	8.30	8.65	10.85	10.70	9.80	10.02	0.84
C16:1 Hexadecenoic acid (palmitoleic acid) (C16:1 n7)	0.40	0.40	0.40	0.40	0.40	0.40	0.40	0.40	0.40	0.50	0.40	0.41	0.03
C17:0 Heptadecanoic acid (margaric acid)	0.10	0.10	0.10	0.10	0.10	0.10	0.10	0.10	0.10	0.10	0.10	0.10	0.00
C18:0 Octadecanoic acid (stearic acid)	9.20	8.75	9.00	9.95	10.35	9.15	7.70	7.60	9.45	8.10	8.95	8.93	0.86
C18:1 Octadecenoic (oleic acid, w-9) (C18:1n9c)	59.80	60.55	60.50	59.60	59.75	59.15	63.80	64.25	59.80	60.85	59.65	60.70	1.72
Elaidic acid (C18:1n9t)	n/d	n/d	n/d	0.10	n/d	n/d	0.05	0.05	0.10	n/d	n/d	0.03	0.04
C18:1 (Vaccenic acid) (C18:1-11)	0.40	0.40	0.40	0.40	0.40	0.40	0.50	0.40	0.40	0.40	0.40	0.41	0.03
C18:2 Octadecadienoic acid (linoleic acid) (w-6)	18.50	17.50	17.70	17.50	16.65	19.15	17.80	16.95	17.10	17.70	18.90	17.77	0.79
C18:3 Octadecatrienoic acid (linolenic acid) (w-3)	0.10	0.10	0.10	0.15	0.10	0.10	0.10	0.15	0.10	0.20	0.20	0.13	0.04
C20:0 Eicosanoic acid (arachidic acid)	0.70	0.60	0.60	0.70	0.70	0.70	0.50	0.55	0.70	0.60	0.60	0.63	0.07
C20:1 Eicosenoic acid (gadoleic acid)	0.20	0.20	0.20	0.20	0.20	0.20	0.20	0.20	0.20	0.20	0.20	0.20	0.00
C22:0 Docosanoic acid (behenic acid)	0.20	0.10	0.10	0.10	0.10	0.10	0.10	0.10	0.20	0.10	0.10	0.12	0.04
C24:0 Tetracosanoic acid (lignoceric acid)	0.20	0.20	0.20	0.20	0.20	0.20	0.20	0.20	0.20	0.20	0.20	0.20	0.00

n/d: Not detected.

Table 3. Total energy content and carbohydrate composition of the different cashew samples.

	Central West India—Goa origin	South West India—Kerala origin 1	South West India—Kerala origin 2	South East India—Panruti origin	Central East India—Andhra Pradesh origin	Central India—Maharashtra origin	Ivory Coast	Brazil	Viet Nam	Kenya	Mozambique	Mean	SD
Total dietary fiber (g/100 g)	3.4	3.2	3.5	3.7	3.4	3.9	3.8	3.6	3.7	3.7	3.7	3.6	0.2
Sucrose (g/100 g)	6.3	6.1	6.0	6.4	5.8	6.0	6.3	7.3	6.8	5.7	6.6	6.3	0.5
Carbohydrate calculated (diff.) (g/100 g)	21.7	20.1	20.2	20.2	19.6	19.9	19.6	20.9	23.6	18.1	22.2	20.5	1.5
Energy (kJ/100 g)	2551	2531	2516	2542	2553	2545	2549	2482	2453	2566	2490	2525	35.8
Energy (kcal/100 g)	615	610	607	613	616	614	615	598	591	619	600	609	8.9

followed by δ-5-avenasterol with a 7.5 ± 1.1%, campesterol with a 6.2 ± 0.5%, cholesterol with 0.7 ± 0.4%, and δ-5,24-stigmastadienol with a 0.7 ± 0.3% of total sterols. On the other hand, 24-methylene-cholesterol with 0.13 ± 0.1% and δ-7-campesterol with 0.08 ± 0.15 were the sterols with lower concentration (Table 4).

Glutamic acid, with 4.60 ± 0.23 g/100 g, was the amino acid with the highest presence in all the samples, followed by arginine (2.22 ± 0.13 g/100 g), aspartic acid (1.89 ± 0.05 g/100 g), leucine (1.47 ± 0.09 g/100 g), and valine (1.12 ± 0.05 g/100 g). Cysteine + Cystine with 0.40 ± 0.02 g/100 g, methionine with 0.37 ± 0.01 g/100 g, and tryptophan with 0.31 ± 0.02 g/100 g were the amino acids with lower presence (Table 5).

With an average of 5.80 ± 1.0 mg/100 g, vitamin E (sum of tocopherols) was the most found vitamin in cashew samples. Vitamin B3 (total niacin) was the second one with 1.31 ± 0.19 mg/100 g and vitamin B5 the third with 0.77 ± 0.28 mg/100 g. Provitamin A with 7.63 ± 2.50 μg/100 g and vitamin B12 with 0.06 ± 0.04 μg/100 g were the vitamins with lowest amount found in the samples (Table 6).

Potassium with a mean value of 622 ± 59 mg/100 g was the most abundant mineral present in cashew samples, followed by phosphorus with 503 ± 50 mg/100 g, magnesium with 249 ± 12 mg/100 g, and calcium with 41 ± 10 mg/100 g. Sodium with 10.0 ± 3.2 mg/100 g, iron with 5.7 ± 1.1 mg/100 g, zinc with 5.3 ± 0.5 mg/100 g, and selenium with 0.039 ± 0.045 mg/100 g were the heavy metals with lower content (Table 7).

This is the first study analyzing the nutritional profile of cashew kernel samples from all the largest worldwide growing regions. Although we could observe differences among all samples, in general, the variance found between the nutritional compositions of the analyzed samples was not of great significance.

However, some important differences can be found between the nutritional estimates of our samples and those published by other authors in the literature. In 2010, Trox et al. reported a 66.21 ± 7.87 g/100 g mean content of total fat in nine cashew samples from Indonesia which is considerably higher than our findings 48.3 ± 1.6 g/100 g. None of our samples showed more than 50 g/100 g of total fat. In addition, a higher standard deviation is observed on their results in relation to the fat content. On the other hand, Venkatachalam and Sathe (2006) found slightly lower values for total fat content (43.71 ± 1.13 g/100 g) in three samples from US grocery stores, and Ryan et al. (2006) reported 40.4 ± 2.0 g/100 g (n = 3) of total fat in cashews from a local health food store in Cork (Ireland) which are the closest values to our findings. Differences related to the origin of the samples, the processes (storage and

Table 4. Sterol profile of the different cashew samples.

	Vietnamese cashew kernels	Indian cashew kernels Kerala origin	Brazilian cashew kernels	Ivory Coast cashew kernels	Mean	SD
Total sterols in fat (mg/kg fat)	3170	2700	2920	2640	2858	241
% Total sterols						
Cholesterol	0.40	0.60	0.50	0.40	0.48	0.10
24-methylene-cholesterol	<0.1	0.20	0.20	0.10	0.13	0.10
Campesterol	6.20	6.80	6.30	5.60	6.23	0.49
Stigmasterol	0.20	0.30	0.30	<0.1	0.20	0.06
δ-7-campesterol	<0.1	0.30	<0.1	<0.1	0.08	0.15
δ-5,23-stigmastadienol	1.20	<0.1	0.30	0.30	0.45	0.52
Chlerosterol	0.30	0.40	1.10	1.10	0.73	0.43
β-Sitosterol	83.90	82.30	81.80	85.10	83.28	1.51
Sitostanol	0.50	0.30	0.40	0.50	0.43	0.10
δ-5-avenasterol	6.50	8.60	8.30	6.70	7.53	1.08
δ-5,24-stigmastadienol	0.70	0.90	0.90	0.30	0.70	0.28

[Correction added on 15 December 2015, after first online publication: the word "Cholesterol" has been revised to "Chlerosterol" in Table 4, column 1, row 9.]

manipulation), and the methods used for lipid extraction for its gravity determination may explain these differences observed between studies.

Results on fatty acid composition expressed as percent on total FA were very similar to the previous mentioned studies. Ryan et al. (2006) who found 9 g/100 g less total FA than our results, found a mean concentration of 57.2 g/100 g of oleic acid (18:1), 20.8 g/100 g of linoleic acid (18:2), and 8.7 g/100 g of stearic acid (18:0), in front of 60.7 g/100 g, 17.8 g/100 g, and 8.9 g/100 g of total FA in our study. More closely, Venkatachalam and Sathe (2006) found 61.1 g/100 g, 16.9 g/100 g, and 9.3 g/100 g of total FA of the above FA.

Huge discrepancies in the results of the cashew's sterol content were found in the literature. Ryan et al. (2006) reported 1768.0 ± 210.6 mg/g of fat of β-sitosterol compared to our results of 2380 ± 4 mg/kg. The same occurred with the amount of campesterol reported, they found 105.3 ± 16.0 mg/g fat against 178 ± 1 mg/kg fat of our results, and of stigmasterol, 116.7 ± 12.6 mg/g fat in front of 5.72 ± 0.34 mg/kg fat in our study. Large differences were also observed between the results of Ryan et al. (2006) and ours in relation to the tocopherol content. Their results showed 57.2 ± 6.2 mg/g of γ-tocopherol, much higher than the 5.07 ± 1.06 mg/100 g found in our study. In relation to the α-tocopherol content, Ryan

Table 5. Amino acid profile of cashews of different origin.

	Vietnamese cashew kernels	Indian cashew kernels Kerala origin	Brazilian cashew kernels	Ivory Coast cashew kernels	Mean	SD
Amino acids g/100 g						
Alanine	0.812	0.792	0.846	0.810	0.815	0.023
Aspartic acid	1.900	1.850	1.960	1.860	1.893	0.050
Arginine	2.240	2.030	2.340	2.250	2.215	0.131
Cysteine + Cystine	0.396	0.381	0.394	0.429	0.400	0.020
Glutamic acid	4.580	4.320	4.890	4.600	4.598	0.233
Glycine	0.902	0.862	0.902	0.897	0.891	0.019
Histidine	0.475	0.454	0.471	0.471	0.468	0.009
Isoleucine	0.781	0.759	0.828	0.820	0.797	0.033
Leucine	1.440	1.390	1.590	1.470	1.473	0.085
Lysine	0.974	0.924	1.000	0.984	0.971	0.033
Methionine	0.377	0.352	0.367	0.381	0.369	0.013
Phenylalanine	0.916	0.880	0.990	0.945	0.933	0.047
Proline	0.767	0.715	0.753	0.759	0.749	0.023
Serine	1.090	1.050	1.190	1.090	1.105	0.060
Tryptophan (total)	0.307	0.300	0.322	0.337	0.317	0.016
Tyrosine	0.616	0.570	0.691	0.638	0.629	0.050
Valine	1.110	1.060	1.170	1.120	1.115	0.045
Threonine	0.704	0.701	0.813	0.729	0.737	0.052

Table 6. Vitamin profile of cashews of different origin.

	Unit	Vietnamese cashew kernels	Indian cashew kernels Kerala origin	Brazilian cashew kernels	Ivory Coast cashew kernels	Mean	SD
Vitamin B1	mg/100 g	0.426	0.487	0.369	0.624	0.477	0.110
Vitamin B12	μg/100 g	0.073	0.038	0.111	0.025	0.062	0.039
Vitamin C (ascorbic acid + dehydroascorbic acid)	mg/100 g	<5 (LOQ)	0.500	<0.5	<0.5	0.125	0.250
Vitamin B2—riboflavin	mg/100 g	0.029	0.030	0.020	0.034	0.028	0.006
Vitamin B5—pantothenic acid, microbiological (mg/100 g)	mg/100 g	0.519	0.577	0.872	1.120	0.772	0.279
Vitamin B8—biotin, microbiological	μg/100 g	61.100	34.100	16.300	22.900	33.600	19.751
Vitamin B9—total folate, microbiological	μg/100 g	35.400	33.400	42.500	45.200	39.125	5.626
Vitamin E (tocopherol profile)							
Vitamin E (α-tocopherol)	mg/100 g	0.850	0.289	0.384	0.289	0.453	0.268
Vitamin E (γ-tocopherol)	mg/100 g	3.720	6.210	5.510	4.840	5.070	1.060
δ-Tocopherol	mg/100 g	0.572	0.701	<0.5	<0.5	0.318	0.371
Sum of tocopherols	mg/100 g	4.970	7.200	5.890	5.130	5.798	1.017
Vitamin B6	mg/100 g	0.389	0.414	0.255	0.511	0.392	0.106
Vitamin B3 (total niacin)	mg/100 g	1.180	1.140	1.400	1.530	1.313	0.185
β-Carotene fat containing samples provitamin A	μg/100 g	5.350	5.590	9.950	9.630	7.630	2.499
Vitamin K1	μg/100 g	5.350	16.500	25.000	14.200	15.263	8.077

et al. (2006) reported 3.6 ± 1.4 mg/g fat, an amount also higher than in our study, 0.453 ± 0.268 mg/100 g.

The amount of γ-tocopherol (1.10 ± 0.12 mg/100 g) and α-tocopherol (0.29 ± 0.04 mg/100 g) reported by Trox et al. (2010) was similar to that found in our study.

Considerable differences in the amino acid composition were also found from previous studies. In 2007, Adeyeye et al. showed approximately 30% lower amount of amino acids than in our study with the highest differences in proline (0.82 g/100 g crude protein found by Adeyeye et al. [2007], in front of 3.514 g/100 g crude protein found in our study), and threonine contents (1.694 g/100g crude protein found by Adeyeye et al. and 3.459 g/100g crude protein found in our study, respectively). However, slight differences were found in the amino acid profile between the Venkatachalam and Sathe (2006) study and our results.

Among vitamins, the amount of tocopherol content reported by Ryan et al. (2006) was much higher than that found in our study, showing our findings 0.453 mg/100 g of α-tocopherol in front of 360 mg/100 g of oil found by Ryan et al. and 5.07 mg/100 g against 5720 mg/100 g of oil for γ-tocopherol, respectively. Trox et al. (2010) found 0.29 mg/100 g of α-tocopherol and 1.10 mg/100 g of γ-tocopherol. In 2006 Kornsteiner et al. showed 5.1 mg/100g extracted oil for the sum of β- and γ-tocopherol. Our results on β-carotene were close to the ones found for Trox et al. (2010) (9.57 μg/100 g).

Several differences were also found in mineral composition between our study and others previously published.

Table 7. Mineral profile in cashew of different origins.

	Vietnamese cashew kernels	Indian cashew kernels Kerala origin	Brazilian cashew kernels	Ivory Coast cashew kernels	Mean	SD
Iron (mg/100 g)	6.1	4.5	5.1	7.1	5.7	1.1
Zinc (mg/100 g)	4.9	5.5	5.0	5.9	5.3	0.5
Sodium (mg/100 g)	8.3	11.0	14.0	6.6	10.0	3.2
Potassium (mg/100 g)	660.0	620.0	540.0	670.0	622.5	59.1
Magnesium (mg/100 g)	240.0	250.0	240.0	265.0	248.8	11.8
Calcium (mg/100 g)	38.0	46.0	28.0	52.0	41.0	10.4
Phosphorus (mg/100 g)	460.0	510.0	470.0	570.0	502.5	49.9
Selenium (mg/100 g)	<0.2	0.08	0.075	<0.2	0.04	0.04

Compared to our study, Fagbemi (2008) reported in cashew nut flours higher amounts of sodium (19.1 vs. 10.0 mg/100 g), phosphorus (509.8 vs. 502.5 mg/100 g), zinc (8.3 vs. 5.3 mg/100 g), and iron (15.8 vs. 5.7 mg/100 g); and lower amounts of calcium (12.8 vs. 41.0 mg/100 g), potassium (466.8 vs. 622.5 mg/100 g), magnesium (172.2 vs. 248.8 mg/100 g), and selenium (0.0024 vs. 0.04 mg/100 g). On the other hand, compared to the present study, Ijarotimi et al. (2012) reported lower amounts of potassium, magnesium, phosphorus, zinc, and iron and higher amounts of sodium and calcium in cashew nut flour.

The differences observed between studies could be explained from the different methodology used in each study. Nevertheless, most of our results were consistent with the previous published studies. The differences found among samples from different producing regions were not of great significance and could be the result of the soil composition in each area, the climate conditions, and the genetic evolution of the trees in each region (Cheng et al. 2014; Giorgi et al. 2010; Ahmed et al., 2014). Therefore, the nutritional composition of raw cashew kernels is very similar to whatever its growth region. Raw cashew kernels shows equilibrate and high nutritional composition, full of healthy fats and considerable amounts of sterols, amino acids, vitamins, and minerals that have been considered to have beneficial effect on health (Wight et al. 2012; Gupta and Prakash 2014; Ras et al. 2014; Agnew-Blais et al. 2015).

Cashew nuts represent a good source of unsaturated FA, fiber, sterols, vitamins, and amino acids whatever its grown region, suggesting that their intake contribute to the widely known beneficial roles in health of these nutrients.

One of the limitations of our study is that the determination of total dietary fiber, sugars, protein, lipid profile, salt, and energy contents was carried out in 11 cashew samples from different origins by duplicate and the analysis of the sterol profile and amino acid, vitamin, and mineral content were just conducted in only four samples of different origins with only one determination for each analysis, which limits the reproducibility of our results. However, this is the first study where all the determinations were carried with samples from the worldwide most important growing regions, which makes a much better approximation of the real nutrition content of raw cashew kernels.

Acknowledgments

We thank African Cashew Alliance, Olam International, The Cashew Export Promotion Council of India (CEPCI), Sindicato das Indústrias de Beneficiamento de Castanha de Caju e Amêndoas Vegetais do Estado do Ceará (SINDICAJU), The Richard Franco Agency, Inc., and Vietnam Cashew Association for providing the cashew samples.

Conflict of Interest

Jordi Salas-Salvadó serves at the INC World Forum for Nutrition Research and Dissemination and has received grant support from the International Nut and Dried Fruit Council. Mònica Bulló has received a grant support for one of her projects from the American Pistachio Growers and Paramount Frams (USA). Ricardo Rico received grant support from the International Nut and Dried Fruit Council.

References

Adeyeye, E. I., S. S. Asaolu, and A. O. Aluko. 2007. Amino acid composition of two masticatory nuts (Cola acuminate and Garcinia kola) and a snack nut (*Anacardium occidentale*). Int. J. Food Sci. Nutr. 58:241–249.

Agnew-Blais, J. C., S. Wassertheil-Smoller, J. H. Kang, P. E. Hogan, L. H. Coker, L. G. Snetselaar, et al. 2015. Folate., vitamin B-6., and vitamin B-12 intake and mild cognitive impairment and probable dementia in the women's health initiative memory study. J. Acad. Nutr. Diet. 115:231–241.

Ahmed, S. O., A. W. Abdalla, T. Inoue, A. Ping, and E. E. Babiker. 2014. Nutritional quality of grains of sorghum cultivar grown under different levels of micronutrients fertilization. Food Chem. 159:374–380.

Aiyadurai, S. G. 1966. A review of Research on Spices and Cashew nut in India. *Agriculture Commission, Government of India, Indian Council of Agriculture Research.*

Asogwa, E. U., L. A. Hammed, and T. C. N. Ndubuaku. 2008. Integrated production and protection practices of cashew (*Anacardium occidentale*) in Nigeria. Afr. J. Biotechnol. 7:4868–4873.

Bes-Rastrollo, M., N. M. Wedick, M. A. Martinez-Gonzalez, T. Y. Li, L. Sampson, and F. B. Hu. 2009. Prospective study of nut consumption., long-term weight change and obesity risk in women. Am. J. Clin. Nutr. 89:1913–1919.

Carey, A. N., S. M. Poulose, and B. Shukitt-Hale. 2012. The beneficial effects of tree nuts on the aging brain. Nutr. Aging 1:55–67.

Cheng, G., Y. N. He, T. X. Yue, J. Wang, and Z. W. Zhang. 2014. Effects of climatic conditions and soil properties on cabernet sauvignon berry growth and anthocyanin profiles. Molecules 19:13683–13703.

Davis, K.. 1999. Cashew echo technical note. Available at http://c.ymcdn.com/sites/members.echocommunity.org/resource/collection/49b3d109-0de9-458e-915b-11aaf1a67e20/Cashew.pdf?hhSearchTerms=%22cashew+and+echo+and+technical+and+note%22.

Davis, L., W. Stonehouse, T. du Loots, J. Mukuddem-Petersen, F. H. van der Westhuizen, S. M. Hanekom, et al. 2007. The effects of high walnut and cashew nut diets on the antioxidant status of subjects with metabolic syndrome. Eur. J. Nutr. 46:155–164.

Estruch, R., E. Ros, M. I. Covas, D. Corella, F. Arós, E. Gómez-Gracia, et al. 2013. Primary prevention of cardiovascular disease with a Mediterranean diet. N. Engl. J. Med. 368:1279–1290.

Fagbemi, T. N. 2008. The influence of processing techniques on the energy, ash properties and elemental composition of cashew nut (Anacardiumoccidentale Linn). Nutri. Food Sci. 38:136–145.

Fernández-Montero, A., M. Bes-Rastrollo, J. J. Beunza, M. T. Barrio-Lopez, C. de la Fuente-Arrillaga, L. Moreno-Galarraga, et al. 2013. Nut consumption and incidence of metabolic syndrome after 6-year follow-up: the SUN (Seguimiento Universidad de Navarra., University of Navarra Follow-up) cohort. Public Health Nutr. 16:2064–2072.

Flores-Mateo, G., D. Rojas-Rueda, J. Basora, E. Ros, and J. Salas-Salvadó. 2013. Nut intake and adiposity: meta-analysis of clinical trials. Am. J. Clin. Nutr. 97:1346–1355.

Giorgi, A., M. Madeo, G. Speranza, and M. Cocucci. 2010. Influence of environmental factors on composition of phenolic antioxidants of Achillea collina Becker ex Rchb. Nat. Prod. Res. 24:1546–1559.

Gupta, C., and D. Prakash. 2014. Phytonutrients as therapeutic agents. J. Comp. Integr. Med. 11:151–169.

Herbison, C. E., S. Hickling, K. L. Allen, T. A. O'Sullivan, M. Robinson, A. P. Bremner, et al. 2012. Low intake of B-vitamins is associated with poor adolescent mental health and behavior. Prev. Med. 55:634–638.

Ijarotimi, O. S., I. B. Oluwalana, and M. O. Ogunedojutimi. 2012. Nutrient composition., functional., sensory and microbial status of popcorn-based (*Zea may* everta) complementary foods enriched with cashew nut (anacardiumoccidentale l.) flour. Afr. J. Food Agri. Nutri. Dev. 12:6424–6446.

Kendall, C. W., A. Esfahani, A. R. Josse, L. S. Augustin, E. Vidgen, and D. J. Jenkins. 2011. The glycemic effect of nut-enriched meals in healthy and diabetic subjects. Nutr. Metab. Cardiovasc. Dis. 21(Suppl 1):S34–S39.

Kornsteiner, M., K.-H. Wagner, and I. Elmadfa. 2006. Tocopherols and total phenolics in 10 different nut types. Food Chem. 98:381–387.

Kris-Etherton, P. M., F. B. Hu, E. Ros, and J. Sabate. 2008. The role of tree nuts and peanuts in the prevention of coronary heart disease: multiple potential mechanisms. J. Nutr. 138:1746S–1751S.

Mitjavila, M. T., M. Fandos, J. Salas-Salvadó, M. I. Covas, S. Borrego, R. Estruch, et al. 2013. The Mediterranean diet improves the systemic lipid and DNA oxidative damage in metabolic syndrome individuals. A randomized, controlled, trial. Clin. Nutr. 32:172–178.

Ras, R. T., J. M. Geleijnse, and E. A. Trautwein. 2014. LDL-cholesterol-lowering effect of plant sterols and stanols across different dose ranges: a meta-analysis of randomised controlled studies. Br. J. Nutr. 112:214–219.

Rivas, A., A. Romero, M. Mariscal-Arcas, C. Monteagudo, B. Feriche, M. L. Lorenzo, et al. 2013. Mediterranean diet and bone mineral density in two age groups of women. Int. J. Food Sci. Nutr. 64:155–161.

Ros, E., L. C. Tapsell, and J. Sabate. 2010. Nuts and berries for heart health. Curr. Atheroscler Rep. 12:397–406.

Ryan, E., K. Galvin, T. P. O'Connor, A. R. Maguire, and N. M. O'Brien. 2006. Fatty acid profile., tocopherol., squalene and phytosterol content of Brazil., pecan., pine., pistachio and cashew nuts. Int. J. Food Sci. Nutr. 57:219–228.

Sanhueza, C., L. Ryan, and D. R. Foxcroft. 2013. Diet and the risk of unipolar depression in adults: systematic review of cohort studies. J. Hum. Nutr. Diet. 26:56–70.

Shobha, S. V., P. R. Krishnaswamy, and B. Ravindranath. 1992. Phenolic lipid composition during development of cashew. Phytochem 31:2295–2297.

Trox, J., V. Vadivel, W. Vetter, W. Stuetz, V. Scherbaum, U. Gola, et al. 2010. Bioactive compounds in cashew nut (*Anacardium occidentale* L.) kernels: effect of different shelling methods. J. Agric. Food Chem. 58:5341–5346.

Venkatachalam, M., and S. K. Sathe. 2006. Chemical composition of selected edible nut seeds. J. Agric. Food Chem. 54:4705–4714.

Wight, R. D., C. A. Tull, M. W. Deel, B. L. Stroope, A. G. Eubanks, J. A. Chavis, et al. 2012. Resveratrol effects on astrocyte function: relevance to neurodegenerative diseases. Biochem. Biophys. Res. Commun. 426:112–115.

13

Effect of green Spanish-style Manzanilla packaging conditions on the prevalence of the putative probiotic bacteria *Lactobacillus pentosus* TOMC-LAB2

Francisco Rodríguez-Gómez, Verónica Romero-Gil, Pedro García-García, Francisco Noé Arroyo-López & Antonio Garrido-Fernández

Food Biotechnology Department, Instituto de la Grasa (Agencia Estatal Consejo Superior de Investigaciones Científicas, CSIC) Campus Pablo de Olavide, Building 46. Ctra. Utrera, km 1., 41013 Seville, Spain

Keywords
Lactic acid bacteria, packaging conditions, probiotic, table olives, yeasts

Correspondence
Francisco Noé Arroyo-López, Food Biotechnology Department, Instituto de la Grasa (Agencia Estatal Consejo Superior de Investigaciones Científicas CSIC), Campus Pablo de Olavide, Building 46. Ctra. Utrera km 1, 41013 Seville, Spain.

E-mail: fnarroyo@cica.es

Funding Information
The research leading to these results has received funding from the EU's Seventh Framework Program (FP7/2007-2013) under grant agreement n°243471 (PROBIOLIVES) and the Junta de Andalucía (through financial support to group AGR-125).

Abstract

This work focuses on the persistence of the putative probiotic bacteria *Lactobacillus pentosus* TOMC-LAB2 on green Spanish-style Manzanilla olives according to different packaging conditions and storage temperatures. The lactic acid bacteria population decreased with time but the highest survival counts (and lowest yeasts) at the end of storage (8 months) were observed in plastic pouches under nitrogen atmosphere and glass jars with brine stored at 20°C. Molecular techniques showed a 100% presence of the putative probiotic bacteria in biofilms adhered to olive epidermis, while it was absent in PPB (plastic pouches with brine) and in olives stored at 7°C. No changes in NaCl, pH or combined acidity were observed during the storage except for a slight increase in titratable acidity at 20°C. The color of the fruits was stable but degraded at 20°C for olives in plastic pouches with brine.

Introduction

The production of green Spanish-style table olive is a traditional process which is usually achieved by spontaneous fermentation at ambient temperature. The main group of microorganism involved in the fermentation process is LAB (lactic acid bacteria), but yeasts are always present throughout processing (Garrido-Fernández et al. 1997; Arroyo-López et al. 2012a). In general, the genus *Lactobacillus* is recognized as the most characteristic of the indigenous LAB involved in green Spanish-style fermentation (Hurtado et al. 2012; Doulgeraki et al. 2013). On the contrary, the most frequent yeast genera isolated from table olive processing have been *Candida, Pichia, Debaryomyces*, and *Saccharomyces* (Arroyo-López et al. 2012a; Botta and Cocolin 2012).

Table olives were a convenient carrier for delivering probiotic bacteria to humans (Lavermicocca et al. 2005)

and their abilities in this aspect are comprehensively discussed in a recent review (Peres et al. 2012). Initial studies were based on the adhesion and survival of non-native lactobacilli and bifidobacteria species. In this way, *Lactobacillus paracasei* IMPC2.1 (isolated from humans) had a lengthy survival on olives and could be recovered from the fecal samples of consumers (Lavermicocca et al. 2005). This organism survived in olive fermentations but olives showed a considerably genetic diversity of LAB species (De Bellis et al. 2010). However, autochthonous microorganisms may also colonize the olives during fermentation and, in principle, due to their origin, have a major survival and imposition (Nychas et al. 2002). The formation of bacteria-yeast communities (true biofilms) on Gordal olives during fermentation has been described (Domínguez-Manzano et al. 2012). Several LAB strains selected by their potential probiotic characteristics not only fermented the olives but formed mixed biofilms (composed of LAB and yeasts) on Manzanilla olives (Arroyo-López et al. 2012b; Bautista-Gallego et al. 2013). Further studies reported that inoculation assured a favorable competition with the wild strains but did not guarantee per se the complete imposition (Rodríguez-Gómez et al. 2013). Blana et al. (2014) has reported high colonization (80–90%) of *Lactobacillus pentosus* B281 and B282 at 8% NaCl but the second was unable to establish on the olive surface. In heat-shocked olives, the former exhibited higher percentages of recovery (Argyri et al. 2014). Other examples on the use of starter cultures for the production of probiotic vegetables are sauerkraut, Irish brassica, or cereal-based substrates (Charalampopoulus et al. 2003; Verganović et al. 2011; Jaiswal et al. 2012).

But not only the survival and imposition of the probiotic LAB in the polymicrobial biofilms at the end of the fermentative process is important, but also its presence at the end of the storage and packaging. The effect of packaging material, storage conditions, or the food/LAB relationships may affect the functional efficacy (Ranadhera et al. 2010; Rodríguez-Gómez et al. 2015). Natural black Conservolea olives packaged in polyethylene pouches showed a high heterogeneity among LAB but the species were, as usual, *L. pentosus* and *Lactobacillus platarum*. The composition of the packaging atmosphere (aerobic or modified) influenced the yeast activity of natural black Conservolea olives packaged in polyethylene pouches (Doulgeraki et al. 2012). The putative probiotic *L. pentosus* TOMC-LAB2 strain showed a high survival for a long period of time (>6 months) in fortified green Spanish-style olives (Rodríguez-Gómez et al. 2014a). However, scarce work has been carried out with the objective of linking the olive biofilm formed during fermentation to the microbial population at the end of larger periods of the packaged products, although this information is essential for producing probiotic olives by controlled fermentation which guarantees, after the adequate packaging conditions, the delivering of the potential functional LAB to consumers.

Therefore, the objective of the present work was to study the changes in the polymicrobial biofilms formed during fermentation (and particularly the presence of the putative probiotic bacteria *L. pentosus* TOMC-LAB2, henceforth LAB2), throughout a lengthy storage of packaged green Spanish-style Manzanilla table olives, according to different packaging conditions and storage temperature. The level of imposition of the bacterium at the end of this period was also analyzed. In addition, the evolution during storage of the physicochemical characteristics of brines and the olive color of the previously LAB2-fermented products were also monitored. The results can contribute to improving information about the changes that the microbial population adhered to olives during fermentation may suffer from packaging until the product reaches the consumer. Eventually, they may also help to redesign current packaging practices or to develop new specific technologies to produce probiotic olives.

Materials and Methods

Selected olives

The olives used in this study were from the Manzanilla cultivar, fermented as Spanish-style during the 2010/2011 season using LAB2 as starter culture. The characteristics of the fermentations have been described elsewhere (Rodríguez-Gómez et al. 2014b). After fermentation, fruits were manually selected to separate defective olives, washed with sterile water to remove the microbial load not integrated into the olive biofilm, and finally packaged according to the conditions described below.

Packaging conditions

Packaging was achieved in GJB (glass jars with brine), plastic pouches (composed of a high barrier polyester and polyethylene with a thickness of 109 μm and oxygen permeability of less than 8.5 $cm^3/m^2/24$ h, SP Group, Villarrubia, Spain) with brine (PPB), or plastic pouches under N_2 atmosphere without brine (PPN). These packaging conditions were selected due to their promising behavior in previous studies on overall LAB survival during packaging (Rodríguez-Gómez et al. 2015); however, a longer study and the presence of the inoculated strain in the final product require further confirmation. The GJB containers were filled with 125 g of olives and 125 mL of sterile brine. The PPB pouches were filled with 75 g olives which were covered with 75 mL of sterile brine. The PPN pouches were filled with 75 g olives and 30% of its displaced free volume replaced with N_2. Plastic pouches were closed manually using a Tecnotrip mod EVT7G (Terrassa, Spain) closing machine.

In this work, the physicochemical conditions developed by Borbolla y Alcalá and González Pellissó (1972) for long-term green Spanish-style table olive preservation and the limits established in the Trade Standard Applying to Table Olives (IOC, 2004) for packaging of this product were used. Accordingly, the equilibrium concentrations were fixed at 5 g NaCl 100 mL^{-1} and 0.5 g lactic acid 100 mL^{-1}. The use of the minimum allowed salt level is compulsory due to the LAB sensitivity to salt (Romero-Gil et al. 2013). Before packaging, the cover brines were sterilized (121°C, 15 psi for 15 min) to prevent any contamination of the packaged olive microbiota. Olives packaged under nitrogen atmosphere were previously equilibrated at the above-mentioned conditions in sterilized glass containers stored for 20 days in a cold-storage room at 7°C. Packaged olives from all treatments (GJB, PPB, and PPN) were divided into two sublots which were stored at 7 ± 1°C (to mimic conditions prevailing during a possible distribution of the product throughout a cold chain) and 20 ± 2°C (for mimicking distribution at environmental temperature). Therefore, the experiment consisted of a full factorial design with a total of six treatments (3 packaging methods × 2 storage temperatures). Duplicated samples from each treatment were periodically withdrawn (without replacement) during 8 months.

Microbiological analysis

Brine samples were diluted, if necessary, in a sterile saline solution (0.9 g 100 mL^{-1} NaCl) and plated using a Spiral System model dwScientific (Dow Whitley Scientific Limited, Shipley, West Yorkshire, England) on appropriate media. *Enterobacteriaceae* were counted on Crystal-violet Neutral-Red bile glucose agar (Merck, Darmstadt, Germany), LAB were spread onto de Man-Rogosa and Sharpe agar (Oxoid, Cambridge, UK) supplemented with 0.02% (wt/vol) sodium azide (Sigma, St. Luis, MO), and yeasts were grown on a YM (yeast–malt–peptone–glucose medium) agar (Difco, Becton and Dickinson Company, Sparks, MD) supplemented with oxytetracycline and gentamicin sulfate (0.005%, wt/vol) as selective agents for yeasts. The plates were incubated at 30°C for 24 *(Enterobacteriaceae)* or 72 h (yeasts and LAB) and counted using a CounterMat v.3.10 (IUL, Barcelona, Spain) image analysis system. Brine counts were expressed as $\log_{10}$ CFU mL^{-1}.

The microbial population dynamics on olives was followed by determining the microorganisms adhered to the olive epidermis, using the enzymatic protocol developed by Böckelmann et al. (2003) for the detachment of biofilms. Briefly, three fruits from each packaging vessel were randomly taken and washed for 1 h with 250 mL of a sterile PBS buffer solution. Then, the olives were transferred to 50 mL of a PBS solution with the following enzymes: 14.8 mg L^{-1} lipase (L3126), 12.8 mg L^{-1} β-galactosidase (G-5160), and 21 μL L^{-1} α-glucosidase (G-0660) (Sigma-Aldrich, St. Louis, MO). To achieve biofilm disintegration and removal of the adhered cells, the fruits were incubated at 30°C in this enzyme cocktail with slight shaking (150 rpm). After 12 h, the olives were removed and the resulting suspension was centrifuged at 9000 × g for 10 min at 4°C. Finally, the pellet was resuspended in 2 mL of PBS and spread onto the different culture media described above. Olive counts were expressed as $\log_{10}$ CFU $olive^{-1}$. Expression in other units can easily be achieved considering an average (obtained from 50 fruits) weight of 4.08 ± 0.46 g and an olive surface of 10.99 ± 1.01 cm^2 per fruit.

The analyses were performed, in duplicate (two packages) and simultaneously, for brines and olives from each treatments at 0, 60, 120, 180, and 240 days (8 months).

Characterization of the lactic acid bacteria population

For characterization of the lactobacilli population, repetitive bacterial DNA element fingerprinting analysis (rep-PCR) with primer GTG_5 was followed (Gevers et al. 2001). The PCR reaction in a final volume of 25 μL contained: 5 μL of 5× MyTaq reaction buffer (5 mmol L^{-1} dNTPs and 15 mmol L^{-1} $MgCl_2$), 0.1 μL of My Taq DNA polymerase (Bioline reactives, London, United Kingdom), 1 μL GTG_5 primer (25 μm), 13.9 μL deionized H_20, and 5 μL DNA (~20 ng μL^{-1}). PCR amplification was carried out in a thermal cycler (Master Cycler Pro; Eppendorf, Hamburg, Germany) with the following program: 95°C for 5 min as initial step, plus 30 cycles at: (1) 95°C for 30 sec; (2) annealing at 40°C for 30 sec; and (3) 65°C for 8 min, with a final step of 65°C for 16 min to conclude the amplification. This methodology was used to determine the recovery frequency of the LAB2 strain at the end of packaging. Firstly, the repeatability of the technique was determined using the same LAB2 strain as the internal control, obtaining 86.9 ± 3.4% of reproducibility (data not shown). Then, diverse isolates (a total of 20) were randomly picked from each treatment at the end of the experiment (8 months), making a total of 120 lactobacilli to analyze (60 isolates at 7°C and 60 isolates at 20°C). They were named according to packaging treatment (GJB, PPB, or PPN). Their pattern profiles of bands (from 100 up to 3000 bp) were compared with the strain used to inoculate initially the fermentation process (LAB2). For this purpose, the PCR products were electrophoresed in a 2% (wt/vol) agarose gel and visualized under ultraviolet light by staining with ethidium bromide. The resulting fingerprints were digitally captured and analyzed with the BioNumerics 6.6 software package (Applied Maths, Kortrijk, Belgium). The similarity among digitalized profiles was calculated using the Pearson product-moment correlation coefficient. Dendrograms were obtained by means of the UPGMA (Unweighted Pair Group Method using the Arithmetic Average) clustering algorithm and the automatic calibration tool for the determination of the optimization and curve smoothing parameters.

Physicochemical analyses

The analyses of cover brines for pH, salt concentration (g NaCl 100 mL^{-1} brine), titratable (expressed as g lactic acid 100 mL^{-1} brine), and combined acidities (expressed as milliequivalents of HCl added to 1 L brine to reach pH 2.6) were carried out using the standard methods developed for table olives (Garrido-Fernández et al. 1997). Each parameter was measured in duplicate and the average recorded.

The firmness of olives was measured at the beginning and at the end of the storage using a Kramer shear compression cell coupled to an Instron Universal Machine (Canton, MA). The crosshead speed was 200 mm min^{-1}. The firmness, expressed as N 100 g^{-1} flesh, was the mean of ten replicate measurements, each of which was performed on three pitted olives.

The instrumental surface color of the fruits was measured using a BYK-Gadner Model 9000 Colour View Spectrophotometer (Silver Spring, MD). Any interference from stray light was minimized by covering the samples with a box, which had a matt black interior. Color was expressed as CI (Colour Index) calculated according to (Sánchez-Gómez et al. 1985):

$$\mathrm{CI} = \frac{-2 * R_{560} + R_{590} + 4 * R_{635}}{3},$$

where R stands for the reflectance at 560, 590, and 635 nm, respectively. Olive color was also determined in terms of the CIE L^*, a^*, b^* parameters. Results were the average of 10 measurements.

Statistical data analysis

Comparisons among variable levels were obtained after General Linear model (GLM) analysis by Least Significant Difference. In the graphs, average means with nonoverlapping confident limits are significantly different at a probability level of $P < 0.05$. Data analysis was carried out using Statistica 8.0 software package (StatSoft Inc, Tulsa, OK).

Results

Microbial population changes

The evolution of the microbial load on olives as a function of time was studied for the three packaging conditions assayed while the changes in brines were monitored only for the GJB and PPB treatments (Figs. 1, 2). On olives, there was a general decrease in the LAB and yeast populations with significant effects due to temperature and packaging conditions on specific sampling points (Fig. 1). The greatest survival of LAB populations on olives was achieved at 20°C with only limited (although significant in some cases) differences among packaging conditions (Fig. 1A, right). Interestingly, at this temperature, PPN had the highest significant population levels at the end of the study (Fig. 1A, right). Overall, changes in LAB population moved from 7.77 ± 0.02 $\log_{10}$ CFU $olive^{-1}$ (at the onset of the experiment) to 5.86 ± 0.50 (PPB) or 6.78 ± 0.23 $\log_{10}$ CFU $olive^{-1}$ (PPN) (after 8 month storage). Hence, storage at 20°C led to a fairly good LAB population survival on olives, particularly in PPN packaging where the counts only decreased 1 log cycle after an 8-month storage (a lengthy period for probiotic olives, and tested in this work for the first time). On the contrary, the decrease was higher at 7°C (Fig. 1A, left), particularly in PPB which showed markedly significant and the lowest averages during the central period of the storage. At this temperature, the olives packaged in PPN also had the best behavior and its curve was, in general, above those of the other packaging conditions (Fig. 1A, left). Therefore, in general, the greatest LAB survival was observed when olives were stored at 20°C, particularly in PPN packaging (only 1 $\log_{10}$ cycle decrease), followed by GJB and PPB (2 $\log_{10}$ cycle decrease).

There was also a marked decrease in the yeast populations on olives (Fig. 1B). At 20°C, the decrease observed in olives packaged in PPN or GJB was very marked and sharp, while in PPB the reduction was moderate and similar to that shown at 7°C (Fig. 1B, right). At 7°C, the decrease was noticeably significant, regardless of packaging methods, but the population stabilized during the last storage period at levels between 5.0 (PPN) and 4.0 $\log_{10}$ CFU $olive^{-1}$ (GJB and PPB) (Fig. 1B, left). Apparently, there was an apparent inverse relationship between LAB and yeast survival at 20°C which depended on the packaging method. However, the same effect was hardly appreciable at 7°C (Fig. 1B, left) probably because this temperature was more stressing for LAB than for yeasts. Therefore, LAB population survival was better preserved at 20°C but at the expense of a lower yeast population; on the contrary, LAB survival was lower at 7°C and its decrease propitiated a higher yeast survival in the long run.

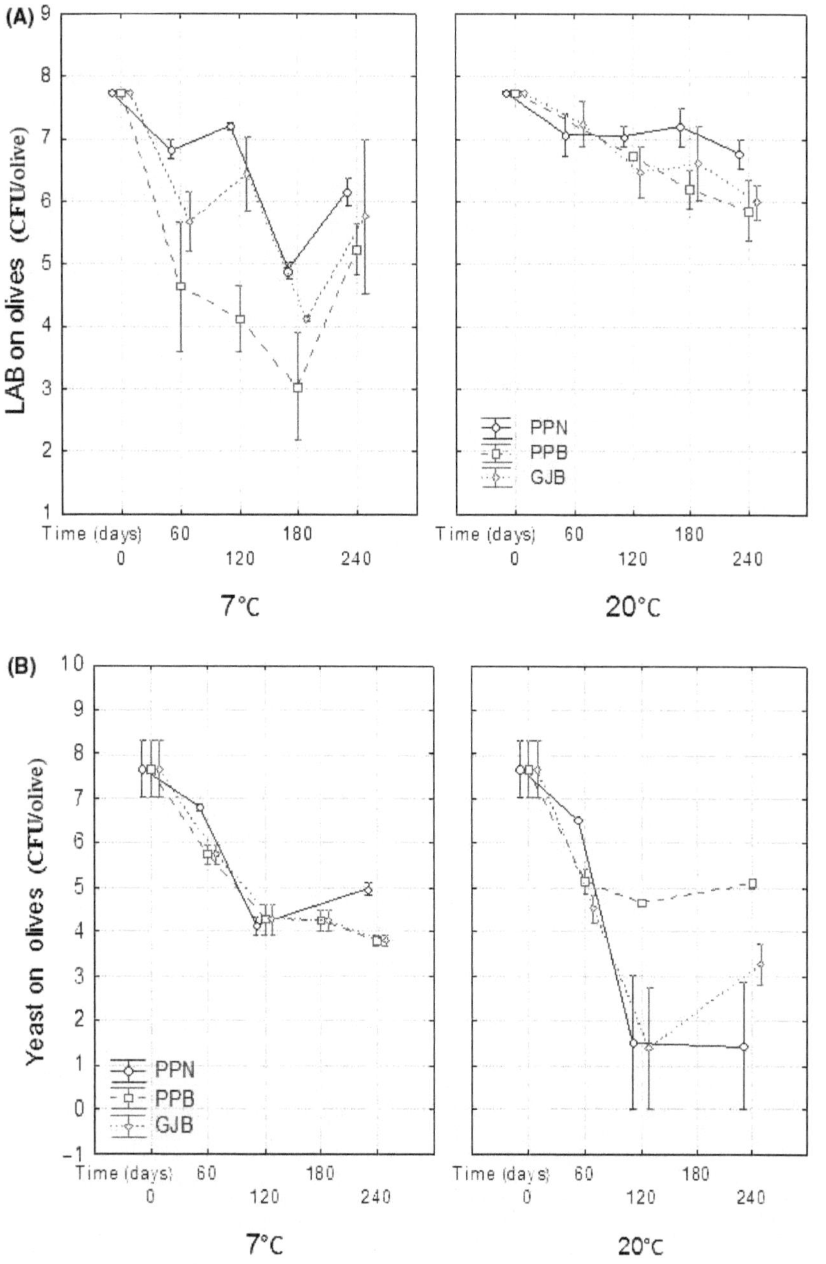

Figure 1. Lactic acid bacteria (panel A) and yeast (panel B) average (n = 2) changes on olive biofilm as a function of time, according to packaging conditions. GJB, packaging in glass jars with brine; PPB, packaging in plastic pouches with brine; PPN, packaging in plastic pouches under nitrogen atmosphere; weighted means; vertical bars denote ± standard errors.

In brines, LAB and yeasts were initially below the detection limits due to the initial sterilization of the packaging brine; later, LAB and yeasts from the olive biofilm were released into the brine, and their populations increased progressively with a significant effect due to packaging conditions and temperature (Fig. 2). The LAB increase was faster and reached higher average populations at 20°C than at 7°C, except at the end of the storage; in most of the sampling points GJB brines also showed the greatest average population (Fig. 2A). On the contrary, the yeasts increased faster and reached their highest initial populations at 7°C, particularly in PPB (Fig. 2B). Therefore, the same opposed behavior between LAB and yeast populations described on olives was also observed in brine; a slower increase in LAB and lower populations led to faster increase and higher populations of yeasts. The effect was particularly evident at 7°C where the LAB increase was rather slow (mainly in PPB) and reached lower averages

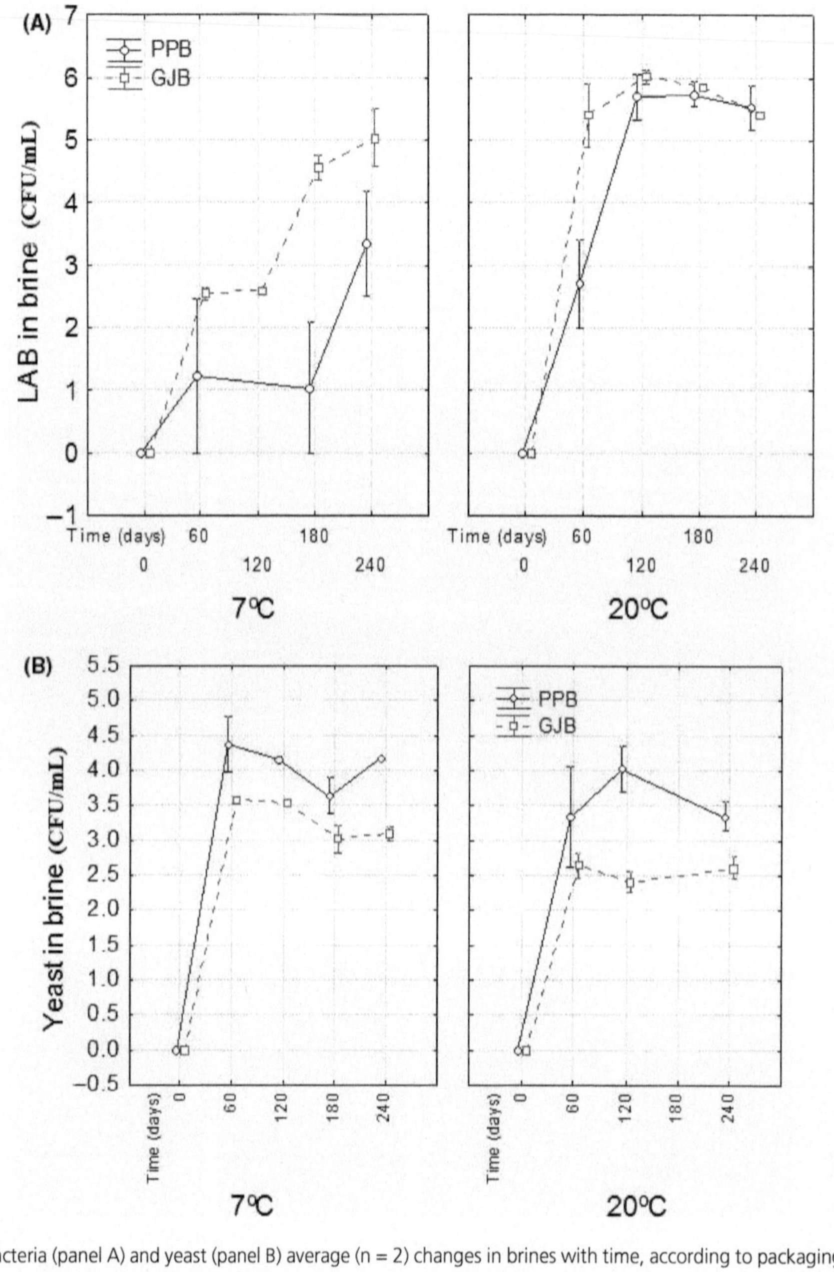

Figure 2. Lactic acid bacteria (panel A) and yeast (panel B) average (n = 2) changes in brines with time, according to packaging conditions. GJB, glass jars with brine; PPB, plastic pouches with brine; weighted means; vertical bars denote ± standard errors.

(Fig. 2A, left). At 20°C, the effect of packaging conditions on LAB increase was appreciated only during the first half period of the storage (Fig. 2A, right) but the position of the yeast curves in the same containers (Fig. 2B, right) were also reversed with respect to the position of those of the LAB and showed a marked lower maximum population in GJB than in PPB. Therefore, the effects of the packaging materials on LAB and yeasts in the brine were also opposed, as on counts on olives, with GJB leading to the highest LAB counts and PPB to the highest yeast populations.

Characterization of the lactobacilli population obtained from olive biofilm at the end of storage

The presence of the LAB2 strain at the end of packaging storage was determined by molecular methods (rep-PCR). Figure 3 shows the dendrogram generated using the pattern profiles of the 60 lactobacilli isolates obtained, after 8 months of packaging, from the treatments stored at 7°C. The cluster analysis showed that a total of nine major groups were differentiated below reproducibility of the

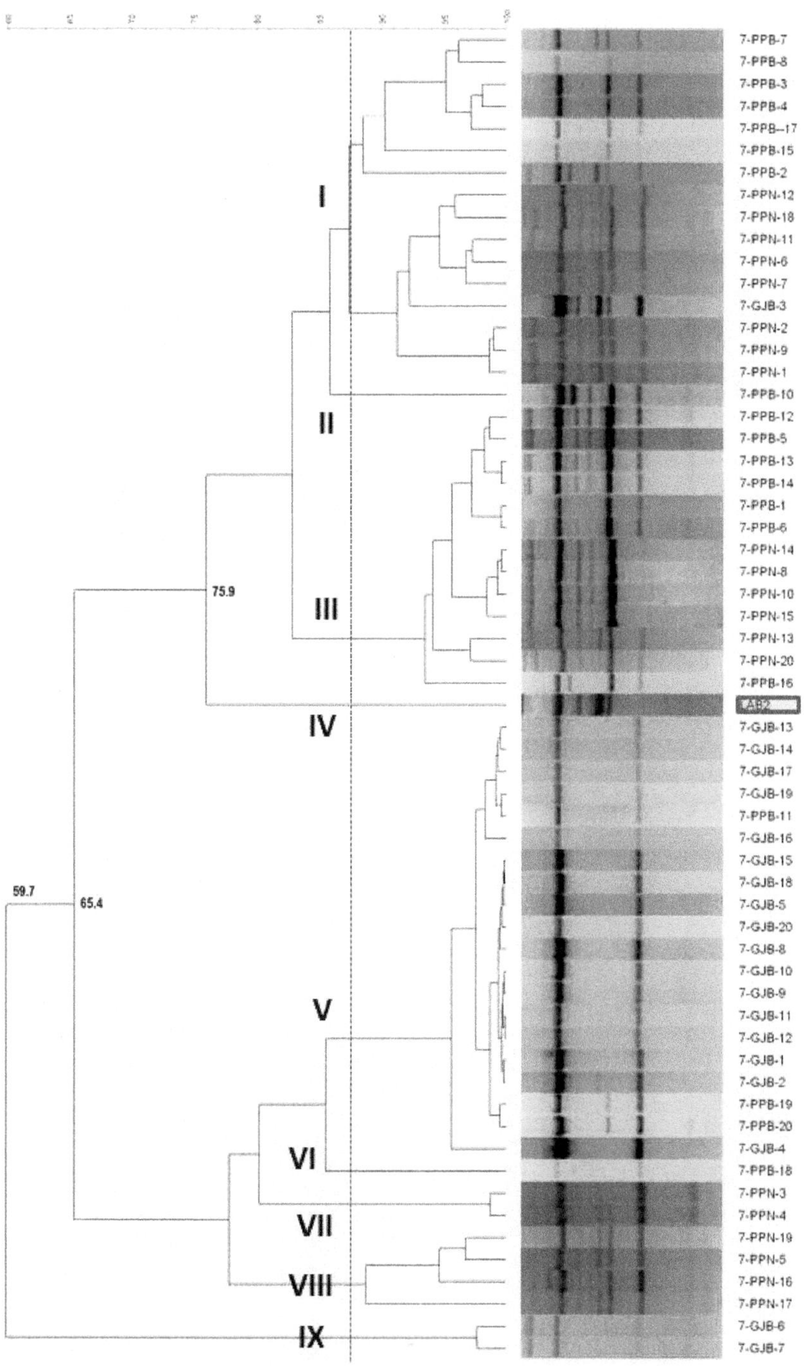

Figure 3. Dendrogram generated after cluster analysis of the digitalized rep-PCR fingerprints with primer GTG_5 of LAB isolates obtained from olives stored at 7°C. Clustering parameters: 0.5% optimization and 3.75% curve smoothing. GJB, glass jars with brine; PPB, plastic pouches with brine; PPN, plastic pouches under nitrogen atmosphere.

technique and associated error (86.9%). The LAB2 isolate used as an internal control formed a cluster (IV) clearly separated from the rest of the lactobacilli. This is indicative that the putative probiotic strain LAB2 is not present at the end of the storage in the treatments stored at 7°C. With respect to the (wild) LAB population on olives at a low temperature, a total of eight different wild genotypes were found among LAB isolates, with the cluster V containing 20 isolates (most of them obtained from GJB treatment) as the most important, while treatments in plastic pouches (PPB and PPN) showed a high biodiversity.

Figure 4 shows the dendrogram generated using the pattern profile of the 60 lactobacilli isolates obtained at the end of storage from the treatments at 20°C. The cluster analysis showed that a total of three major groups were differentiated below reproducibility of the technique. In this case, cluster III included the LAB2 strain used as internal control as well as another 43 isolates. Thereby, storage at room temperature (20°C) had favored considerably the permanence of the LAB2 strain in selected packaging conditions, mainly in treatments with nitrogen atmosphere (PPN) and GJB, where the recovery frequency of the inoculum was 100%. On the contrary, the inoculum was not detected in PPB (plastic

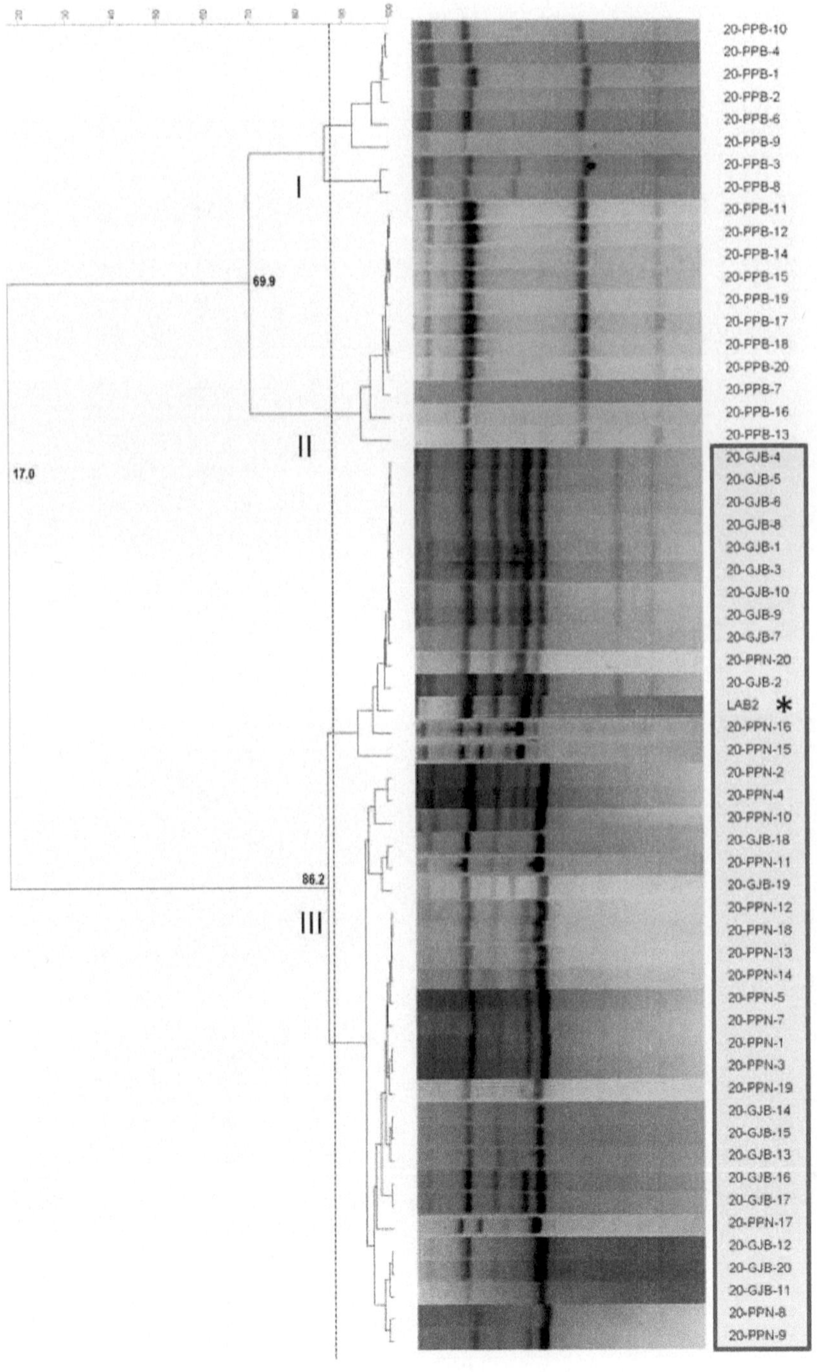

Figure 4. Dendrogram generated after cluster analysis of the digitalized rep-PCR fingerprints with primer GTG_5 of lactic acid bacteria isolates obtained from olives stored at 20°C. Clustering parameters: 2.0% optimization and 3.75% curve smoothing. GJB, glass jars with brine; PPB, plastic pouches with brine; PPN, plastic pouches under nitrogen atmosphere.

pouches with brine) (recovery frequency 0%) and two wild genotypes (clusters I and II) were found.

Effect of the packaging treatments on the physicochemical characteristics

The changes in NaCl, pH, and combined acidity were appreciated only during the first 30 days after packaging; later, due the equilibrium between brine and flesh, the levels remained stable. Final values of the physicochemical characteristics in GJB were: pH 3.68 (average) ± 0.02 (standard error) and 3.74 ± 0.03 for storage at 20 and 7°C, respectively; NaCl, 5.50 ± 0.06 and 5.48 ± 0.07 g 100 mL^{-1}; and combined acidity 57 ± 5 and 57 ± 1 mEq L^{-1}. In PPB, the levels were: pH, 3.52 ± 0.04 and 3.55 ± 0.02; NaCl, 5.57 ± 0.04 and 5.59 ± 0.02 g 100 mL^{-1}; and combined acidity, 48 ± 1 and 46 ± 1 mEq L^{-1}, for 20 and 7°C, respectively. Hence, the values in

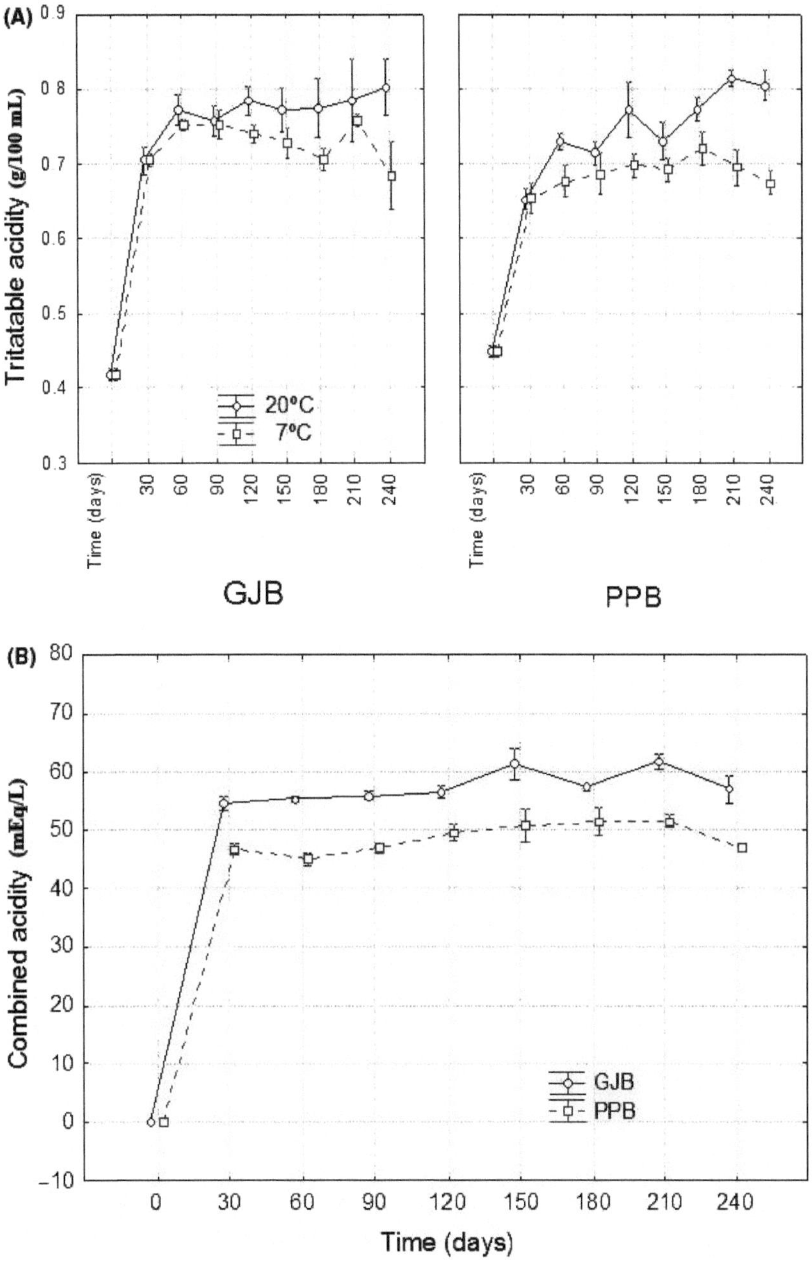

Figure 5. Changes in the averages of titratable (panel A) and combined acidity (panel B) (n = 4) during storage (time), according to packaging conditions and storage temperature. GJB, glass jars with brine; PPB, plastic pouches with brine; weighted means; vertical bars denote ± standard errors.

the equilibrium for the main variables responsible for the preservation of this type of olive were appropriate and the packages remained stable during the 8 months of the experiment monitoring. Titratable acidity was always (and sometimes significantly) higher in packages stored at 20°C and showed a first sharp raise, due to its release from the flesh. Then, this parameter showed a steady slight increasing trend at 20°C in packages containing brine, with significant differences between some sampling points within packaging material. This production of lactic acid indicates a certain LAB activity throughout this period. In principle, these changes do not represent any inconvenience and can contribute to improving the stability and safety of the product during commercialization. Finally, although combined acidity did not change during storage, the levels found in GJB were always significantly greater

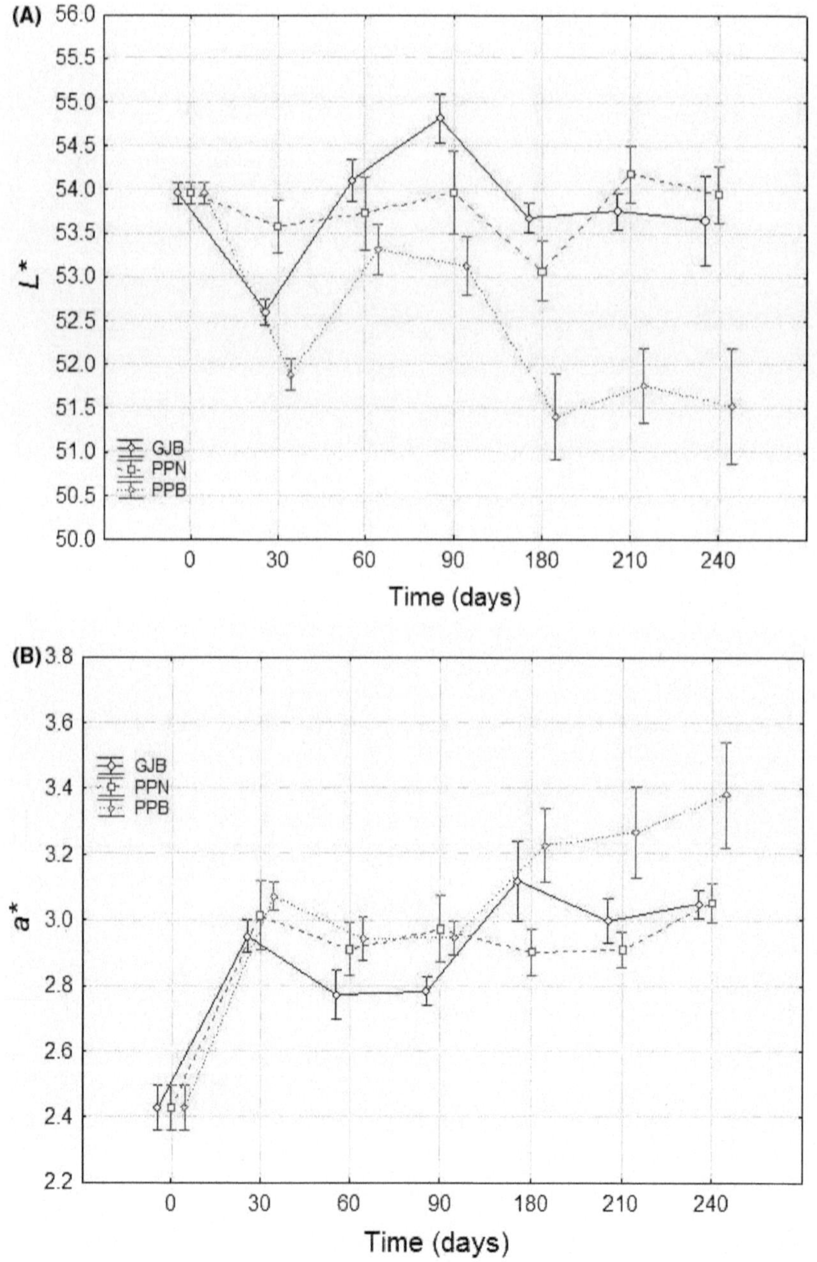

Figure 6. Average (n = 8) changes in L^* (panel A) and a^* (panel B) color parameters during storage (time), according to packaging conditions. Variability due to temperature included in error. GJB, packaging in glass jars with brine; PPB, plastic pouches with brine; PPN, plastic pouches under nitrogen atmosphere; weighted means; vertical bars denote ± standard errors.

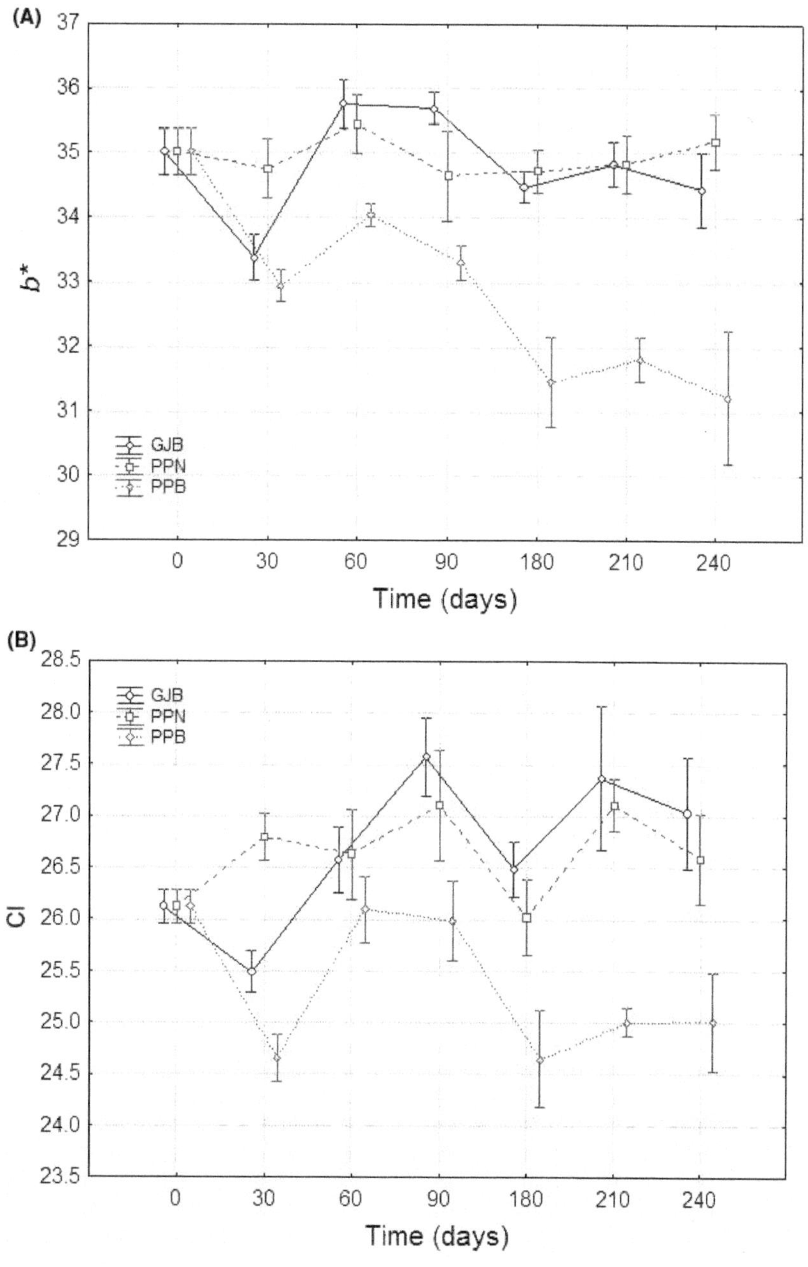

Figure 7. Average (n = 8) changes in b^* (panel A) and Color Index (panel B) color parameters during storage (time), according to packaging conditions. Variability due to temperature included in error. GJB, glass jars with brine; PPB, plastic pouches with brine; PPN, plastic pouches under nitrogen atmosphere; weighted means; vertical bars denote ± standard errors.

than those in PPB (Fig. 5B), but the difference (only about 10 mEq L^{-1}) had a limited influence on the respective storage stabilities.

In the PPN packaging, without brine, the physicochemical characteristics in the flesh after the equilibrium were: NaCl, 5.65 ± 0.03 g 100 g^{-1}; pH, 3.51 ± 0.01; titratable acidity, 0.70 ± 0.01 g lactic acid 100 g^{-1}; and combined acidity, 54.9 ± 0.5 mEq L^{-1} brine. The periodical analysis of the PPN samples throughout the storage period showed that these parameters remained stable during the entire storage period.

The firmness showed a slight decline from the original value (1377 ± 24 N 100 g^{-1} olive flesh) to final levels (1278 ± 20 N 100 g^{-1} olive fresh in GJB; 1257 ± 26 N 100 g^{-1} olive flesh in PPB olives; and 1385 ± 30 N 100 g^{-1} olive flesh in PPN). There were no significant differences among packaging conditions at any sampling time and with only a slightly but not significant higher average in olives packaged in PPN stored at 7°C. Therefore, from the firmness side, because of the lack of effect of the packaging conditions on this quality attribute during the 8 months of storage, any of them could be used.

Therefore, the physicochemical characteristics prevailing during storage were very close to the values expected and allowed the adequate stability of the products, regardless of packaging materials and storage temperature. The results validate the suitability of the packaging conditions previously fixed (Borbolla y Alcalá and González Pellissó 1972; IOC, 2004) and the calculus habitually used for estimating equilibrium conditions (Garrido-Fernández et al. 1997).

Effect of the packaging treatments on the colour parameters

The GLM analysis applied to each parameter and the packaging condition*temperature interaction showed several significant differences at numerous sampling periods. However, this work is mainly interested in investigating general trends. A first, data overview showed that temperature had the lowest influence on color. Hence, a graph of each color parameter versus time, according to packaging conditions, was a convenient option for displaying the interaction; in this case, one must bear in mind that the error includes the variability due to temperature.

The L^* parameter (luminance) (Fig. 6A) was, in general, poorer (lower values) in pouches with brine (PPB) while olives packaged in GJB and PPN followed, in general, a rather similar trend with acceptable color. Therefore, packaging in PPB always led to darker olives. In a^* (Fig. 6B), the three packaging conditions followed similar trends during the first 90 days but, later, the values of this parameter increased progressively in the PPB olives which, in the long run, had significant higher values of a^* (related to more reddish tones and poorer colors). Similarly, values of b^* and CI in olives from PPB (Fig. 7) were below those corresponding to GJB and PPN fruits (with similar behavior and better color) throughout the storage. As a result, olives in PPB have faded (b^* have moved toward bluer tones) and had lower CI; in both cases, these changes are related to color degradation and poorer appearance. Therefore, the values of L^*, a^*, b^*, and CI followed a similar trend with time in GJB and PPN olives which maintained their initial color (or even improved it in some cases) for the 8 months that the study lasted. On the contrary, all the color parameters showed poorer values in PPB shortly after packaging and throughout the entire storage period.

The analysis of the effect of temperature on color can be finished by displaying the packaging condition*temperature interaction (Figs. 8, 9). In these cases, the effect of time is included in the respective errors. According to both figures, when the packaging material was glass (GJB) none of the color parameters was affected by temperature. In olives packaged under nitrogen atmosphere (PPN), L^*, b^*, and CI have significantly higher values at 20°C (better color) while no effect was noticed on the a^* values of these fruits; therefore, olives from PPN had, in general, better color when stored at 20°C. Finally, in olives packaged in PPB, L^*, b^*, and CI had lower values (poorer color) at 20°C while a^* showed higher levels (also poorer colour) at this temperature. Thus, when using PPB, storage at 7°C was more favorable (higher L^*, b^* and CI values and lower a^* level) owing to the lower oxygen content in the brines of the pouches at this temperature. As a result, GJB and PPN had a good behavior with respect to color preservation which even improved in PPN when stored at 20°C (a temperature which is also convenient for LAB survival, as mention above). On the contrary, packaging in PPB was markedly affected by temperature and preservation or color improvement required refrigeration (storage at 7°C); but this cannot be considered as a good option because of the lower LAB survival and null LAB2 imposition at this temperature. Undoubtedly, this packaging condition is not recommendable for any type of green Spanish-style table olive where color is the attribute to be preserved.

Discussion

In table olives, research has demonstrated that the packaging conditions can significantly influence the physicochemical and microbiological characteristics of the final products (Panagou 2004; Doulgeraki et al. 2012; Rodríguez-Gómez et al. 2015). In the case of olives fermented with potential probiotic strains, packaging requires a compatible stabilization/preservation of the packaged products with the optimization of the LAB survival. A first approach to achieving these objectives could be the use of proper physicochemical conditions (Borbolla y Alcalá and González Pellissó 1972). The method is simple and the characteristics of the packaging brines can be estimated easily by means of mass balance, once the equilibrium conditions have been set (Garrido-Fernández et al. 1997). However, this strategy was developed for the stabilization of packages (that is, at least, for preventing the growth of live organisms) but there is limited experience in its application to potential probiotic olives (e.g., for preserving the olive biofilm). An exploratory research has disclosed promising results and shown that packaging conditions and storage temperature may play an essential role in this aim (Rodríguez-Gómez et al. 2015). The objective of this work is to go further into these aspects (longer

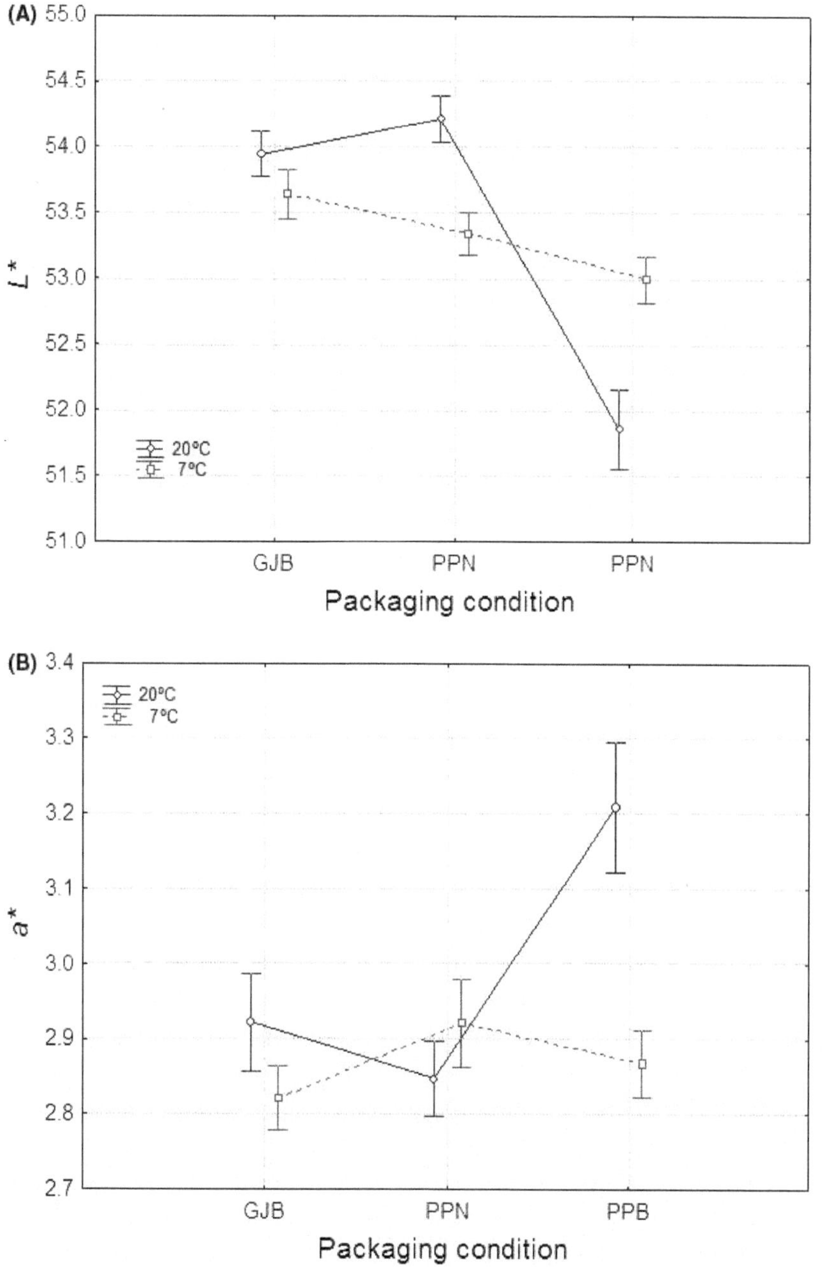

Figure 8. Overall average ($n = 28$) changes in L^* (panel A) and a^* (panel B) as a function of the packaging conditions, according to temperature. GJB, glass jars with brine; PPB, plastic pouches with brine; PPN, plastic pouches under nitrogen atmosphere; weighted means; vertical bars denote ± standard errors.

storage period and presence in the final product of the specific putative probiotic strain (LAB2) used to ferment the olives. Apparently, the products have remained stable (physicochemical characteristics) during a period of 8 months, except for titratable acidity which increased in some treatments. In principle, such an effect cannot be considered as a problem but a convenient circumstance for strengthening the product safety, provided it will not produce a markedly negative impact on LAB survival (as observed in GJB). Furthermore, it may be associated with LAB survival and vitality, in agreement with the objectives of the work, because of the strong association between both phenomena in GJB at 20°C. Color is among the most sensible attributes of green Spanish-style table olives (Sánchez-Gómez et al. 2013). In this work, the GJB and PPN were the most reliable options with respect to color owing to their favorable effect on its preservation at room temperature. On the contrary, the results advise against

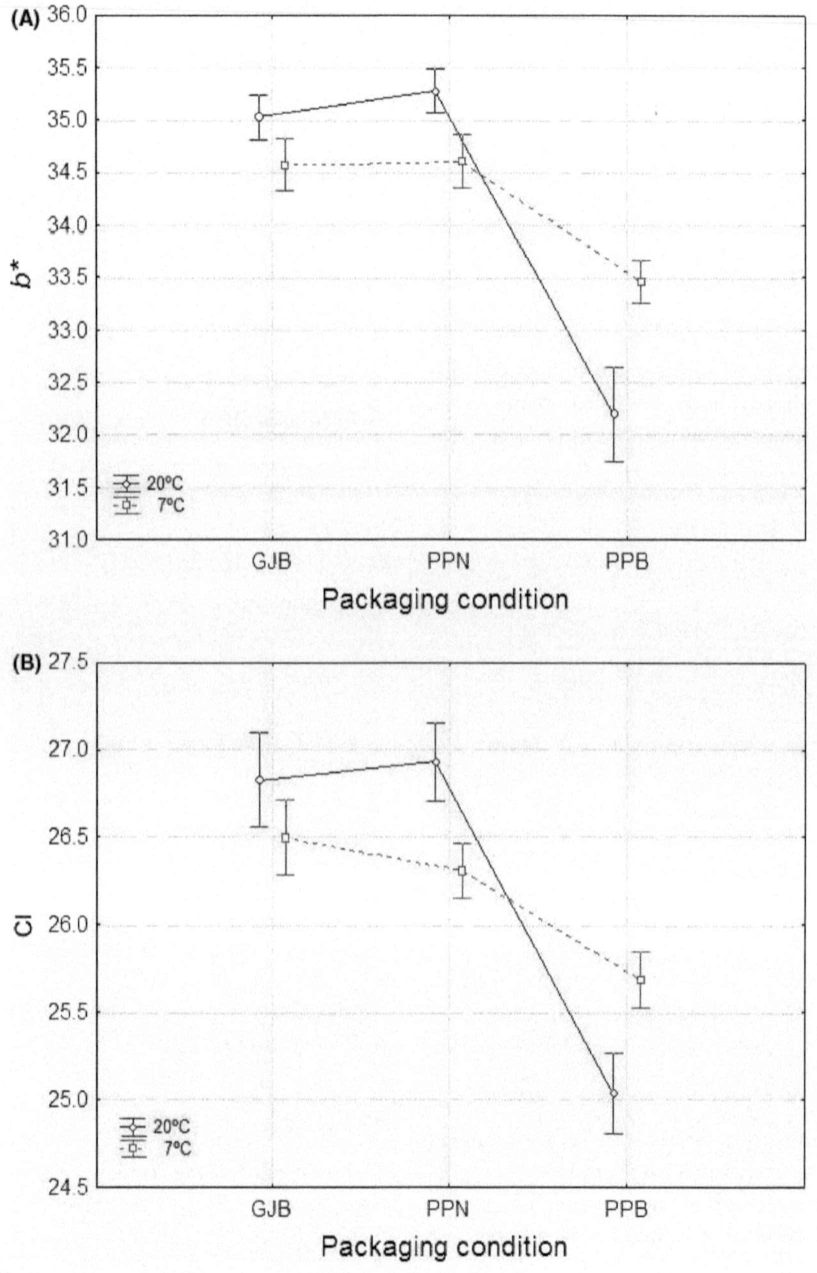

Figure 9. Overall average (n = 28) changes in b^* (panel A) and Color Index (panel B) as a function of the packaging conditions, according to temperature. GJB, packaging in glass jars with brine; PPB, packaging in plastic pouches with brine; PPN, packaging in plastic pouches under nitrogen atmosphere; weighted means; vertical bars denote ± standard errors.

the use of PPB in olive packaging in general because it resulted in an important degradation of the color (all parameters) in the long run, due to its permeability to oxygen.

The most important objective when producing probiotic table olives is the preservation of a high LAB population on fruits from fermentation to intake. A progressive decline of both LAB and yeast populations on olives throughout storage is usual (Rodríguez-Gómez et al. 2015). Based on previous results, this work has controlled the packaging conditions and temperature in order to minimize this effect. In this way, GJB and PPN were able to retain high putative probiotic LAB2 strain populations at 20°C. On the contrary, refrigeration temperatures produced unassumable LAB decreases. Furthermore, the most important and, possibly, critical conclusion has been derived from the interaction of packaging conditions*storage and the temperature effect on LAB2 presence. At room temperature, LAB2 (used for fermentation) constituted 100% of the LAB populations on the olives from GJB and PPN, while it was completely absent in those from PPB. At refrigeration temperature (7°C), LAB2 was also absent, regardless of treatments. Apparently, low temperature and PPB favored the replacement of LAB2 by wild strains better adapted to such environmental conditions. It is the first time that such a determinant effect of storage temperature and packaging conditions is reported to so radically affect the imposition of a selected strain (LAB2). It is obvious that this effect requires further confirmation but diverse responses to environmental conditions of different strains have already been informed. Blana et al. (2014) reported high colonization (80–90%) of *L. pentosus* B281 and B282 on olive fermentation at 8% NaCl but the second microorganism was unable to establish itself on the olive biofilm. The strong negative effect of storage at 7°C on LAB2 presence in the olive biofilm at the end of storage is remarkable and contrasts with the usual distribution throughout the cold chain of probiotic dairy products; in fact, reports about distribution under non-refrigerated conditions are the exception (Liu and Tsao 2009). Furthermore, temperature abuse is supposed to spoil the products because of the growth of yeasts (Viljoen et al. 2003). In this way, the response of LAB2 to temperature is rather peculiar. In this work, the eventual storage was extended to 8 months. Lavermicocca et al. (2005) recommended a 3-month period, with a high viability in LAB population. A longer period (270 days) was observed for probiotic LAB in cheddar cheese (Ganesan et al. 2014) but, in general, the survival in cheese is variable and is usually shorter (Karimi et al. 2011). Therefore, the 8-month table olive storage is a prolonged period which would be longer than most assigned to many other probiotic products.

At room temperature, the decrease in yeasts on olives was very pronounced, except in PPB (because of the possible growth promoting effect of the presence of oxygen, due to plastic permeability) and represents a serious drawback for the development of products containing simultaneously functional LAB and yeast strains. At refrigeration temperature 7°C, the yeast survival was moderate and might be adequate for storing eventual yeast probiotic olives.

There are also other strategies to improve the survival of probiotics in foods. Charalampopoulus et al. (2003) reported the use of malt, wheat, and barley extracts with this objective. Bevilacqua et al. (2010) and Altieri et al. (2011) suggested the addition of amino-acids and prebiotics, respectively. However, these compounds are hardly applicable to the case of probiotic table olives, where brine transparency and the absence of strange materials are very influential for consumer acceptance. Possibly, a more convenient strategy in table olives would be the enhancement of LAB survival by selected yeasts but, in light of the sensibility shown by the yeasts habitually present in olives, new less common species or strains should be checked. In other products, this option has been successfully applied. The stability of probiotics in fermented milk was improved by *Williopsis saturnus* var. *saturnus* presence (Liu and Tsao 2009, 2010). Furthermore, the addition of *Saccharomyces cerevisiae* had a favorable effect on *Lactobacillus rhamnosus* viability in fermented milk (Suharja et al. 2014).

Conclusions

In summary, this work has demonstrated that olives initially fermented with potential probiotic bacteria (LAB2) can be packaged for at least for 8 months without apparent product spoilage and quality preservation. Furthermore, the putative probiotic bacteria, used as inoculum in fermentation, was also present at the end of the commercialization period (100% imposition at the end of storage), provided the proper packaging conditions (GJB and PPN) and storage temperature (20°C) were applied. This behavior, which corroborates other previous works on LAB survival for a shorter period of time, may allow an eventual distribution of the new probiotic LAB2 products in common packaging containers without refrigeration. On the contrary, the eventual use of mixture cultures (LAB and yeasts) for the production of potential probiotic olives is not straightforward due to a possible opposed response to packaging conditions and storage temperatures between both groups of microorganisms.

Acknowledgments

The research leading to these results has received funding from the EU's Seventh Framework Program (FP7/2007-2013) under grant agreement n°243471 (PROBIOLIVES) and the Junta de Andalucía (through financial support to group AGR-125). Thanks to JOLCA for supplying the fruits and the packages and to ASEMESA for its support. FNAL thanks the Spanish Government and CSIC for his Ramón y Cajal postdoctoral research contract, while VRG wishes to thank the AgriFood Campus of International Excellence (ceiA3), Bank of Santander, Spanish Government, and 'Aloreña de Málaga' Olive Manufacturing Association for her predoctoral fellowship (training program of PhD in companies).

Conflict of Interest

The authors declare no conflict of interest.

References

Altieri, C., C. Bevilacqua, and M. Sinigaglia. 2011. Prolonging the viability of *Lactobacillus plantarum* throught the addition of prebiotic into the medium. J. Food Sci. 76:M336–M345.

Argyri, A. A., A. A. Nisiotou, A. Mallouchos, E. Z. Panagou, and C. C. Tassou. 2014. Performance of two potential probiotic *Lactobacillus* strains from the olive microbiota as starters in the fermentation of the heat shocked green olives. Int. J. Food Microbiol. 171:68–76.

Arroyo-López, F. N., V. Romero-Gil, J. Bautista-Gallego, F. Rodríguez-Gómez, R. Jiménez-Díaz, P. García-García, et al. 2012a. Yeasts in table olive processing: desirable or spoilage microorganisms. Int. J. Food Microbiol. 160:42–49.

Arroyo-López, F. N., J. Bautista Gallego, J. Domínguez Manzano, V. Romero Gil, F. Rodríguez Gómez, P. García García, et al. 2012b. Formation of lactic acid bacteria-yeasts communities on the olive surface during Spanish-style Manzanilla fermentations. Food Microbiol. 32:295–301.

Bautista-Gallego, J., F. N. Arroyo López, K. Rantsiou, R. Jiménez Díaz, A. Garrido Fernández, and L. Cocolin. 2013. Screening of lactic acid bacteria isolated from fermented table olives with probiotic potential. Food Res. Int. 50:135–142.

Bevilacqua, A., M. Sinigaglia, and M. R. Corbo. 2010. Ana cid/alakline stress and the addition of amino acids induce a prolonged viability of *Lactobacillus plantarum* loaded into alginate gel. Int. J. Food Microbiol. 142:242–246.

Blana, V. A., A. Grounta, C. C. Tassou, G. J. E. Nychas, and E. Z. Panagou. 2014. Inoculated fermentation of green olives with potential probiotic *Lactobacillus plantarum* starter cultures isolated from industrially fermented olives. Food Microbiol. 38:208–218.

Böckelmann, U., U. Szewzyk, and E. Grohmann. 2003. A new enzymatic method for the detachment of particle associated soil bacteria. J. Microbiol. Methods 55:201–211.

Borbolla y Alcalá, J. M. R., and F. González Pellissó. 1972. Estudios sobre aceitunas envasadas. XI. La inhibicion del sedimento. Grasas Aceites, 23:107–117.

Botta, C., and L. Cocolin. 2012. Microbial dynamics and biodiversity in table olive fermentation: culture-dependent and –independent approaches. Front. Microbiol. 3:1–9.

Charalampopoulus, D., S. S. Pandiella, and C. Webb. 2003. Evaluation of the effect of malt, wheat, and barley extracts on the viability of potentially probiotic lactic acid bacteria under acidic conditions. Int. J. Food Microbiol. 82:113–141.

De Bellis, P., F. Valerio, A. Sisto, S. L. Lonigro, and P. Lavermicocca. 2010. Probiotic table olives: microbial populations adhering on olive surface in fermentations sets inoculated with the probiotic strain *Lactobacillus paracasei* IMPC2.1 in an industrial plant. Int. J. Food Microbiol. 140:6–13.

Domínguez-Manzano, J., A. León Romero, C. Olmo-Ruiz, J. Bautista Gallego, F. N. Arroyo López, A. Garrido-Fernández, et al. 2012. Biofilm formation on abiotic and biotic surfaces during Spanish-style green table olive fermentation. Int. J. Food Microbiol. 157:230–238.

Doulgeraki, A. I., O. Hondrodimou, V. Iliopoulos, and E. Z. Panagou. 2012. Lactic acid bacteria and yeasts heterogeneity during aerobic and modified atmosphere packaging storage of natural black Conservolea olives olive in polyethylene pouches. FoodxControl 26:49–57.

Doulgeraki, A. I., P. Pramateftaki, A. A. Argyri, G. J. E. Nychas, C. C. Tassou, and E. Z. Panagou. 2013. Molecular characterization of lactic acid bacteria isolated from industrially fermented Greek olives. LWT Food Sci. Technol. 50:353–356.

Ganesan, B., B. C. Weimer, J. Pinzon, N. Dao Kong, G. Rompato, C. Brothersen, et al. 2014. Probiotic bacteria survive in cheddar cheese and modify populations of other lactic acid bacteria. J. Appl. Microbiol. 116:1642–1656.

Garrido-Fernández, A., M. J. Fernández-Díez, and R. M. Adams. 1997. Table olives. Production and processing. Chapman and Hall, London.

Gevers, D., G. Huys, and J. Swings. 2001. Applicability of rep-PCR fingerprinting for identification of *Lactobacillus* species. FEMS Microbiol. Lett. 205:31–36.

Hurtado, A., C. Requant, A. Bordons, and N. Rozes. 2012. Lactic acid bacteria from fermented olives. Food Microbiol. 31:1–8.

IOC (International Olive Oil Council). 2004. Trade Standards Applying to Table Olives. Document number COI/OT/NC no1. Madrid, Spain.

Jaiswal, A. K., S. Gupta, and N. Abu-Ghannam. 2012. Optimization of lactic acid fermentation of York cabbage for the development of potential probiotic products. Int. J. Food Sci. Technol. 47:1605–1612.

Karimi, R., A. M. Mortazavian, and A. G. Da Cruz. 2011. Viability of probiotic microorganisms in cheese during production and storage. A review. Dairy Sci. Technol. 91:283–308.

Lavermicocca, P., F. Valerio, S. L. Lonigro, M. De Angelis, L. Morelli, M. L. Callegari, et al. 2005. Study of the adhesion and survival of Lactobacilli and Bifidobacteria on table olives with the aim of formulating a new probiotic food. Appl. Environ. Microbiol. 71:4233–4240.

Liu, S. Q., and M. Tsao. 2009. Enhancement of survival of probiotic and non probiotic lactic acid bacteria by yeasts in fermented milks under non-refrigerated conditions. Int. J. Food Microbiol. 135:34–38.

Liu, S. Q., and M. Tsao. 2010. Enhancing stability of lactic acid bacteria and probiotics by *Williopsis saturnus* var. *saturnus* in fermented milks. Nutr. Food Sci. 40:314–322.

Nychas, G. J. E., E. Z. Panagou, M. L. Parker, K. W. Waldron, and C. C. Tassou. 2002. Microbial colonization of naturally black olives during fermentation and associated biochemical activities in the cover brine. Lett. Appl. Microbiol. 34:173–177.

Panagou, E. Z. 2004. Effect of different packaging treatments on the microbiological and physicochemical characteristics of untreated green olives on the Conservolea cultivar. J. Sci. Food Agricult. 84:757–764.

Peres, C. M., C. Peres, A. Hernández-Mendoza, and F. X. Malcata. 2012. Review on fermented plant materials as carriers and sources of potentially probiotic lactic acid bacteria-with an emphasis in table olives. Trends Food Sci. Technol. 26:31–42.

Ranadhera, R. D. C. S., S. K. Baines, and M. C. Adams. 2010. Importance of food in probiotic efficacy. Food Res. Int. 43:1–7.

Rodríguez-Gómez, F., J. Bautista-Gallego, F. N. Arroyo-López, V. Romero-Gil, R. Jiménez-Díaz, P. García-García, et al. 2013. Table olive fermentation with multifunctional *Lactobacillus pentosus* strains. Food Control 34:96–105.

Rodríguez-Gómez, F., V. Romero-Gil, P. García-García, A. Garrido-Fernández, and F. N. Arroyo-López. 2014a. Fortification of table olive packaging with the potential probiotic bacteria *Lactobacillus pentosus* TOMC-LAB2. Front. Microbiol. 5:1–9.

Rodríguez-Gómez, F., V. Romero-Gil, J. Bautista-Gallego, P. García-García, A. Garrido-Fernández, and F. N. Arroyo-López. 2014b. Production of potential probiotic Spanish-style green table olives at pilot plant scale using multifunctional starters. Food Microbiol. 44:278–287.

Rodríguez-Gómez, F., V. Romero-Gil, F. N. Arroyo-López, P. García-García, and A. Garrido Fernández. 2015. Effect of packaging and storage conditions on microbial survival, physicochemical characteristics and colour of non-thermally preserved green Spanish-style Manzanilla olives. LWT Food Sci. Technol. 63:367–375.

Romero-Gil, V., J. Bautista Gallego, F. Rodríguez Gómez, P. García García, R. Jiménez Díaz, A. Garrido Fernández, et al. 2013. Evaluating the individual effects of temperature and salt on table olive related microorganisms. Food Microbiol. 22:178–184.

Sánchez-Gómez, A. H., L. Rejano Navarro, and A. Montaño Asquerino. 1985. Colour determination on green Spanish-style Manzanilla olives. Grasas Aceites 36:258–261.

Sánchez-Gómez, A. H., P. García-García, and A. Garrido-Fernández. 2013. Spanish-style green table olive shelf-life. Int. J. Food Sci. Technol. 48:1559–1568.

Suharja, A. A. S., A. Henriksson, and S. Q. Liu. 2014. Impact of *Saccharomyces cerevisiae* on viability of probiotic *Lactobacillus rhamnosus* in fermented milk under ambient conditions. J. Food Process. Preserv. 38:326–337.

Verganović, J., A. L. Pavunc, K. Gjuraćić, M. Špoljarec, J. Šušković, and B. Kos. 2011. Improved sauerkraut production with probiotic strain *Lactobacillus plantarum L4* and *Leuconostoc mesenteroides* LMG 7954. J. Food Sci. 76:M124–M129.

Viljoen, B., A. Lourens-Hattingh, B. Ikalafen, and G. Peter. 2003. Temperature abuse initiated yeast growth in yoghurt. Food Res. Int. 36:193–197.

14

Effects of maturity on physicochemical properties of Gac fruit (*Momordica cochinchinensis* Spreng.)

Xuan T. Tran[1], Sophie E. Parks[1,2], Paul D. Roach[1], John B. Golding[1,2] & Minh H. Nguyen[1,3]

[1]School of Environmental and Life Sciences, University of Newcastle, Ourimbah, NSW 2258, Australia
[2]NSW Department Primary Industries, Central Coast Primary Industries Centre, Ourimbah, NSW 2258, Australia
[3]School of Science and Health, University of Western Sydney, Penrith, NSW 2751, Australia

Keywords
β-carotene, Gac fruit, lycopene, maturation, oil content

Correspondence
Xuan T. Tran, School of Environmental and Life Sciences, The University of Newcastle, PO BOX 127, Ourimbah, NSW 2258, Australia.

E-mail: thixuan.tran@uon.edu.au

Funding Information
The authors acknowledge the Vietnamese Government and the University of Newcastle, Australia for financial support through a PhD scholarship for Xuan Thi Tran. We also thank Joshua Jarvis and Dr. Shashirekha Satyan at Central Coast Primary Industries Centre, NSW Department Primary Industries for their assistance with this study.

Abstract

The aril around the seeds of Gac fruit is rich in fatty acids and carotenoids (lycopene and β-carotene). Understanding how these qualities are affected by fruit maturity at harvest may identify indices for quality assessment. Some physical and chemical properties of Gac fruit were determined for fruit harvested between 8 and 16 weeks after pollination (WAP). Fruit respiration rates and ethylene production rates were assessed after harvest and up to 20 days in storage at 20°C. Fruit harvested at 14 WAP had the highest oil (0.27 ± 0.02 g/g DW), lycopene content (0.45 ± 0.09 mg/g FW), and β-carotene content (0.33 ± 0.05 mg/g FW) which declined by 16 WAP. External skin color and aril TSS were indicative of oil and carotenoid contents in aril. Skin color, TSS and potentially firmness were good indices of fruit quality. Harvesting less mature fruit at 12 WAP would be practical as the fruit were firmer and more capable of transport; however, quality during postharvest ripening may be limited. Fruits continued to ripen after they were harvested and an ethylene peak in the least mature fruit may reflect a climacteric behavior but this needs further investigation.

Introduction

Gac (*Momordica cochinchinensis* Spreng.) is a tropical fruit that is used as a food and as traditional medicine in East and Southeast Asia (Iwamoto et al. 1985). The red aril which surrounds the seeds of mature Gac fruit is consumed in the traditional recipe Vietnamese "Xoi Gac", a popular sticky rice dish that is eaten at weddings and New Year celebrations. In addition, the immature green fruit is also used as a vegetable in Thailand (Kubola and Siriamornpun 2011) and India (Joseph and Bharathi 2008). The ripe aril has a very high content of lycopene and *β*-carotene and is a natural red colorant. The highest content of lycopene in fresh aril in fully ripe fruit was reported as 3.728 mg/g while *β*-carotene levels were 0.379 mg/g (Nhung et al. 2010). These levels are at least five times higher than the lycopene content that is reported in the tomatoes (Rao and Agarwal 1999; Lenucci et al. 2009) and eight times higher than the *β*-carotene content reported in the carrots (Cefola et al. 2012).

External subjective measures of fruit quality such as skin color, firmness, and fruit size influence consumer acceptance of some fruits, but many consumers are also interested in nutritional quality (Iglesias et al. 2012). For Gac fruit, the major consumer quality attributes include fruit size and weight, skin color, firmness, aril thickness, and color. Traditionally, Vietnam consumers generally prefer Gac fruits to be about 1.2–2 kg with good firmness and to have red skin with thick dark-red aril around the seeds. Fruits that are very soft are considered "too old" and of a poorer quality, which attract lower prices. Understanding the relationships between the external measures of fruit quality such as skin color and firmness and the nutritional qualities of the aril inside the fruit will lead to simple and quantifiable indicators of fruit quality.

The quality of Gac fruit is strongly affected by its maturity at harvest. Fruit harvested at the full maturity level has shown to contain the highest concentration of carotenoids (lycopene and β-carotene content) in the aril compared with green and semi-ripe fruits (Nhung et al. 2010; Kubola and Siriamornpun 2011). A previous study has also shown that fruit size can affect the thickness of aril which increases with increasing fruit size (Parks et al. 2013). However, these previous studies are limited as they only considered up to three stages of fruit maturity, which were poorly defined and did not explore the relationships between other important physical characteristics such as fruit weight or skin color and the nutritional quality of the aril. Using well-defined maturity stages, such as the number of weeks after the time of pollination (WAP), provide a clear definition of maturity and allow a clear comparison between multiple maturity stages.

In this study, the relationships between a number of physical properties (fruit weight, size, skin color, and flesh firmness) and chemical properties (concentration of carotenoids, total soluble solid (TSS), pH, titratable acidity (TA), and oil content) of Gac fruit harvested at five maturity stages were made. The aim of this study was to determine if any of these properties could be used as an indirect measure of aril quality. Indirect measures of quality would be of great benefit to growers, consumers, and processors to make informed decisions about when to harvest, sell, and consume Gac fruits with an optimum nutritional content.

Materials and Method

Crop production

A Gac crop was produced in greenhouses at the NSW Department of Primary Industries at Ourimbah, NSW, Australia (151°22′E, 33°21′S). The 18 plants (12 female and six male plants) were grown from seed in February 2013. The seed was sourced from fruit grown locally in Sydney, Australia. The environmental parameters and growing conditions for the Gac crop are described by Parks et al. (2013). The greenhouse temperature and the relative humidity were maintained between 18 to 25°C and 60 to 80% respectively. A hydroponic system provided water and fertilisers with a complete nutrient solution with a target electrical conductivity (EC) of 1.2 dS/m, and a pH of 5–6.5. At the flowering stage, the target EC of the nutrient solution was increased to 2.4 dS/m. The female flowers were hand pollinated using fresh pollen collected from the male flowers.

Fruit harvest

Gac fruits were harvested, between 12 November 2013 (first fruit) and 16 March 2014 (last fruit) from 12 female plants at five stages of maturity: 8, 10, 12, 14, and 16 weeks after the day of pollination (WAP) and each stage included eight fruits. The fruit characteristics at the five stages of maturity are described in Table 1.

Two to four fruits were harvested per plant and every fruit from the same plant was assigned to a different stage of maturity. The eight fruit for each maturity stage were sampled on different dates with three fruits used for quality measurements (weight, size, color, firmness, TSS, pH, oil content, lycopene, and β-carotene content) and five fruits used for respiration and ethylene production measurements at 20°C for up to 20 days after harvest. The Gac fruits were all harvested in the morning and delivered to the laboratory within 30 min for analysis.

Fruit morphology and moisture content

The weight of the whole fruit and its components (skin, pulp, aril and seed (mature black seed and immature white seed)) were determined using an electronic balance. Fruit length (polar axis-distance between the apex and the stem) and fruit diameter (the maximum width perpendicular to the polar axis) were measured. Skin color was measured using a Minolta Chroma Meter CR-400/410 (Minolta Corp, Osaka, Japan) where 10 measurements (L^*, a^*, b^*) were taken along the equatorial axis of each fruit for three fruits per maturity stage. The color

Table 1. Description of Gac fruit at five stages of maturity.

Stages	WAP	Description of maturity stages
M1	8	Fully green skin, white pulp, light yellow aril
M2	10	Green skin, spines turning yellow at the top of fruit, white pulp, yellow or pink aril
M3	12	Semi-ripe, skin starting to yellow or orange in patches, light yellow pulp, red aril
M4	14	Ripened, fully orange or red skin, yellow pulp, red aril
M5	16	Fully ripe, dark-red skin, dark yellow pulp, dark-red aril

WAP, weeks after pollination.

parameters chroma ($C^* = (a^{*2}+b^{*2})^{1/2}$) and hue angle ($h° = \arctan(b^*/a^*)$) were calculated for fruit skin color as described by McLellan et al. (1995). The flesh firmness was determined using a drill-mounted penetrometer (Facchini, Alfonsine, Italy) and measuring the force to manually lower a flat penetrometer tip (8-mm diameter) under constant force to penetrate into the fruit to a depth of 8 mm, corresponding to a mark inscribed on the shaft of the probe (Harker et al. 1996). The value of fruit firmness was an average of 10 points per fruit for three replicate fruits. The results were expressed as load in kilograms force (kgf). The moisture content of the fruit components was measured by drying at 70°C in a vacuum oven (Vord-46OD; Australasian Scientific Marketing Group, Kotara, NSW, Australia) until a constant weight was obtained.

Respiration rate and ethylene measurements

Approximately 1 h after harvest, the respiration rate and the ethylene production of the fruit were determined by measuring the concentration of CO_2 and ethylene accumulated from each Gac fruit placed in a 4 L sealed container previously equilibrated for 24 h in a controlled room at 20°C and 80–85% RH for at least 30 min. Five replicate fruits were used for this experiment. The respiration rate and the ethylene production rates were determined daily for each fruit for 20 days after harvest at 20°C.

Respiration rate

A gas sample (5 mL) of the headspace was withdrawn from each sealed container, containing a single Gac fruit, the level of CO_2 within the sample were measured with ICA gas analyser (ICA 40 system; Tonbridge, Kent, UK) and the respiration rate were calculated.

Ethylene production

A gas sample (1 mL) of the headspace was withdrawn from each sealed containers, containing a single Gac fruit, and the concentration of ethylene determined with Gas Chromatograph (Gow-Mac-580 Instrument Co., Bethlehem, PA, USA) equipped with a stainless steel column (190 mm × 216 mm) packed with activated alumina (80–100 mesh; Alltech, Sydney, NSW, Australia) and a flame ionization detector. The operation temperatures were 70, 90, and 100°C for the injector, column and detector respectively. The gas flow rates were 20, 30, and 300 mL/min for nitrogen, hydrogen and air respectively.

Ethylene production rate for each fruit were determined daily for 20 days after harvest at 20°C.

The aril quality of the Gac fruit

Total soluble solids, pH, and titratable acidity of the aril

The red aril was separated from the seed then blended and filtered with cheese cloth to determine TSS, pH, and TA on the juice. The TSS was measured using a digital refractometer (Atago Co.Ltd, Tokyo, Japan) and the pH was determined at room temperature using a pH meter (Hanna Instruments Inc., Woonsocket, RI, USA). The TA was measured using an automatic titrator (Mettler Toledo T50, Schwerzenbach, Switzerland) against 0.1 N NaOH to an end-point of pH 8.2 and the results were expressed as g citric acid (CA) per 100 mL.

HPLC analysis of β-carotene and lycopene content

The content of *β*-carotene and lycopene in Gac aril was evaluated at each maturity stage using high performance liquid chromatography (HPLC) as described by Kha et al. (2013b). Two grams of fresh aril were crushed and extracted with 60 mL of ethanol: hexane (4:3 v/v) at room temperature until there was no color left in the aril material. The extracted solution was filtered using a 0.45 μm syringe filter (Grace Davison, Rowville, Vic., Australia) prior to injection onto the Agilent 1200 HPLC system and Shimadzu LC-10AD HPLC system equipped with a Luna C18 (100 × 46 mm) coupled to a Jupiter C18 (250 × 46 mm) column (Phenomenex, Lane Cove, NSW, Australia). The mobile phase consisted of acetonitrile (ACN), dichloromethane (DCM) and methanol (MeOH) (5:4:1, v/v/v). The injection volume was 20 μL, the flow rate was 1.0 mL/min, and detection was at 450 nm. The *β*-carotene and lycopene were quantified based on the retention times and standard curves of authentic standards (Sigma-Aldrich, Castle Hill, NSW, Australia) and their content was expressed as mg/g of fresh aril weight (FW).

Determination of total oil content

The total oil content of the Gac fruit aril was measured using the Soxhlet extraction method as described by Kha et al. (2013b). First, 200 g of the fresh aril was dried using microwave oven (Model R42BST; Sharp Corporation, Artarmon, Australia) and 3 g of the dried-aril was placed in a cellulose thimble, which was inserted into the Soxhlet apparatus and extracted with 300 mL of boiling hexane until the sample was colorless. The extracted Gac sample was left at room temperature for 15 min in a fumehood to evaporate any remaining hexane and then dried at 70°C in a vacuum oven (Vord-46OD; Australasian Scientific Marketing Group) until a constant weight was obtained.

The oil content was then calculated by difference and expressed as weight percentage (g/g of dry weight, DW).

Statistical analyses

All chemical characteristic measurements were done in triplicate. The values were expressed as means ± standard deviations (SD) and statistical analyses were performed using the Statistical Package for the Social Sciences (SPSS) software version 22 (IBM Corp., Armonk, NY, USA). Analysis of variance (ANOVA), followed by the least significant difference (LSD), post hoc test, was performed to determine statistical significance between the five stages of maturity (M1 to M5). Pearson's correlation test was used to determine whether there were any significant associations between the mean values for the variables. Statistical significance was given at $P < 0.05$.

Results

Fruit morphology

As expected, as the Gac fruits grew on the plant, the fruit from each maturity stage were larger and heavier. The results presented in Table 2 show that the fruit harvested at stages M4 and M5 were larger (length and diameter) and heavier compared to fruit harvested at stage M1. Gac fruit weight increased during the developmental stages, increasing 66% from stage M1 to stage M5. Although the fruit length and diameter increased as the fruit matured, the ratio of length/diameter remained similar during the five stages at 0.5 (Table 2).

The development of the seeds within the Gac fruit was affected by the harvest maturity stage, where there was a significant difference in the number of immature white seeds relative to fully mature black seeds between stage M1 and the other stages (Table 2). At stage M1, the seeds were almost all white (98%) and they were not completely developed, whereas at the other stages they were mostly black (86–93%) and well formed.

The external color of the Gac fruit skin as measured with the Minolta color meter showed a distinct progression through the five distinct stages described in Table 1. Skin color at M1 was dark green but changed as the fruit matured to green with some yellowing (M2), to yellow and orange (M3), to orange and red (M4), and finally dark red (M5). The changes of skin color were clearly reflected by the Chroma meter a* value (which indicates "greenness" when it is negative and "redness" when it is positive), increasing progressively from being negative at stage M1, M2 and M3 to being highly positive at stage M4 with no further increase at the last stage (M5) (Table 2). Where there were significant increases between stage M1, M3 and stage M4, fruit skin changed from fully green at M1 to semi-ripe at M3 and fully ripen at M4. The L* value (which indicates the lightness or darkness of fruit), remained stable at the five maturity stages and the positive values indicated that the Gac fruit remained fairly light in color throughout. Conversely, the hue angle (h° value, which integrates both a* and b* values) decreased significantly between stage M3 (in the yellow range) and M4 (in the red range). There was no hue angle color differences between M1 to M2 (in the green range) and between M4 to M5 (in the red range).

Flesh firmness could not be determined with the M1 and M2 stages as the fruits were too hard (>15 kgf), the maximum value on the penetrometer. However, during the growth and maturity, flesh firmness declined by ≥70%

Table 2. Physical properties of Gac fruit at five maturity stages.

Fruit Attributes	Fruit maturity stages M1	M2	M3	M4	M5
Weight (g)	1040.42 ± 294^{a}	1276.62 ± 269^{ab}	1586.64 ± 174^{ab}	1665.76 ± 185^{b}	1729.74 ± 227^{b}
Length (cm)	21.33 ± 1.22^{a}	22.67 ± 1.44^{ab}	24.50 ± 1.67^{ab}	25.33 ± 1.44^{b}	26.33 ± 1.56^{b}
Diameter (cm)	42.50 ± 3.00^{a}	44.67 ± 2.78^{a}	48.67 ± 1.44^{b}	49.17 ± 1.78^{b}	50.83 ± 2.22^{b}
Length/diameter	0.50 ± 0.01^{a}	0.51 ± 0.00^{a}	0.50 ± 0.02^{a}	0.51 ± 0.02^{a}	0.52 ± 0.01^{a}
Total seeds	32.67 ± 9.11^{a}	33.00 ± 2.67^{a}	36.00 ± 4.67^{a}	37.67 ± 1.56^{a}	34.00 ± 8.67^{a}
Immature seeds	32.00 ± 9.33^{b}	4.67 ± 6.22^{a}	3.00 ± 1.33^{a}	4.67 ± 2.44^{a}	2.33 ± 1.56^{a}
Mature seeds	0.67 ± 0.89^{a}	28.33 ± 4.89^{b}	33.00 ± 4.67^{b}	33.00 ± 2.00^{b}	31.67 ± 9.78^{b}
Color					
*a**	-18.25 ± 3.72^{a}	-8.14 ± 6.83^{ab}	-4.76 ± 6.12^{b}	40.11 ± 3.60^{c}	44.08 ± 6.07^{c}
*b**	39.87 ± 5.14^{a}	40.27 ± 4.45^{a}	49.03 ± 5.67^{ab}	51.55 ± 11.17^{ab}	58.66 ± 6.06^{b}
*L**	37.39 ± 1.28^{a}	38.50 ± 3.11^{a}	46.06 ± 3.22^{a}	42.17 ± 3.83^{a}	43.05 ± 5.55^{a}
h°	114.38 ± 2.87^{c}	100.97 ± 9.43^{bc}	96.41 ± 7.20^{b}	51.52 ± 3.20^{a}	53.02 ± 5.54^{a}
Firmness (kgf)	>15	>15	9.67 ± 3.30^{b}	2.96 ± 0.10^{a}	2.28 ± 0.09^{a}

The values are means ± SD ($n = 3$) and those not sharing the same letter superscripts in a row are significantly different ($P < 0.05$) as determined using the ANOVA and the LSD post hoc test. The different stages of fruit maturity (M1 to M5) are defined in Table 1.

Table 3. The components of Gac fruit and moisture contents at five maturity stages (n = 3).

	Maturity stages				
Parameters (%)	M1	M2	M3	M4	M5
Percentage of fruit					
Skin	19.08 ± 5.39^{e}	16.86 ± 4.80^{e}	15.70 ± 2.49^{e}	13.89 ± 2.32^{e}	15.16 ± 0.17^{e}
Pulp	38.00 ± 2.11^{f}	36.99 ± 3.35^{f}	36.20 ± 1.23^{f}	43.86 ± 4.99^{f}	42.74 ± 3.85^{f}
Aril	24.92 ± 1.57^{g}	26.64 ± 2.35^{g}	29.17 ± 2.21^{g}	30.00 ± 3.78^{g}	29.50 ± 4.37^{g}
Seed	12.24 ± 1.85^{h}	9.77 ± 1.65^{h}	10.20 ± 1.52^{h}	9.33 ± 0.67^{h}	9.84 ± 1.73^{h}
Moisture content					
Skin	86.94 ± 0.33^{c}	85.34 ± 0.89^{c}	78.11 ± 1.81^{a}	83.97 ± 0.29^{c}	79.11 ± 1.89^{b}
Pulp	93.96 ± 0.06^{d}	91.15 ± 0.23^{c}	89.61 ± 0.73^{b}	91.42 ± 0.17^{c}	88.68 ± 0.28^{a}
Aril	89.66 ± 0.37^{e}	76.28 ± 0.46^{b}	78.91 ± 0.75^{c}	82.31 ± 0.25^{d}	72.51 ± 1.61^{a}
Seed	64.77 ± 1.17^{d}	30.65 ± 0.70^{b}	37.90 ± 2.11^{c}	30.36 ± 0.56^{b}	25.91 ± 0.98^{a}

The values are means ± SD (n = 3) and those not sharing the same letter superscripts for the proportion of fruit or for the moisture content are significantly different (P < 0.05) as determined using the ANOVA and the LSD post hoc test. The different stages of fruit maturity (M1 to M5) are defined in Table 1.

between the M3 stage and the M4 and M5 stages (Table 2), whereby the final maturity stage (M5), the fruit were very soft (2 kgf).

The relative weights of the four main fruit components (skin, yellow pulp, aril, and seeds), as a percentage of the whole fruit weight, and their moisture content at the five different maturity stages are presented in Table 3. The results show what the pulp made up the highest component of the fruit (36.2–43.9%) and whereas the seeds comprised were the lowest component (9.3–12.2%). The aril is the component of most interest, accounted for approximately 25–30% of the total fruit weight whist the skin contributed 14–19% to the total weight of the fruit. The results showed that although the total weight increased during growth (Table 2), the relative amounts of the fruit components were not affected by the maturity stages (Table 3).

In contrast, the moisture content of the five components was influenced by the harvest maturity stage. A significant difference in the moisture content of the aril was observed at all five maturity stages, where the moisture content of the four components were higher at stage M1 and decreased through the other stages to be 9% lower for the skin, 5.6% lower for the pulp, 19% lower for the aril, and 60% lower for the seeds at stage M5.

Physiological properties

Respiration rate

The results of the respiration rates of the Gac fruit from the different harvest maturity stages are presented in Figure 1 and show that the respiration rate of fruit at the first day after harvest depended on the stage of maturity. The results showed that fruit from the early harvest maturities had higher respiration rates than those fruit at the more mature stages (Fig. 1). The maximum respiration rate was obtained on the first day after harvest for the M1 stage (71 mL CO_2/kg/h) and it was lower for the M2 (46 mL CO_2/kg/h), M3 (51 mL CO_2/kg/h), M4 (36 mL CO_2/kg/h), and M5 stages (10 mL CO_2/kg/h).

The respiration rates over time after fruit harvest from the different harvest maturities are presented in Figure 2 and show that the production of carbon dioxide generally declined during postharvest storage at 20°C.

Ethylene production

The levels of ethylene production on the first day after harvest in fruit at the M2 stage were higher than all other maturity stages (Fig. 1). Conversely, the ethylene production rates of fruit harvested at the final maturity stage, M5 was the lowest ethylene production rate (Fig. 1).

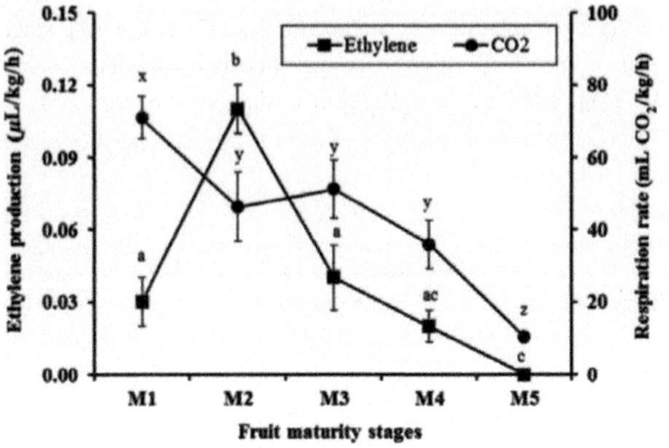

Figure 1. The respiration rate and ethylene production of Gac fruits harvested at five stage of maturity. Measurements were taken 1 day following harvest. The values are means ± SD (n = 5) and those not sharing a letter (a–d for ethylene, x–z for respiration) are significantly different (P < 0.05).

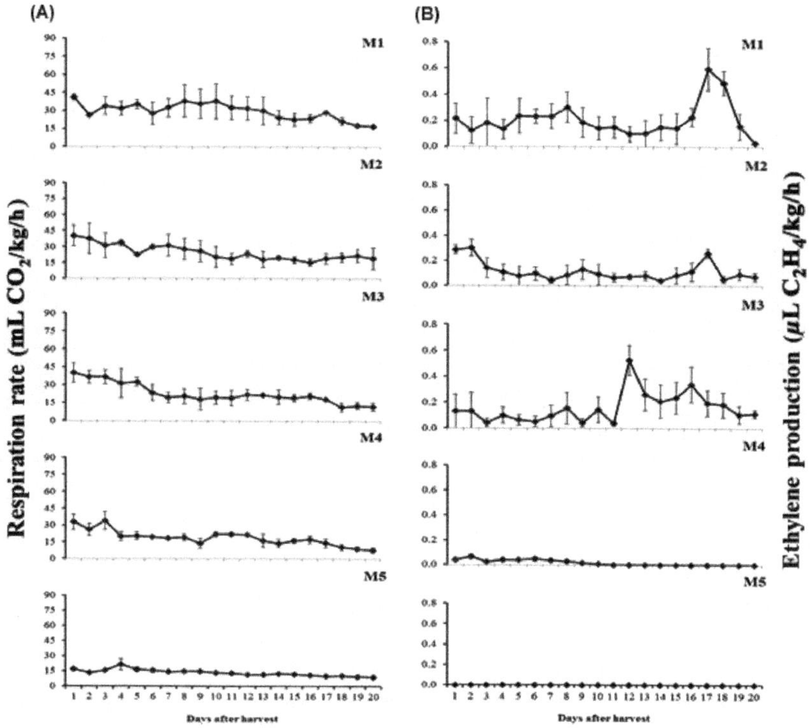

Figure 2. The respiration rate and ethylene production of Gac fruit during 20 days after harvest at the five stages of maturity: (A) respiration rate; (B) ethylene production. The values are means ± SD; (n = 5).

During the 20 days of storage at 20°C, a peak of ethylene production was observed on different days for different maturity stages (Fig. 2). At stage M1, the highest level of ethylene (0.59 μL C_2H_4/kg/h) was obtained 17 days after harvesting. Similarly, the peak ethylene production rate for the M2 stage (0.26 μL C_2H_4/kg/h) was observed 17 days after harvest (Fig. 2). Unfortunately, skin color was not monitored during the postharvest storage life at 20°C, but it was observed that the color of fruit's skin had completely changed from green to yellow at day 17 at the M1 stage.

In contrast, the highest concentration of ethylene for the M3 stage was 0.52 μL C_2H_4/kg/h 12 days after harvest (Fig. 2). Very low levels were observed for the M4 stage, with a peak of 0.06 μL C_2H_4/kg/h 2 days after harvesting and no ethylene production was detected for the M5 stage (Fig. 2).

Fruit quality

Total soluble solids and pH of the aril

A close relationship between harvest maturity and TSS in the aril of the Gac fruit was observed. The results in Table 4 show that the TSS of the Gac aril was significantly different at each of the five maturity stages with the highest levels of TSS measured at the M4 stage. There was an increase in the TSS of the Gac aril from the M1 stage

Table 4. Chemical properties of Gac aril juice at different maturity stages.

	Fruit maturity stages				
Attributes	M1	M2	M3	M4	M5
Total soluble solid, TSS (°Brix)	4.93 ± 0.38^{a}	6.30 ± 0.07^{b}	12.43 ± 0.42^{c}	15.80 ± 0.13^{d}	13.90 ± 0.87^{e}
pH	6.54 ± 0.11^{a}	6.74 ± 0.10^{a}	6.56 ± 0.18^{a}	6.73 ± 0.13^{a}	6.52 ± 0.14^{a}
TA (g CA per 100 mL)	0.24 ± 0.01^{bc}	0.18 ± 0.01^{a}	0.29 ± 0.05^{c}	0.26 ± 0.01^{bc}	0.21 ± 0.01^{ab}
TSS:TA	20.88 ± 1.68^{a}	36.11 ± 1.97^{b}	44.64 ± 6.71^{b}	59.72 ± 0.97^{c}	65.97 ± 2.87^{c}

The values are means ± SD (n = 3) and those not sharing the same letter superscripts in a row are significantly different ($P < 0.05$) as determined using the ANOVA and the LSD post hoc test.

Table 5. The oil, lycopene, and *β*-carotene content of Gac fruit at the five maturity stages.

	Fruit maturity stages				
Attributes	M1	M2	M3	M4	M5
Oil content (g/g DW)	0.03 ± 0.01^{a}	0.12 ± 0.01^{b}	0.23 ± 0.02^{c}	0.27 ± 0.02^{c}	0.25 ± 0.01^{c}
Lycopene (mg/g FW)	0.02 ± 0.00^{a}	0.23 ± 0.04^{b}	0.31 ± 0.04^{b}	0.45 ± 0.09^{c}	0.28 ± 0.00^{b}
β-carotene (mg/g FW)	0.02 ± 0.00^{a}	0.13 ± 0.04^{b}	0.22 ± 0.06^{cd}	0.33 ± 0.05^{d}	0.21 ± 0.02^{bc}
Total carotenoids (mg/g FW)	0.05 ± 0.01^{a}	0.36 ± 0.06^{b}	0.53 ± 0.06^{b}	0.78 ± 0.12^{c}	0.49 ± 0.02^{b}

The values are means ± SD ($n = 3$) and those not sharing the same letter superscripts in a row are significantly different ($P < 0.05$) as determined using the ANOVA and the LSD post hoc test; FW, fresh aril weight.

(4.9%) to the M4 stage (15.8%) but these levels declined to 13.9% at the final maturity stage (M5 stage) (Table 4).

As the TSS of the Gac aril increased during maturation, the pH of the aril remained stable (Table 4). Titratable acidity (TA) were generally low across all the maturity stages, but were lowest at M2 stages then followed by an increase at semi-mature stage (M3). A gradual decrease in TA was observed with advancing fruit maturity (M3 to M5). The TSS/TA ratio increased from 20.9 at the M1 stage to 66.0 at the M5 stage.

Oil, lycopene and β-carotene contents in the aril

The harvest maturity stages strongly influenced the oil content of Gac aril (Table 5). The oil content increased significantly from 0.03 g/g DW at M1 stage to a maximum level of 0.27 g/g DW at M4; the M5, the oil content was 0.25 g/g DW and was not different from the values measured at M3 and M4 (Table 5).

The content of lycopene and *β*-carotene in the aril increased with fruit maturity, similar to the increase for oil content (Table 5). At the fully green stage, the lycopene and *β*-carotene contents were at their lowest values (0.02 and 0.02 mg/g FW respectively). The lycopene content was highest at the M4 stage (0.45 mg/g FW) before it decreased to at the M5 harvest maturity stage (0.28 mg/g FW). Similarly, the *β*-carotene content increased at the M4 stage (0.33 mg/g FW) but decreased at the M5 stage (0.21 mg/g FW). While, the lycopene content in the aril was not different at the three stages M2, M3, and M5 and the *β*-carotene content at the M5 stage was not different from its contents at the M3 and M4 stages. The total carotenoids content (total of lycopene and *β*-carotene content) was highest at M4 stage (0.78 mg/g FW), where there were no differences between the M2, M3, and M5 maturity stages.

Multivariate analysis

The relationships between the morphological properties and the quality parameters of the Gac fruit during fruit development were investigated using the Pearson correlation and the results are presented in Table 6. The results showed that there were positive correlations ($r > 0.65$, $P < 0.01$) between the fruit size parameters (weight, length, and diameter) and the aril TSS and oil content. Fruit diameter possessed the highest correlations ($r > 0.70$, $P < 0.01$). Fruit length and diameter also had strong inverse correlations with the respiration rate after harvest ($r = -0.68$ and $r = -0.67$, $P < 0.01$, respectively) but there was no correlation with ethylene production after harvest.

There was a positive correlation between the color of the skin fruit (a* value) and the quality indices (TSS, oil content, lycopene, and *β*-carotene, $r > 0.575$, $P < 0.05$) while the inverse correlation between a* value and firmness ($r = -0.884$, $P < 0.01$) and respiration rate ($r = -0.939$, $P < 0.01$) were observed. Significant ($P < 0.01$) negative correlation was observed between TSS and respiration rate ($r = -0.776$, $P < 0.01$).

Strong relationships ($P < 0.01$) between the TSS of the aril and the content of oil, lycopene and *β*-carotene in the aril were observed (oil: $r = 0.941$, lycopene: $r = 0.810$, *β*-carotene: $r = 0.835$). Although significant ($P < 0.05$), the correlations between the fruit size parameters (weight, length, and diameter) and the lycopene and *β*-carotene content of the aril were less strong ($r < 0.62$) than for the aril TSS and oil content. There was an inverse correlation between the hue angle and the TSS, the oil, lycopene, and *β*-carotene content of the aril (TSS: $r = -0.84$, oil: $r = -0.78$, lycopene: $r = -0.71$, *β*-carotene: $r = -0.74$, $P < 0.01$) and this showed that the TSS, oil, lycopene, and *β*-carotene content of the aril increased as the fruit matured.

Discussion

This study clearly demonstrated some of the important changes in several physical and chemical properties in Gac fruit harvested at increasing stages of maturity and provides the first comprehensive account of maturation and ripening in Gac fruit. Ripening of Gac fruit was defined by the changes of skin color (green to orange

Table 6. Correlations between the morphological properties and the quality parameter of the Gac during fruit development.

Parameters	1	2	3	4	5	6	7	8	9	10	11	12	13	14
1. Weight	1													
2. Length	0.952**	1												
3. Diameter	0.983**	0.948**	1											
4. L*	0.553*	0.618*	0.611*	1										
5. a*	0.569*	0.637*	0.614*	0.334	1									
6. Hue angle	−0.535*	−0.580*	−0.573*	−0.303	−0.985**	1								
7. Firmness	−0.043	−0.043	−0.152	0.261	−0.884**	0.893*	1							
8. CO_2	−0.617*	−0.676**	−0.671**	−0.292	−0.939**	0.912**	0.832**	1						
9. C_2H_4	−0.333	−0.335	−0.410	−0.129	−0.569*	0.529*	0.892**	0.553*	1					
10. TSS	0.678**	0.671**	0.709**	0.413	0.817**	−0.841**	−0.539	−0.776**	−0.568*	1				
11. TA	0.057	−0.049	0.093	0.159	0.047	−0.083	0.278	0.105	−0.442	0.423	1			
12. Oil	0.686**	0.657**	0.710**	0.421	0.736**	−0.780**	−0.240	−0.719**	−0.363	0.941**	0.352	1		
13. Lycopene	0.618*	0.575*	0.599*	0.456	0.638*	−0.705**	−0.032	−0.565*	−0.103	0.810**	0.175	0.862**	1	
14. β-carotene	0.553*	0.477*	0.578*	0.385	0.575*	−0.740**	−0.422	−0.655**	−0.318	0.835**	0.281	0.858**	0.855**	1

*$P < 0.05$ (2-tailed); **$P < 0.01$ (2-tailed).

and red), aril color (yellow to red), pulp color (white to yellow), seed color (white to black), and firmness of fruit (firm to soft). Ripening commenced on the vine in the fruit harvested at a mature stage (M3) and following harvest in less mature fruit (M2). The appearance of yellowing on the fruit skin spines (M2) was a sign that the maturation process had commenced. Fruit harvested at this stage of maturity had a prominent level of ethylene production relative to the other fruit maturities (Fig. 1). For fruits harvested green (M1), a peak of ethylene production occurred 17 days following harvest (Fig. 2). This production peak is evidence of ethylene climacteric behavior but this needs further investigation as respiration rates did not peak and were not characteristic of climacteric fruit. Nonetheless, respiration declined during storage at all maturity stages. Fruit rots did not occur at any stage of the experiment and thus did not exacerbate ethylene or respiration observations. Fruit ripening was characterized by fruit softening and increases in TSS, oil, and carotenoid contents.

The proportion of aril did not change as a function of maturity or fruit size, the larger the fruit size, the greater the internal aril volume. The aril, the most utilized part of the fruit, and the other components declined in moisture content with maturity (Table 3). Although the proportion of aril did not relate to fruit size, these data contrasted to another Gac study with more limited data by Parks et al. (2013). This study suggests that the customer would not be disadvantaged by purchasing smaller fruit at prices based on weight. The total number of seeds was not related to fruit quality (Table 2). Mature and immature seed number did not relate to fruit quality for fruit between M2 to M5 stages and thus do not provide a good index of quality. A significant increase in mature seeds from M1 to M2 and corresponding decrease in immature seeds reflects the maturation of these seeds between these stages of fruit maturity. Further work is required to investigate the potential effect of the mature seed number on the storage life of Gac.

Between M3 and M4 stages, the firmness of Gac fruit significantly declined (>70%) and this suggests that this characteristic may be a good indicator of quality as M4 fruit was of the best quality. As fruit firmness could not be measured in M1 and M2, data were limited and more research is required to evaluate this hypothesis.

Fruit maturity at harvest had a strong effect on the carotenoid contents in the aril, where increasing carotenoids were measured in the later maturity stages. The highest lycopene (0.454 mg/g FW) and β-carotene (0.326 mg/g FW) contents were obtained in M4 fruit. The most advanced stage of ripeness (completely dark-red skin, M5 stage) had lower levels of carotenoids than completely orange fruit (M4 stage) indicating that the fruit were over-ripening. Kha et al. (2013a) reviewed the carotenoid contents in Gac fruit reported the contents were variable. The carotenoid contents obtained in this study are within the range reported by others (Aoki et al. 2002; Ishida et al. 2004; Vuong et al. 2006; Nhung et al. 2010) but clearly showed differences in the stage of fruit maturity at harvest. However, other variables such as variety, techniques used for analysis, and variable production conditions will also have an effect on the quality and carotenoid contents and should be further evaluated.

The skin color of Gac fruit showed a positive correlation with quality indices (TSS, carotenoid and oil contents) (Table 6). Growers and consumers could use this simple parameter to identify fully mature fruits with high quality. Although objective parameters of color (Minolta) and firmness (penetrometer) did not significantly separate the two most mature categories, the difference in color was apparent to the eye highlighting the large variability in the Minolta color measurements. Thus skin color, a parameter already used by consumers, when choosing fruits for purchase or when deciding if a fruit is ready to eat (Opara et al. 2009) is appropriate for Gac fruit.

As more mature Gac fruits were harvested, the TSS of the Gac aril considerably increased from 4.9% Brix at M1 to 15.8% Brix at M4. Such increases in the TSS level are common with fruit maturation and it has been observed in many fruit types (Salvador et al. 2007; Wanitchang et al. 2010; Fawole Olaniyi and Opara 2013). In addition, is likely that TSS also increases in Gac fruit as it ripens after harvest. We have previously observed TSS in the Gac aril increase during storage for Gac fruit harvested at a stage between M3 and M4 (Xuan et al., unpublished data). As TSS is strongly correlated with the oil and carotenoid contents ($r > 0.81$; $P < 0.01$) (Table 6), the simple measurement of TSS with a refractometer maybe a practical and simple tool to use as an indicator of fruit quality. However, more research is required to verify this relationship in different varieties and growing situations.

The increase in the ratio TSS/TA of Gac aril juice during fruit maturation was similar to other fruits (Pinillos et al. 2011; Fawole Olaniyi and Opara 2013) and is also a reliable indicator of quality (Table 4). The TSS represents the total soluble solids such as sugars, acids and other components (Bailen et al. 2006). The relatively high level of TSS in Gac aril (15.8% Brix at M4) is interesting, as the informal assessment of taste of Gac fruit is not sweet (unpublished data) like other fruits with similar levels. Although taste is a complex interaction of many characteristics, this may reflect that sugar levels may be a small proportion of the TSS but this needs further investigation.

Conclusions

This study has identified several measures that provide an index of maturity which relates to Gac fruit quality in terms of high contents of oil and carotenoids. The objective indices useful for identifying high-quality fruit are skin color, TSS, the TSS: TA ratio and most likely firmness. Those measures identified as not being suitable are total seed number and TA. Gac fruits harvested at the M4 stage were ripe and soft, had completely orange or red skin with a yellow pulp and red aril. These were of the highest quality which could be considered best for consumption. However, we propose that Gac fruits can be picked at the M3 stage for transportation and distribution to the consumer. The fruit described at the M3 stage were semi-ripe and firm with skin starting to yellow or orange in patches and with light yellow pulp and red aril. Whether or not fruits harvested at the M2 and M3 stage can be ripened in postharvest to obtain acceptable levels of carotenoids and oil contents needs to be clarified. In addition, confirming the climacteric nature of Gac fruit needs further investigation.

Acknowledgments

The authors acknowledge the Vietnamese Government and the University of Newcastle, Australia for financial support through a PhD scholarship for Xuan Thi Tran. We also thank Joshua Jarvis and Dr. Shashirekha Satyan at Central Coast Primary Industries Centre, NSW Department Primary Industries for their assistance with this study.

Conflict of Interest

None declared.

References

Aoki, H., N. T. M. Kieu, N. Kuze, K. Tomisaka, and N. V. Chuyen. 2002. Carotenoid pigments in gac fruit (*Momordica cochinchinensis* Spreng.). Biosci. Biotechnol. Biochem. 66:2479–2482.

Bailen, G., F. Guillen, S. Castillo, M. Serrano, D. Valero, and D. Martinez-Romero. 2006. Use of activated carbon inside modified atmosphere packages to maintain tomato fruit quality during cold storage. J. Agric. Food Chem. 54:2229–2235.

Cefola, M., B. Pace, M. Renna, P. Santamaria, A. Signore, and F. Serio. 2012. Compositional analysis ans antioxidant profile of yellow, orange and purple polignano carrots Italian. J. Food Sci. 24:284–291.

Fawole Olaniyi, A., and U. L. Opara. 2013. Changes in physical properties, chemical and elemental composition and antioxidant capacity of pomegranate (cv. Ruby) fruit at five maturity stages. Sci. Hortic. 150:37–46.

Harker, F. R., J. H. Maindonald, and P. J. Jackson. 1996. Penetrometer measurement of apple and kiwifruit firmness: operator and instrument differences. J. Am. Soc. Hortic. Sci. 121:927–936.

Iglesias, I., G. Echeverría, and M. L. Lopez. 2012. Fruit color development, anthocyanin content, standard quality, volatile compound emissions and consumer acceptability of several 'Fuji' apple strains. Sci. Hortic. 137:138–147.

Ishida, B. K., C. Turner, M. H. Chapman, and T. A. McKeon. 2004. Fatty acid and carotenoid composition of gac (*Momordica cochinchinensis* Spreng.) fruit. J. Agric. Food Chem. 52:274–279.

Iwamoto, M., H. Okabe, T. Yamauchi, M. Tanaka, Y. Rokutani, S. Hara, et al. 1985. Studies on the constituents of *Momordica cochinchinensis* Spreng. I. Isolation and characterization of the seed saponins, momordica saponins I and II. Chem. Pharm. Bull. 33:1–7.

Joseph, J. K., and L. K. Bharathi. 2008. Sweet gourd (*Momordica cochinchinensis* (Lour) Spreng.). Underutilized Underexploited Hortic. Crops 4:185–191.

Kha, T. C., M. H. Nguyen, P. D. Roach, S. E. Parks, and C. Stathopoulos. 2013a. Gac fruit: nutrient and phytochemical composition, and options for processing. Food Rev. Int. 29:92–106.

Kha, T. C., M. H. Nguyen, P. D. Roach, and C. E. Stathopoulos. 2013b. Effects of Gac aril microwave processing conditions on oil extraction efficiency, and-*β*carotene and lycopene contents. J. Food Eng. 117:486–491.

Kubola, J., and S. Siriamornpun. 2011. Phytochemicals and antioxidant activity of different fruit fractions (peel, pulp, aril and seed) of Thai gac (*Momordica cochinchinensis* Spreng.). Food Chem. 127:1138–1145.

Lenucci, M. S., A. Caccioppola, M. Durante, L. Serone, M. De Caroli, G. Piro, et al. 2009. Carotenoid content during tomato (*Solanum lycopersicum* L.) fruit ripening in traditional and high-pigment cultivars Italian. J. Food Sci. 21:461–472.

McLellan, M. R., L. R. Lind, and R. W. Kime. 1995. Hue angle determinations and statistical analysis for multiquadrant hunter L, a, b data. J. Food Qual. 18:235–240.

Nhung, D. T. T., P. N. Bung, N. T. Ha, and T. K. Phong. 2010. Changes in lycopene and beta carotene contents in aril and oil of gac fruit during storage. Food Chem. 121:326–331.

Opara, L. U., M. R. Al-Ani, and Y. S. Al-Shuaibi. 2009. Physico-chemical properties, vitamin C content, and antimicrobial properties of pomegranate fruit (*Punica granatum* L.). Food Bioprocess Technol. 2:315–321.

Parks, S. E., C. T. Murray, D. L. Gale, B. Al-Khawaldeh, and L. J. Spohr. 2013. Propagation and production of Gac (*Momordica cochinchinensis* Spreng.), a greenhouse case study. Exp. Agric. 49:234–243.

Pinillos, V., J. J. Hueso, M. Filho, L. Jose, and J. Cuevas. 2011. Changes in fruit maturity indices along the harvest season in 'Algerie' loquat. Sci. Hortic. 129:769–776.

Rao, A. V., and S. Agarwal. 1999. Review: role of lycopene as antioxidant carotenoid in the prevention of chronic diseases: a review. Nutr. Res. 19:305–323.

Salvador, A., L. Arnal, C. Besada, V. Larrea, A. Quiles, and I. Pérez-Munuera. 2007. Physiological and structural changes during ripening and deastringency treatment of persimmon fruit cv. 'Rojo Brillante'. Postharvest Biol. Technol. 46:181–188.

Vuong, L. T., A. A. Franke, L. J. Custer, and S. P. Murphy. 2006. *Momordica cochinchinensis* Spreng. (gac) fruit carotenoids reevaluated. J. Food Compos. Anal. 19:664–668.

Wanitchang, J., A. Terdwongworakul, P. Wanitchang, and S. Noypitak. 2010. Maturity sorting index of dragon fruit: *Hylocereus polyrhizus*. J. Food Eng. 100:409–416.

15

Influence of extraction methods on antioxidant and antimicrobial properties of essential oil from *Thymua danesis* subsp. *Lancifolius*

Yousef Tavakolpour[1], Marzieh Moosavi-Nasab[1,2], Mehrdad Niakousari[1,3] & Soroush Haghighi-Manesh[4]

[1]Department of Food Science and Technology, College of Agriculture, Shiraz University, Shiraz, Iran
[2]Seafood Processing Research Group, College of Agriculture, Shiraz University, Shiraz, Iran
[3]Nanotechnology Institute, Shiraz University, Shiraz, Iran
[4]Department of Food Science and Technology, School of Agriculture, Tarbiat Modares University, Tehran, Iran

Keywords
Antimicrobial, antioxidant, essential oil, extraction, *Thymua danesis*

Correspondence
Marzieh Moosavi-Nasab, Seafood Processing Research Group and Department of Food Science and Technology, College of Agriculture, Shiraz University, Shiraz, Iran.

E-mail: marzieh.moosavi-nasab@mail.mcgill.ca

Funding Information
No funding information provided.

Abstract

The essential oil (EO) from dried ground powder leaves and stems of Thymua danesis was extracted using hydrodistillation (HD), ohmic extraction (OE), ultrasound-assisted HD and ultrasound-assisted OE methods. Then, the antioxidant, antimicrobial, and sensory properties of the EO were investigated both in vitro and in food systems. Thyme EO extracted by ultrasound-assisted HD method had promising antibacterial activities against Escherichia coli and Staphylococcus aureus and had the best antioxidant properties when tested in vitro. In food systems, higher concentrations of the EO were needed to exert similar antibacterial and antioxidant effects. Furthermore, thyme EO added yogurt and drink yogurt revealed better sensory properties than the control and fresh samples. Essential oil from Thymua danesis has a good potential to be used as an antioxidant, antimicrobial, and flavoring agent in food systems and the extraction method effects on the antioxidant and antimicrobial properties of the thyme extract.

Introduction

Oxidation of lipids, which occurs during raw material storage, processing, heat treatment, and further storage of final products is one of the major reasons for deterioration of food products during processing and storage (Tomaino et al. 2005). On the other hand, it has been estimated that as many as 30% of people in industrialized countries suffer from a food borne disease each year. Therefore, investigation of new methods for reduction in foodborne pathogens and lipid oxidation of food products is needed. At the same time, there is an increasing trend of "green" consumerism, with lower side effects on consumers and environments (Burt 2004).

Plant EOs have been long recognized for their antibacterial, antifungal, antiviral, insecticidal, and antioxidant properties. They are widely used in medicine and the food industry for these purposes (Khosravi et al. 2009; Bassolé and Juliani 2012). Antioxidants are the compounds that, when added to lipid-containing foods, can increase shelf life by retarding the process of lipid oxidation (Goli et al. 2005). Synthetic antioxidants have been used in food industry since the late 1940s. However, some physical properties of synthetic antioxidants, such as their instability at elevated temperatures, strict legislation on the use of synthetic food additives and consumer preferences have shifted the attention of manufacturers from synthetic to natural antioxidants from spices and herbs (Dapkevicius et al. 1998). Especially worthy of note are spices and herbs used for many years to enhance the sensory features of food (Tomaino et al. 2005).

The aim of this study was to compare the effect of four different extraction methods on antioxidant and antimicrobial properties of EO from *Thymua danesis* subsp. *Lancifolius* when tested in vitro and to investigate its antioxidant, antimicrobial, and sensory properties in food systems.

Experimental

Materials

Thymua danesis subsp. *Lancifolius* (Herbarium No. 23271) was collected from Fars province and verified by the Institute of Medicinal Plants, Shiraz, Iran. Sodium thiosulfate, sodium sulfate, methanol, acetic acid, chloroform, and hexane were all from Merck (Darmstadt, Germany).

Plant sample preparation

At full flowering stage, the aerial parts of the plant (contained 900 g kg^{-1} leaves and 100 g kg^{-1} fine stems) were air dried at ambient temperature in the shade and powdered.

Yogurt and drink yogurt sample preparation

Yogurt and drink yogurt samples were kindly provided by Mahdam Dairy Factory, 200 kilometers from Shiraz to Bushehr, Iran. For preparation of thyme-added yogurt and thyme-added drink yogurt samples, 5 ppm of EO from thyme was added to each of the yogurt and drink yogurt samples before filling and incubating.

Hydrodistillation

For extracting EO via hydrodistillation (HD) process, 25 g of the sample was submitted to water distillation in a Clevenger-type apparatus with 500 mL water for 2.5 h at distillation rate of 3–3.5 mL min^{-1} according to the European Pharmacopoeia. After cooling, the oil was collected by use of a syringe. Dry sodium sulfate was added to remove water from the oil and after vigorous shaking and filtration, the EO was transferred into a brown, capped bottle, and stored in under refrigeration (Pharmacopoeia 1998).

Ultrasound-assisted hydrodistillation

Ultrasound irradiation was applied by means of a Hielscher ultrasonic device (UP100H, 100 W, 30 kHz) equipped with a titanium sonotrode (tip diameter 10 mm) was used to sonicate the samples. The extraction unit was also equipped with an all glass clevenger-type apparatus. The extraction process was performed by adding 25 g of the sample into 500 mL distilled water in a volumetric flask. The flask was then sonicated for 5 min which caused a 5°C temperature increase. Next, the sample was hydrodistillated for 80 min based on the HD procedure described above. After this period the temperature was decreased to 50°C and the second sonication process was performed for 5 min which caused a temperature increase in 6°C. Finally, the sample was hydrodistillated again for another 80 min. The EO was collected, dried under anhydrous sodium sulphate, and transferred into a brown, capped bottle and stored at 4°C until used (Palma and Barroso 2002; Hromadkova and Ebringerová 2003).

Ohmic extraction

The ohmic extractor unit consisted of a cylindrical Teflon chamber (0.07 m internal diameter and 0.25 m length) which was equipped with two Titanium electrodes. The system was fully automated for which the voltage (0–300 V) and current (0–16 A) and temperature could be controlled, monitored, and recorded to a data sheet throughout the experiment. In this extraction process 25 g of the sample was added to 500 mL brine (NaCl) solution (3 g L^{-1}) and charged into the chamber (sodium chloride will provide sufficient electrical conductivity between two electrodes for the heat up process to be swift). The ohmic system was then switched on. A constant voltage of 250 V was applied between the two electrodes for 5 min boil the sample. The temperature rise was recorded at about 20°C min^{-1}. After this period, the voltage was reduced to 120 V and kept constant for 25 min. Dry sodium sulfate was added to the extract and the purified EO was stored in sealed brown vials at refrigerator (Knirsch et al. 2010; Hashemi et al. 2011a; Lili et al. 2011).

Ultrasound-assisted ohmic extraction

The extraction process was performed by adding 25 g of the sample to 500 mL brine (NaCl) solution (3 g L^{-1}) in a volumetric flask and sonication for 5 min (100 W) by the cited ultrasonic device. Afterward, the flask's contents were poured into the chamber of ohmic extractor unit and after onset of boiling (250 V, 5 min), a constant voltage of 150 V was applied for 25 min. The EO was collected, dried under anhydrous sodium sulphate and transferred into a brown, capped bottle and stored in under refrigeration (Hashemi et al. 2011a).

Gas chromatography-mass spectrometry

The samples of thyme EO obtained by four different extraction methods were analyzed using gas chromatography–mass spectrometry (GC–MS). The analysis was carried out on a Agilent 6890 GC–MS instrument equipped with a HP-5MS fused silica column (30 m long, 0.25 mm i.d., 0.25 mm film thickness); Helium was used as the carrier gas at a flow rate of 0.8 mL/min with a split ratio equal to 1:50 and 1 μL of the obtained EO was injected. The injector and detector temperatures were kept at 250 and 280°C, respectively. The column temperature increased from 50 to 240°C at a rate of 3°C min^{-1} and from 240 to 300°C at a rate of 15°C min^{-1}. The retention time at 50 and 300°C was 5 and 3 min, respectively. The mass ratio analyzed was 33 to 500 m z^{-1}. The identification of compounds was based on retention times of n-alkanes (C6–C24) that were injected after the oil at the same temperature and conditions. Compounds were identified by comparison of their RI with those reported in the literature and their mass spectrum was compared with the Wiley Library (Hudaib et al. 2002; Hashemi et al. 2011b).

DPPH free radical scavenging activity

The radical scavenging capacity of EO from *Thymua danesis* for DPPH was monitored according to the method described by Burits and Bucar (Burits and Bucar 2000). Fifty microliters of different concentrations of the EO samples in methanol (10–60 mg/mL) were added to 5 mL of a 0.04 g L^{-1} methanol solution of DPPH. After a 30 min incubation period at room temperature under dark condition, the absorbance of the samples was read against a blank at 517 nm. Inhibition of free radical DPPH in percent (*I*%) was calculated in following way:

$$I\,(\%) = (A_{blank} - A_{sample}/A_{blank}) \times 100$$

where A_{blank} is the absorbance of the control reaction (containing all reagent except the test compound), and A_{sample} is the absorbance of the test compound. EO concentration providing 50% inhibition (IC_{50}) was calculated from the graph plotting inhibition percentage against EO concentration (Safaei-Ghomi et al. 2009; Hashemi et al. 2011a).

In vitro antimicrobial activity of the EO

Antibacterial activity of the EO against bacteria was assessed on *Escherichia coli* O157:H7 ATCC 35150 and *Staphylococcus aureus* ATCC 25923 by applying the standard disks diffusion technique. For reaching the stationary phase of growth, the bacterial cultures were activated 24 h before the onset of the assays and to reach the microorganism concentration of 10^5 CFU mL^{-1}, Petri dishes from the cultures were inoculated with proper sterile media. An aliquot of dimethylsulfoxide (DMSO) was added to the EOs in order to obtain a 0.0235–0.75 mL mL^{-1} concentration range. After dropping sequential dilutions of the DMSO (700 g L^{-1})/EO solution on sterile paper disks they were placed on the center of the inoculated petri dishes. Accordingly, the petri dishes were incubated at 37°C for 24 h and subsequently were checked for the minimum inhibitory concentration (MIC) of the EO (Kačániová et al. 2012). The rest of experiments was performed by applying the EO which had the best in vitro antioxidant and antimicrobial properties.

Antioxidant activity in sunflower oil

To determine the antioxidant properties of the EO, 3 g L^{-1} and 6 g L^{-1} of the EO were added to the sunflower oil and its effect on fatty acid composition of sunflower oil was compared to the control and native samples after a period of 4 days at 60°C. Gas chromatography (Agilent Technologies model 6890N, Germany) was used for fatty acid analysis (Lee et al. 2005).

Antimicrobial activity of the EO in yogurt and drink yogurt samples

Pour plate technique was used for coliform counts and surface (spread) plate technique was done for yeast and mold counts (Mohammad and El-Zubeir 2011). For enumeration of Total Yeast and Mold (TYM), and Coliform Bacteria, samples of yogurt and drink yogurt (10 g without and with 6 g L^{-1} EO) were dispersed in 90 mL sterile Ringer's solutions and appropriate decimal dilutions were prepared under the aseptic conditions. Yeast Extract Glucose Chloramphenicol Agar (YGC Agar) was used for TYM enumeration and plates were incubated at 25°C for 5 days. Coliform group bacteria were enumerated in Violet Red Bile Agar (Oxoid) after incubation at 37°C for 24 h (Karagozlu et al. 2008; Mohammad and El-Zubeir 2011).

Sensory analysis

Twelve trained panelists (six males and six females) were chosen from students of School of Agriculture of Shiraz University for the assessment of the sensory attributes of the yogurt and drink yogurt samples. In order to achieve similar conditions the samples were tempered at 4°C for 24 h before their sensory assessment. Each sample was coded using a three-digit random number and served successively to the panelists in individually partitioned booths. Palatable attribute was used to rate the overall acceptability of the samples. Taste and odor evaluation was assessed by introducing five sensory numbering descriptors including: 1 to 5, wherein which number 5 presents the best quality. Panelists were motivated to express any criticisms on the score sheets used for the sensory evaluation.

Table 1. IC_{50} of the EO extracted by different extraction methods

Method of EO extraction	IC_{50} mg mL^{-1} (Mean ± SD)
HD	24.3^b ± 0.3*
UAHD	24.1^b ± 0.2[1]
OE	23.9^b ± 0.6
UAOE	27.8^a ± 0.7

*In this column different superscript letters indicate significant differences ($P < 0.05$).
[1]Each point is the average of three replicates.

Table 2. MIC of the EO extracted by different extraction methods.

Method of EO extraction	MIC mg mL^{-1} for *Escherichia coli* (Mean ± SD)	MIC mg mL^{-1} for *Staphylococcus aureus* (Mean ± SD)
HD	130.8^a ± 4.4*	117.8^a ± 4.6
UAHD	132.1^a ± 6.1[1]	118.2^a ± 5.2
OE	132.9^a ± 4.5	119.1^a ± 3.8
UAOE	125.5^b ± 5.6	110.3^b ± 6.1

*In each column different superscript letters indicate significant differences ($P < 0.05$).
[1]Each point is the average of three replicates.

Experimental design and data analysis

For this research a completely randomized design (CRD) was used. The data were subjected to the analysis of variance (ANOVA) using SPSS (Abaus Concepts, Berkeley, California, U.S.A.) version 16.0. Significant differences between the means were determined using Duncan's new multiple range test at $\alpha < 0.05$.

Results and Discussion

Antioxidant properties of the EO from *Thymua danesis*

DPPH test

As it is indicated in Table 1, the EO extracted by each of the four extraction methods has very good antiradical power and its IC_{50} is comparable to IC_{50} of BHT (18.2 ± 0.8 mg mL^{-1}). The thyme EO antioxidant activity was depended on the extraction method and its antiradical power can be attributed to the phenolic compounds such as thymol and carvacrol which can scavenge the free radicals (Youdim et al. 2002).

In vitro Antimicrobial activity

As it is represented in Table 2 the minimum inhibitory concentration of the thyme EO for *Escherichia coli* and *Staphylococcus aureus* was depended on the extraction method. Thyme EO contains antibacterial compounds such as thymol and carvacrol which can prevent bacterial growth by making changes in ionic slope of the ion channels of bacterial cell walls (Burt 2004; Oussalah et al. 2007).

It can be inferred from the information on Tables 1 and 2 that the thyme EO extracted by UAOE method had the best in vitro antioxidant and antimicrobial properties among the thyme extracts which were obtained by the other three cited extraction methods; therefore, the thyme EO was produced in bulk by UAOE method for performing the rest of the assays.

Table 3. Changes in fatty acid profile of sunflower oil after 4 days of storage at 60°C.

Fatty acids	Native oil (Mean g L^{-1} ± SD)	Control (Mean g L^{-1} ± SD)	Sample 1 (Mean g L^{-1} ± SD)	Sample 2 (Mean g L^{-1} ± SD)
C14:0	0.11^a ± 0.03*	0.12^a ± 0.03	0.12^a ± 0.02	0.11^a ± 0.04
C16:0	9.43^b ± 0.21[1]	9.62^a ± 0.35	9.65^a ± 0.41	9.45^b ± 0.01
C16:1	0.07^a ± 0.01	0.10^a ± 0.23	0.10^a ± 0.44	0.08^a ± 0.03
C17:0	0.04^a ± 0.02	0.06^a ± 0.03	0.06^a ± 0.02	0.04^a ± 0.01
C18:0	3.33^b ± 0.13	4.03^a ± 0.22	4.00^a ± 0.19	3.35^b ± 0.13
T-C18:1	0^b ± 0.00	0.06^a ± 0.01	0.07^a ± 0.01	0.07^a ± 0.01
C18:1	23.80^b ± 0.62	24.83^a ± 0.41	24.85^a ± 0.59	23.81^b ± 0.38
Iso-C18:1	1.75^a ± 0.20	1.18^b ± 0.16	1.25^c ± 0.15	1.72^a ± 0.19
T-C18:2	0.25^c ± 0.01	0.43^a ± 0.01	0.37^b ± 0.01	0.25^c ± 0.01
C18:2	58.00^a ± 0.80	55.54^c ± 0.44	55.56^c ± 0.68	57.95^b ± 0.55
C20:0	0.20^b ± 0.02	0.31^a ± 0.04	0.30^a ± 0.02	0.22^b ± 0.01
T-C18:3	0.18^b ± 0.01	0.28^a ± 0.01	0.24^a ± 0.01	0.19^b ± 0.01
C18:3	2.42^a ± 0.01	2.37^b ± 0.01	2.39^b ± 0.01	2.41^a ± 0.01
Iso-C18:3	ND^b	ND^b	ND^b	0.02^a ± 0.01
Ga-C18:3	0.10^b ± 0.01	0.17^a ± 0.02	0.16^a ± 0.02	0.10^b ± 0.00
C22:0	0.23^b ± 0.03	0.72^a ± 0.05	0.69^a ± 0.04	0.23^b ± 0.04

ND, not detected.
*In each row different superscript letters indicate significant differences ($P < 0.05$).
[1]Each point is the average of three replicates.

Effect of addition of the thyme EO on the stability of sunflower oil

Oxidation of sunflower oil results in alteration of fatty acid profile of the oil and these alterations monitored by GC (Table 3). To have a good perception of the effect of EO (extracted by UAOE method) added to sunflower oil samples (sample 1 = 3 g L^{-1} EO added and sample 2 = 6 g L^{-1} EO added), they were compared to native and control samples. By proceeding with oil oxidation,

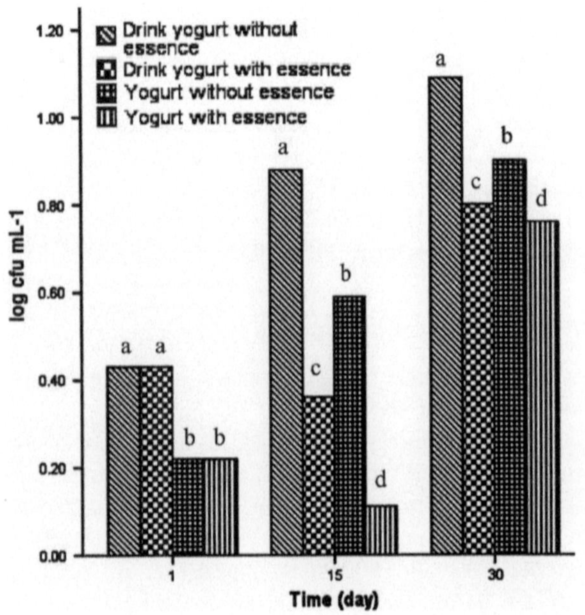

Figure 1. Antimicrobial activity of the EO in yogurt and drink yogurt samples against coliforms. In each column different letters indicate significant differences ($P < 0.05$).

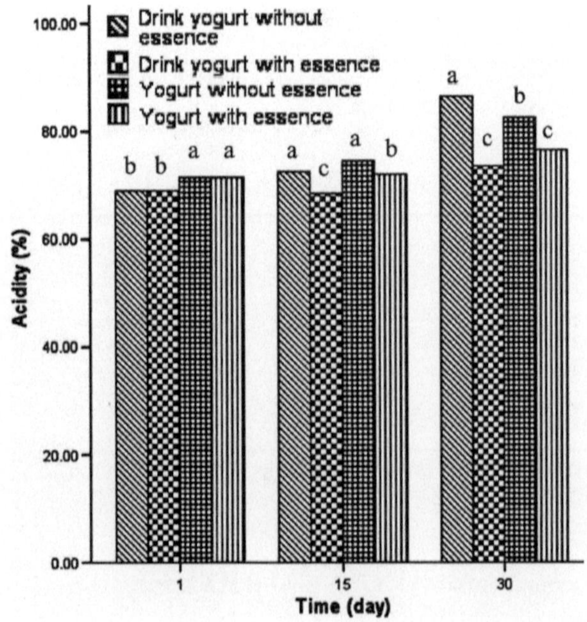

Figure 3. Effect of adding thyme EO on the acidity of the yogurt and drink yogurt samples. In each column different letters indicate significant differences ($P < 0.05$).

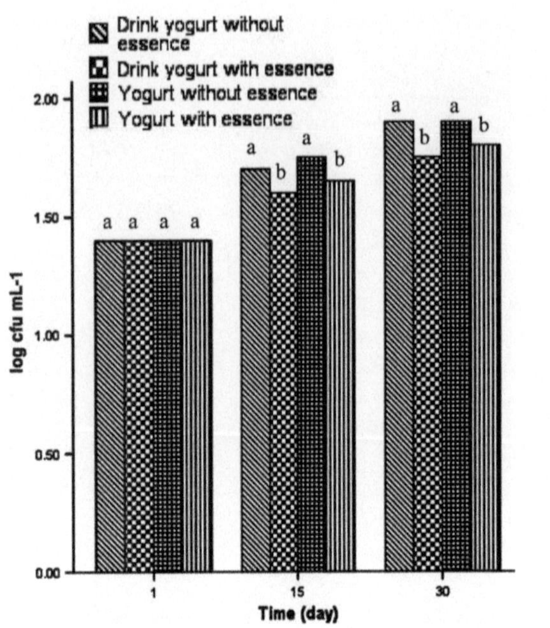

Figure 2. Antimicrobial activity of the EO in yogurt and drink yogurt samples against fungus. In each column different letters indicate significant differences ($P < 0.05$).

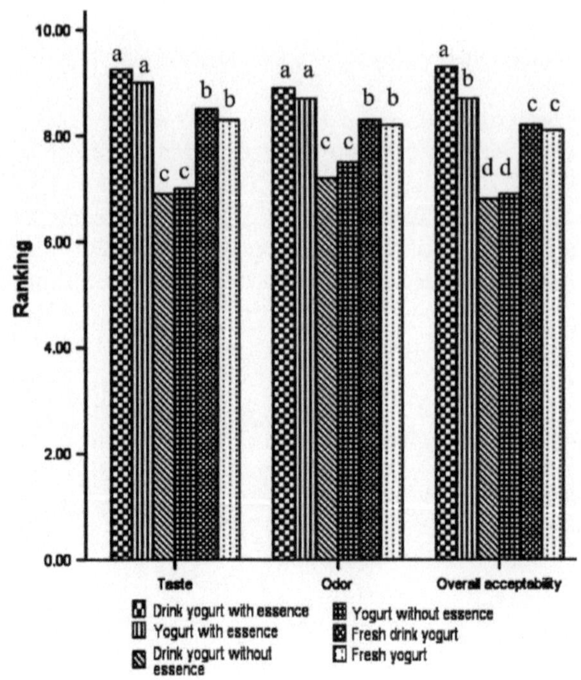

Figure 4. Effect of adding thyme EO on the sensory properties of the yogurt and drink yogurt samples. In each column different letters indicate significant differences ($P < 0.05$).

unsaturated fatty acids (especially linolenic acid and linoleic acid) were converted to saturated ones.

It is clearly seen in Table 3 that addition of EO from Thymua danesis (especially at the level of 6 g L^{-1}) to sunflower oil conserves its unsaturated fatty acids from oxidation.

Antimicrobial activity of the EO in yogurt and drink yogurt samples

Adding 6 g L^{-1} thyme EO (extracted by UAOE method) to the yogurt and drink yogurt samples reduced the overall coliform and fungus counts during the admissible shelf life of these two products (30 days) to the below of their standard levels (10 cfu mL^{-1} for coliforms in each product and 100 cfu mL^{-1} for total yeasts and molds in each product). This antibacterial property which is ascribed to antibacterial compounds of thyme EO (like thymol and carvacrol) was not seen in the samples without EO and their total counts of coliforms and fungus exceeded from the standard level (Figs. 1, 2). The same results were cited in the Burt's review (Burits and Bucar 2000).

Effect of adding thyme EO on the acidity and sensory properties of the yogurt and drink yogurt samples

Figure 3 shows that during 30 days of storage at 4°C the acidity of the samples without EO was increased. However, in samples containing EO (extracted by UAOE method) their acidity remained relatively constant after 15 days of storage and thenceforward during the next 15 days of storage, the rate of increase in the acidity was less than the samples without EO. Prevention of acid production in the thyme EO added samples is ascribed to the antimicrobial properties of the thyme EO which suppresses the extra acid production by microorganisms.

After 30 days of storage at 4°C, the thyme EO-added and control (contained no EO but stored at 4°C for 30 days) samples, were served to panelists to compare them to fresh samples and evaluate their sensory properties. As it is observed in Figure 4 in all cases the samples containing thyme EO have the best taste, flavor, and overall acceptability among the other samples. This is mainly because of excellent sensory properties of thyme EO and controlling of extra acid production by limiting the bacterial growth.

Conclusion

With regard to the excellent results of antioxidant, antibacterial, and sensory tests, it can be inferred that thyme EO can be used as an antioxidant, antimicrobial, and flavoring agent in food systems. Moreover, extraction method can influence the antioxidant and antimicrobial properties of the thyme EO, and in this view, UAOE method is the most effective method of extraction among the other three cited extraction methods.

Conflict of Interest

None declared.

References

Bassolé, I. H. N., and H. R. Juliani. 2012. Essential oils in combination and their antimicrobial properties. Molecules 17:3989–4006.

Burits, M., and F. Bucar. 2000. Antioxidant activity of Nigella sativa essential oil. Phytother. Res. 14:323–328.

Burt, S. 2004. Essential oils: their antibacterial properties and potential applications in foods—a review. Int. J. Food Microbiol. 94:223–253.

Dapkevicius, A., R. Venskutonis, T. A. van Beek, and J. P. Linssen. 1998. Antioxidant activity of extracts obtained by different isolation procedures from some aromatic herbs grown in Lithuania. J. Sci. Food Agr. 77:140–146.

Goli, A. H., M. Barzegar, and M. A. Sahari. 2005. Antioxidant activity and total phenolic compounds of pistachio *Pistachia vera* hull extracts. Food Chem. 92:521–525.

Hashemi, M. B., M. Niakousari, and M. J. Saharkhiz. 2011a. Antioxidant activity of *Satureja bachtiarica Bunge* essential oil in rapeseed oil irradiated with UV rays. Eur. J. Lipid Sci. Tech. 113:1132–1137.

Hashemi, M. B., M. Niakousari, M. J. Saharkhiz, and M. H. Eskandari. 2011b. Influence of Zataria multiflora Boiss. essential oil on oxidative stability of sunflower oil. Eur. J. Lipid Sci. Tech. 113:1520–1526.

Hromadkova, Z., and A. Ebringerová. 2003. Ultrasonic extraction of plant materials—investigation of hemicellulose release from buckwheat hulls. Ultrason. Sonochem. 10:127–133.

Hudaib, M., E. Speroni, A. M. di Pietra, and V. Cavrini. 2002. GC/MS evaluation of thyme (*Thymus vulgaris* L.) oil composition and variations during the vegetative cycle. J. Pharmaceut. Biomed. 29:691–700.

Kačániová, M., N. Vukovic, L. Hleba, A. Bobkova, A. Pavelkova, K. Rovna, et al. 2012. Antimicrobial and antiradicals activity of *Origanum vulgare* L. and *Thymus vulgaris* essential oils. J. Microbiol. Biotech. Food Sci. 2:263–271.

Karagozlu, N., B. Ergonul, and C. Karagozlua. 2008. Microbiological attributes of instant tarhana during fermentation and drying. Bulg. J. Agric. Sci. 14:535–541.

Khosravi, A., H. Shokri, Z. Tootian, M. Alizadeh, and R. Yahyaraeyat. 2009. Comparative efficacies of Zataria multiflora essential oil and itraconazole against disseminated Candida albicans infection in BALB/c mice. Braz. J. Microbiol. 40:439–445.

Knirsch, M. C., C. Alves dos Santos, deMartins Oliveria Soares Vicente A. A., and T. C. Vessoni Penna. 2010. Ohmic heating-a review. Trends. Food Sci. Tech. 21:436–441.

Lee, S.-J., K. Umano, T. Shibamoto, and K.-G. Lee. 2005. Identification of volatile components in basil (*Ocimum basilicum* L.) and thyme leaves (*Thymus vulgaris* L.) and their antioxidant properties. Food Chem. 91:131–137.

Lili, X., Z. Xiaori, Z. Zhaowu, C. Rong, L. Haifeng, X. Tian, et al. 2011. Recent advances on supercritical fluid extraction of essential oils. Afr. J. Pharm. Pharmacolo. 5:1196–1211.

Mohammad, E. E., and I. E. El-Zubeir. 2011. Chemical composition and microbial load of set yoghurt from fresh and recombined milk powder in Khartoum State. Sudan. Int. J. Dairy. Sci. 6:172–180.

Oussalah, M., S. Caillet, L. Saucier, and M. Lacroix. 2007. Inhibitory effects of selected plant essential oils on the growth of four pathogenic bacteria: *E. coli* O157: H7, *Salmonella typhimurium*, *Staphylococcus aureus* and *Listeria monocytogenes*. Food Control 18:414–420.

Palma, M., and C. Barroso. 2002. Ultrasound-assisted extraction and determination of tartaric and malic acids from grapes and winemaking by-products. Anal. Chim. Acta 458:119–130.

Pharmacopoeia, C.o.t.E.o.a.E.. 1998. European Pharmacopoeia: Supplement. Council of Europe.

Safaei-Ghomi, J., A. H. Ebrahimabadi, Z. Djafari-Bidgoli, and H. Batooli. 2009. GC/MS analysis and in vitro antioxidant activity of essential oil and methanol extracts of *Thymus caramanicus Jalas* and its main constituent carvacrol. Food Chem. 115:1524–1528.

Tomaino, A., F. Cimini, V. Zimbalatti, V. Venuti, V. Sulfaro, A. de Pasquale, et al. 2005. Influence of heating on antioxidant activity and the chemical composition of some spice essential oils. Food Chem. 89:549–554.

Youdim, K., S. Deans, and H. Finlayson. 2002. The antioxidant properties of thyme (*Thymus zygis* L.) essential oil: an inhibitor of lipid peroxidation and a free radical scavenger. J. Essent. Oil Res. 14:210–215.

16

Phenolic compounds, antioxidant, and antibacterial properties of pomace extracts from four Virginia-grown grape varieties

Yixiang Xu[1], Sheanell Burton[1,2], Chyer Kim[1] & Edward Sismour[1]

[1]Agricultural Research Station, Virginia State University, Petersburg, Virginia 23806
[2]Department of Biology, Virginia State University, Petersburg, Virginia 23806

Keywords
Antibacterial, antioxidant, extract, grape pomace, phenolic compounds, variety

Correspondence
Yixiang Xu, Agricultural Research Station, Virginia State University, Petersburg, VA 23806.

Funding Information
Funding was provided through the USDA capacity building grant.

Abstract

Grape pomace is a potential source of natural antioxidant and antimicrobial agents. Phenolic compounds, antioxidant, and antibacterial properties of pomace extracts from four Virginia-grown grape varieties were investigated. White grape pomaces had higher ($P < 0.05$) solvent extraction yield than red varieties. Concentrations of total phenolic (TPC), total flavonoid (TFC), total anthocyanin (TAC), tannins, condensed tannins (CT), as well as antioxidant capacities (DPPH• and ABTS•+free radical scavenging) differed ($P < 0.05$) among four pomace extracts. ABTS•+ scavenging capacity was positively correlated with TPC, TFC, tannins, and CT ($P < 0.05$), whereas DPPH• capacity was positively correlated with TAC ($P < 0.05$). Nine flavonoid compounds were identified, of which catechin and epicatechin were the two most abundant. Antibacterial activity was observed against Listeria monocytogenes ATCC 7644 and Staphylococcus aureus ATCC 29213, but not against Escherichia coli O157:H7 ATCC 3510 and Salmonella typhimurium ATCC 14028. L. monocytogenes was more susceptible than S. aureus.

Introduction

Grape pomace refers to the solid remains following pressing of grapes for juice or winemaking, and consists primarily of the skin, pulp, seeds, and stems. Large quantities of grape pomace produced annually, and it has been reported that over 16 million tons of grape by-products were produced in 2010 (González-Centeno et al. 2013). Currently, grape pomace is used mainly for animal feed, organic fertilizers, ethanol production, or is direct disposed as a waste (Ben Rodn et al. 1994; Ferrer et al. 2001; Korkiel et al. 2002).

Grape pomace contains high level of polyphenols, and about 70% phenolic compounds were reported to remain in the pomace (Mazza 1995). Major phenolic compounds in the grape pomace are classified into two groups: flavonoid phenols (anthocyanins, flavanols, flavonols, and tannins) and nonflavonoid phenols (phenolic acids) (Ramirez-Lopez and DeWitt 2014). Anthocyanins are pigments that are localized mainly in red grape skins, whereas flavonoids are localized in seeds and stems (Xia et al. 2010). The phenolic compounds in grape pomace extracts exhibit antioxidant, anticancer, and antidiabetic properties (Ruberto et al. 2007; Hogan et al. 2010; Parry et al. 2011; Zhou and Raffoul 2012; González-Centeno et al. 2013), as well as antibacterial activity against *E. coli, L. monocytogenes,* and *S. aureus* (Ozkan et al. 2004a; Darra et al. 2012). The antioxidant activities exhibited by phenolic compounds are due to their free radical scavenging and metal chelating capacities that are influenced mainly by the number of OH− groups and their position in the phenol ring (Hogan et al. 2009). On the other hand, the antimicrobial activities of the phenolic compounds are attributed to an ability to bind extracellular and soluble proteins enabling complexation with bacterial cell walls (Puupponen-Pimia et al. 2001). Because of these properties, polyphenols are being exploited to extend the shelf life of food products in response to increasing consumer concerns regarding synthetic preservatives (Gyawali and Ibrahim 2014), and to promote human health (Petti & Scully, 2009; Sagdic et al. 2011; Hasani and Hasani 2014; Teixeira et al. 2014).

It is worthy to note that there are varietal differences regarding the concentration and composition of phenolic compounds in grape pomaces and, consequently, in their resultant antioxidant and antimicrobial properties (Teixeira et al. 2014). Furthermore, environmental factors (e.g., geographical location, soil condition, and climate) and agronomic practices play key roles in influencing grape composition and associated properties. Most studies have focused on pomaces derived from red grape varieties, although some recent studies have examined white grape pomaces (González-Centeno et al. 2013; Cerda-Carrasco et al. 2014). Currently, no information is available concerning the pomaces from grape varieties produced in Virginia. Therefore, the objectives of the present study were to (1) quantify the composition and concentrations of phenolic compounds in pomaces from four selected Virginia-grown grape varieties, and (2) assess their antioxidant and antibacterial activities to determine their potential as a source of natural antioxidants and antimicrobials.

Materials and Methods

Materials

Pomaces from four grape varieties widely used in Virginia for wine production were evaluated. Cabernet Franc and Chambourcin are red grape varieties, while Vidal Blanc and Viognier are white grape varieties. Cabernet Franc and Viognier are *Vitis vinifera* species, while Chambourcin and Vidal Blanc are hybrid grape variety. White grape pomaces are separated from the juice prior to winemaking, while red grape pomaces are separated after fermentation. Pomaces were obtained from two Virginia wineries. Chambourcin and Viognier were obtained from a winery in Goochland County, and Cabernet Franc and Vidal Blanc were obtained from a winery in Orange County. All chemicals and reagents were purchased from Fisher Scientific (Pittsburgh, PA) and Sigma-Aldrich (St Louis, MO).

Sample preparation

The pomaces were hand-sorted to remove debris and stems, then freeze-dried, and ground using a micro-mill (IKA, Wilmington, NC) to pass through a size-20 mesh sieve. Extracts were prepared by mixing 10 g of ground sample with 40 mL of aqueous acetone (80% v/v), followed by stirring for 24 h at room temperature, and then centrifugation at 10,000 × g for 20 min at 4°C. Supernatant was decanted into preweighed dishes and dried in a chemical hood with constant air flow. The dried extracts were weighed, resuspended in distilled water, and then filtered through 0.2 μm syringe filters prior to conducting analyses.

Total phenolic and tannins

The contents of total phenolic and tannis were determined using the Folin-Ciocalteu method (Makkar et al. 1993) with some modifications. For total phenolic content (TPC), resuspended extracts were mixed with Folin–Ciocalteu reagent (10%) and sodium carbonate solution (7.5%), and then placed in the dark for 1 h, after which the absorbance was measured at 725 nm using a spectrophotometer (Evolution 60S, Thermo Scientific, Waltham, MA, USA). For simple phenolics, resuspended extract was first mixed with insoluble polyvinylpyrrolidone powder (100 mg) to adsorb tannins. The resulting supernatant was then reacted with Folin reagent as described as above. Tannin content was calculated as the difference between total and simple phenolics. Both TPC and tannins content were expressed as gallic acid equivalent (GAE) (mg/g sample) on a dry weight basis (dwb).

Total flavonoid content

Total flavonoid content (TFC) was determined using the aluminum chloride assay described by Samatha et al. (2012). Briefly, resuspended extracts were mixed with sodium nitrite (5%). After standing for 6 min, aluminum trichloride (10%) was added and incubated for 5 min, followed by the addition of sodium hydroxide (4%) and distilled water. The absorbance was measured against a reagent blank at 510 nm using a spectrophotometer. TFC was expressed as catechin equivalents (CE) (mg/g sample, dwb).

Total monomeric anthocyanins

Total monomeric anthocyanin content (TAC) was determined using the pH-differential method described by Giusti and Wrolstad (2001). Resuspended extracts were diluted to the linear range of absorbance (less than 1.2) at 520 nm using potassium chloride buffer (0.025 M, pH 1.0) and sodium acetate buffer (0.4 M, pH 4.5). Absorbance was measured against a water blank at 520 nm (λvis-max) and 700 nm (to correct the haze) from 15 min to 1 h after sample preparation. TAC was expressed as cyaniding-3-glucoside equivalent (mg/g sample, dwb).

Condensed tannins

Condensed tannins were measured according to Porter et al. (1986). Resuspended extracts were diluted with distilled water, followed by addition of butanol–HCl (95:5) and ferric reagents (2%). The mixtures were vortexed, held in a water bath (100°C) for 60 min, and then cooled to room temperature. Absorbance was measured at 550 nm. Condensed tannins concentration was expressed as leucocyanidin equivalent (% in dry matter).

Antioxidant activity

DPPH• radical scavenging activity was determined according to Sánchez-Moreno et al. (1998) with minor modifications. Briefly, resuspended extract (1.0 mL) was mixed with DPPH• solution (1.0 mL, 0.2 mmol/L, prepared daily) and stirred for 1 h at room temperature. Absorbance was measured at 515 nm. ABTS•+ radical scavenging activity was determined according to Re et al. (1999) with minor modifications. ABTS•+ reagent was prepared by incubating ABTS aqueous solution (7 mmol/L) with potassium persulfate (2.45 mmol/L), and was subsequently stored in the dark at room temperature for 12–16 h. Prior to use, the solution was further diluted to obtain an absorbance of 0.70 ± 0.02 at 734 nm. Resuspended extract (0.1 mL) was then mixed with ABTS•+ reagent (1 mL) for 1 min before measuring the absorbance at 734 nm. Both DPPH• and ABTS•+ radical scavenging activities were expressed as trolox equivalent (μmol/g sample dwb).

Identification of individual flavonoid compounds

Individual flavonoid compounds in the resuspended extracts were identified using HPLC (HP 1090, Agilent Technologies) with integrated a diode array detector. A gradient elution system having two mobile phases was used to separate individual compounds on a Synergy Hydro-RP column (2.4 mm × 250 mm) (Phenomenex, Torrance, CA). Mobile phase "A" contained 100% acetonitrile and mobile phase "B" contained 3% acetic acid. Gradient elution was as follows: 5% A/95% B from 0 to 30 min; 25% A/75% B from 30 to 35 min; 75% A/25% B from 35 to 40 min (end of the run). The injection volume was 10 μL, and the flow rate was 1.0 mL/min. The column temperature was set at 40°C. Absorbance of the elution was measured at 260 nm, 280 nm, 320 nm. Compounds were identified and quantified based on retention times and their peak areas were compared to those of known standards. Concentrations were expressed as mg/100 g grape extract.

Antibacterial activity

Inhibition zones

Two species of pathogenic Gram-positive bacteria (*Listeria monocytogenes* ATCC 7644 and *Staphylococcus aureus* ATCC 29213) and Gram-negative bacteria (*Escherichia coli* O157:H7 ATCC 3510 and *Salmonella typhimurium* ATCC 14028) were used as test organisms. All bacterial cultures were grown separately in Mueller Hinton broth (MHB) for 22 ± 2 h at 36°C to obtain an inoculum concentration (~8 log CFU/mL). An agar-well diffusion method was used to evaluate antibacterial activity of the pomace extracts (Ozkan et al. 2004b). In brief, the aliquots of each extract (100 μL) at two concentrations (150 mg/mL and 300 mg/mL) were added to 7-mm diameter wells cut into Mueller Hinton agar (MHA) plates infused with one of the four test organisms. Distilled water and chloramphenicol (5 mg/mL) were used as negative and positive controls, respectively. Plates were incubated at 36°C for 22 ± 2 h, after which, inhibition zones (mm) were measured to determine antibacterial activity.

Minimum inhibitory concentration and minimum bacteriocidal concentration

Minimum inhibitory concentration (MIC) and minimum bacteriocidal concentration (MBC) of the extracts were determined using a modified broth microdilution method (Nittiema et al. 2012). Resuspended extract (100 μL) was transferred into the first well of a 96-well sterile plate previously filled with MHB (100 μL). Serial twofold dilutions were made by adding MHB and the bacterial inocula into consecutive wells. Test plates were incubated at 36°C for 22 ± 2 h. The serial dilutions were then overlain on plate count agar (PCA) and incubated at 36°C for an additional 22 ± 2 h prior to assaying for bacteriostatic and bacteriocidal activities. The lowest concentration of the extract exhibiting approximately same level of microbial growth as observed for the inoculated level was regarded as the MIC, while the lowest concentration of extract exhibiting no growth of bacteria was regarded as the MBC.

Statistical analyses

Three replications of all assays were used to calculate means and standard deviations. Results were analyzed statistically using IBM© SPSS© Statistics, ver. 22, Armonk, NY: IBM Corp. One-way ANOVA using the Duncan C post hoc test was used to evaluate the statistical significance of differences between grape varieties. Probability (P) ≤0.05 indicates statistical significance. Pearson's correlation coefficient (r) was used to evaluate covariance relationships between contents and antioxidant properties of pomace extracts.

Results and Discussion

Extraction yields and contents of phenolic compounds

Extraction yields differed significantly among grape varieties (Table 1). White grape pomaces had higher extraction yields than their red counterparts. This could be attributed to the different vinification processes for white and red grapes. The skins and seeds of white grapes are not fermented, therefore, most solvent extractable substances remain in the pomace. On the other hand, the skins and seeds of red grapes are fermented with the juice, so that extractable components wind up in the red wine. Additionally, extraction yield varied amonth the pomaces of both white and red grape varieties. Viognier pomace had significantly higher extraction yield than Vidal Blanc, and Cabernet Franc pomace showed a significantly higher yield compared to Chambourcin pomace.

Total phenolic (TPC) and total flavonoid (TFC) differed significantly, while exhibiting the same rank order among the four pomace extracts (Table 1). The extract from Cabernet Franc pomace had the highest TPC and TFC, followed by those from Vioginer, Chambourcin, and Vidal Blanc pomaces. Cabernet Franc pomace extract examined in the present study had higher TPC (153.8 mg GAE/g) and TFC (91.7 mg CE/g), compared to those reported by Hogan et al. (2010), TPC of 30.4 mg GAE/g and TFC of 22.1 mg RE/g. The differences could arise from variations in genetic backgrounds, environmental factors, agronomic practices, or vinification processes (Doshi et al. 2006). Furthermore, Yang et al. (2009) reported fresh Cabernet Franc grape extracts had TPC and TFC of 4.2 mg GAE/g and 1.8 mg CE/g, and fresh Vidal Blanc grape extracts had TPC and TFC of 2.3 mg GAE/g and 1.0 mg CE/g. Significant differences in TPC and TFC between pomaces and fresh grapes are attributed to the localization of phenolic compounds mainly in the skin and seeds of grapes.

Total monomeric anthocyanins (TAC) in the four pomace extracts differed significantly (Table 1). As expected, the red grape pomaces had significantly higher TAC than their white counterparts, since anthocyanins are a major pigment for red, purple, and blue colors, and are present exclusively in the skin of red grapes (He et al. 2012). Of the two red grapes examined, TAC content in the Chambourcin pomace extract was approximately eightfold higher than in the Cabernet Franc. Our results for red grape pomaces are in the agreement with Rockenbach et al. (2011) who reported TAC of four red grape pomaces ranging from 1.84 to 11.2 mg cyaniding-3-glucoside equivalent/g.

Tannin content followed the same trend as TPC, and was the highest for Cabernet Franc pomace extract, followed by Viognier and Chambourcin, and was the lowest for Vidal Blanc (Table 2). Tannins are localized primarily in the skin and seeds of grapes, and can be divided into condensed tannins and hydrolyzable tannins (Alipour and Rouzbehan 2010). Condensed tannins (CT), also known as proanthocyanidins, are highly insoluble and consist of flavan-3-ols monomers subunits, and contribute to bitter and astringent tastes of grapes and wines (Fontoin et al., 2008). Four pomace extracts had CT ranging from 8.61% to 50.5% leucocyanidin equivalent, which is in the agreement with Rondeaua et al. (2013) who reported CT value of 21% to 52% for pomaces from French vineyard grapes. Two red grape pomace extracts had higher CT compared to their two white counterparts. Moreover, CT was significantly higher in the extract of Cabernet Franc pomace compared to that of Chambourcin, while Viognier pomace extract had higher CT compared to that of Vidal Blanc.

Antioxidant activities

Free radical scavenging capacities differed significantly among the four pomace extracts, and diffrened between the DPPH• and ABTS•+ assay systems (Table 2). DPPH• scavenging

Table 1. Total yield, phenolic, flavonoids and anthocyanins contents in the extracts from four grape pomaces.

Varieties	Extraction yield (%)	Total phenolics (TPC) (mg GAE/g extract	Total flavonoids (TFC) (mg CE/g extract	Total anthocyanins (TAC) (mg Cyd-3-glu equivalent/g extract
Viognier	24.9 ± 1.00[a]	99.1 ± 0.29[b]	75.0 ± 0.42[b]	0.02 ± 0.01[c]
Vidal Blanc	20.6 ± 2.57[b]	55.5 ± 0.87[d]	32.8 ± 0.41[d]	0.06 ± 0.01[c]
Cabernet Franc	12.4 ± 0.55[c]	153.8 ± 1.83[a]	91.7 ± 1.00[a]	1.38 ± 0.03[b]
Chambourcin	5.30 ± 0.61[d]	92.0 ± 2.16[c]	38.9 ± 0.74[c]	10.7 ± 0.05[a]

GAE, gallic acid equivalent; CE, catechin equivalent.

Data are expressed as mean ± standard deviation (n = 3).

Means followed by the same letter within a column indicate no significant (P > 0.05) difference among samples.

Table 2. Tannins, condensed tannins and antioxidant activities in the extracts from four grape pomaces.

Varieties	Tannins (mg GAE/g extract)	Condensed Tannins (% leucocyanidin equivalent)	DPPH (μmol TE/g extract)	ABTS (μmol TE/g extract)
Viognier	98.6 ± 0.17^{b}	25.7 ± 2.56^{c}	3.54 ± 0.06^{a}	951 ± 44.4^{b}
Vidal Blanc	54.5 ± 0.85^{d}	8.61 ± 0.95^{d}	7.71 ± 0.02^{b}	334 ± 7.39^{d}
Cabernet Franc	152.2 ± 2.56^{a}	50.5 ± 0.19^{a}	11.2 ± 0.17^{c}	1013 ± 77.3^{a}
Chambourcin	88.5 ± 2.40^{c}	36.3 ± 1.52^{b}	28.2 ± 0.02^{d}	378 ± 11.8^{c}

GAE, gallic acid equivalent; TE, trolox equivalent.
Data are expressed as mean ± standard deviation (n = 3).
Means followed by the same letter within a column indicate no significant ($P > 0.05$) difference among samples.

capacity ranged from 3.54 to 28.2 μmol TE/g among the four pomace extracts, with the highest scavenging capacity exhibited by Chambourcin, followed by Cabernet Franc, Vidal Blanc, and Viognier. Hogan et al. (2009) investigated antioxidant activities of two fresh Virginia-grown Cabernet Franc grapes and found their DPPH• scavenging activities were 5.4 and 8.8 μmol TE/g. The pomace extracts examined in the present study also exhibited significant ABTS•+ scavenging capacity ranging from 334 to 1013 μmol TE/g, with the order of Cabernet Franc > Viognier > Chambourcin >Vidal Branc. ABTS•+ scavenging capacity in the present study are higher than those reported previously for red grape pomaces (193–485 μmol TE/g) and for white grape pomaces (71–134 μmol TE/g) (Rockenbach et al. 2011; González-Centeno et al. 2013).

Relationship between phenolic compounds and antioxidant activity

TPC, TFC, tannins, CT exhibited significant, positive correlations with each other, as well as with ABTS •+ scavenging capacity (Table 3). However, these compounds and ABTS•+ scavenging activity were uncorrelated with either TAC or DPPH• scavenging activity, though TAC and DPPH• exhibited significant, positive correlation with each other. These results suggest that different phenolic compounds are responsible for quenching different free radicals. Flavonoids, tannins, and condensed tannins contribute to ABTS•+ antioxidant capacity, while anthocyanins contribute to DPPH• antioxidant capacity. Elfalleh et al. (2012) found negative correlations between TPC, TFC, TAC, and hydrolyzable tannins with DPPH• scavenging capacity, and no correlation between these phenolic compounds with ABTS •+ scavenging capacity in pomegranate juice. The distinctive structure of each phenolic compound (number of OH groups, side chain on benzoic acid) explains their special capacities to scavenge different free radicals (Tabart et al. 2009).

Individual flavonoid compounds

Nine flavonoid compounds, catechin, epicatechin, epigallocatechin gallate (EGCG), gallocatechin gallate (GCG), epicatechingallate (ECG), quercetin, quercetin-3-rhamnoside, kaempferol, and rutin were identified using HPLC (Fig. 1), and their concentrations are summarized in Table 4. Catechin, epicatechin, quercetin, and rutin were found in all four extracts, though their concentrations differed significantly. Catechin was the most abundant flavonoid compound. This agrees with previous report on phenolic compounds in grape pomace (Rockenbach et al. 2011). Further, white grape pomace extracts had higher catechin and epicatechin concentrations compared to the red ones. This is consistent with the findings of Nile et al. (2013). Catechin and epicatechin were the highest in Viognier pomace extract, and the lowest in Chambourcin pomace extract. Rutin content in the four extracts was in the order of Vidal Blanc > Cabernet Franc > Viognier > Chambourcin. The extracts from red varieties had the highest quercetin contents. Kaempferol was

Table 3. Correlation coefficients between the contents of phenolics and antioxidant activity.

	TPC	TFC	TAC	Tannins	CT	DPPH	ABTS
TPC	1.000	0.889***	0.132	0.999***	0.931***	0.018	0.798**
TFC			−0.292	0.902***	0.686*	−0.409	0.977***
TAC		1.000	1.000	0.101	0.330	0.991***	−0.386
Tannis				1.000	0.919***	−0.013	0.815**
CT					1.000	0.369	0.577*
DPPH						1.000	−0.501
ABTS							1.000

Significant correlations are indicated as: *(0.05 > P > 0.01), ** (0.01 > P > 0.001), *** (0.001 > P).

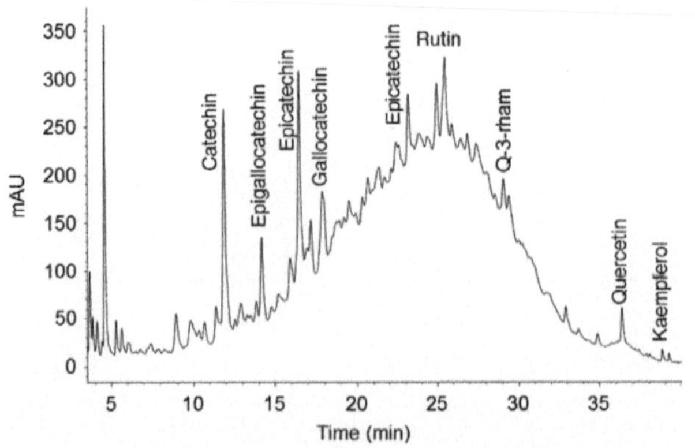

Figure 1. A typical HPLC chromatogram of grape pomace extract at 280 nm.

found only in the red varieties, whereas quercetin-3-rhamnoside was found only in the white varieties. Vuorinen et al. (2000) investigated flavonol contents of different types of grape wines and did not detect quercetin or kaempferol in white wines. Of three catechin and gallic acid esters, EGCG was highest in Cabernet Franc, followed by Viognier and Vidal Blanc, but was not quantified in Chambourcin. Cabernet Franc had the highest GCG followed by Chambourcin and Viognier, whereas Viognier had the highest ECG, GCG, and ECG were not detected in Vidal Blanc.

Antibacterial activity

The antibacterial activity of four grape pomace extracts is presented in terms of size of inhibition zone (mm) (Table 5). All extracts exhibited antibacterial activity against *L. monocytogenes* and *S. aureus* (Fig. 2), but no antibacterial activity was dected against *E. coli* O157:H7 and S. typhimurium. Our results agree partially with previous studies of whole grape or grape pomace extracts that found antibacterial activity against both Gram-positive and Gram-negative bacteria, and that extracts were more effective against Gram-positive bacteria (Darra et al. 2012; Oliveira et al. 2013). The difference between our results and these others could be associated with different interpretations of the inhibition zone. The unique cell structure (two layer cell membrane and strong hydrophilicity of the outer membranres) of the Gram-negative bacteria explains their strong resistance to pomace extracts (Smith-Palmer et al. 1998).

Among the Gram-positive strains, *L. monocytogenes* was more susceptible than *S. aureus*, but susceptibility was influenced by grape variety and extract concentration. At an extract concentration of 150 mg/mL, the susceptibility of *L. monocytogenes* was the highest for Viognier, followed by Vidal Blanc, Cabernet Franc, and Chambourcin. Inhibition increased significantly with increasing extract concentration to 300 mg/mL for Vidal Blanc and Cabernet Franc, but not for Viognier. In comparison, at an extract concentration of 150 mg/mL, Viognier had the highest inhibition activity against *S. aureus*, followed by Cabernet Franc, Chambourcin, and Vidal Blanc. As with *L. monocytogenes*, inhibition of *S. aureus* increased significantly with increasing concentration to 300 mg/mL for Vidal Blanc and Cabernet Franc, but not for Viognier.

The agar diffusion method is considered as a qualitative test for initial screening of the antibacterial activity of a substance to provide indication for further quantitative evaluation of minimum inhibition (MIC) and minimum bactericidal concentration (MBC) (Oliveira et al. 2013). MIC and MBC of our four pomace extracts against *L. monocytogenes* ranged from 4.69 to 18.8 mg/mL and from 9.38 to 37.5 mg/mL, respectively (Table 6). Cabernet Franc pomace extract showed the lowest MIC (4.69 mg/mL) and MBC (9.38 mg/mL). On the other hand, higher MIC (40.6 to 250 mg/mL) was observed for the extracts against *S. aureus* ATCC 29213, and this strain even survived while extract concentration excedding 250 mg/mL for Vidal Blanc pomace. The MIC and MBC results indicated that the grape

Table 4. Major individual flavonoid compounds in the extracts from four grape pomaces.

Flavonoid compounds (mg/g extract)	Viognier	Vidal Blanc	Cabernet Franc	Chambourcin
Catechin	910 ± 10.5^{a}	631 ± 13.4^{b}	560 ± 4537^{b}	214 ± 4.80^{c}
Epicatechin	625 ± 9.20^{a}	451 ± 22.2^{b}	215 ± 4.67^{c}	109 ± 4.17^{d}
Epigallocatechin gallate	96.1 ± 3.47^{b}	62.8 ± 0.78^{b}	171 ± 7.26^{a}	–
Gallocatechin gallate	99.1 ± 1.29^{c}	–	232 ± 3.19^{a}	146 ± 3.37^{b}
Epicatechingallate	427 ± 11.7^{a}	–	122 ± 2.995^{b}	56.9 ± 5.36^{c}
Quercetin-3-rhamnoside	27.1 ± 2.59^{a}	33.5 ± 1.57^{a}	–	–
Quercetin	17.3 ± 0.38^{c}	20.7 ± 0.01^{c}	56.5 ± 1.95^{a}	31.2 ± 2.26^{b}
Kaempferol	–	–	8.69 ± 0.38^{a}	3.28 ± 0.14^{b}
Rutin	255 ± 16.7^{c}	435 ± 14.0^{a}	343 ± 11.0^{b}	99.5 ± 0.39^{d}

Data are expressed as mean ± standard deviation ($n = 2$).
Means followed by the same letter within a row indicate no significant ($P > 0.05$) difference among samples.
–, stands for not detectable.

Table 5. Antibacterial activity of the extracts from four grape pomaces.

		Diameters of inhibition zone (mm)			
		Gram-positive		Gram-negative	
Varieties	Conc. (mg/mL)	*Listeria monocytogenes* ATCC 7644	*Staphylococcus aureus* ATCC 29213	*Escherichia coli* O157:H7 ATCC 3510	*Salmonella Typhimurium* ATCC 14028
Viognier	150	23.6 ± 0.6^{a}	7.8 ± 0.5^{b}	Nd	Nd
	300	25.0 ± 0.6^{a}	8.6 ± 0.4^{b}	Nd	Nd
Vidal Blanc	150	21.2 ± 0.9^{b}	1.2 ± 0.0^{e}	Nd	Nd
	300	25.1 ± 0.4^{a}	2.9 ± 0.6^{d}	Nd	Nd
Cabernet Franc	150	16.4 ± 1.0^{c}	6.9 ± 0.4^{c}	Nd	Nd
	300	21.6 ± 0.6^{b}	11.7 ± 0.3^{a}	Nd	Nd
Chambourcin	150	14.0 ± 1.0^{c}	5.7 ± 0.1^{c}	Nd	Nd
	300	N/A	N/A	Nd	Nd

N/A, not available; Nd, not detectable.
Data are expressed as mean ± standard deviation ($n = 3$).
Means followed by the same letter within a column indicate no significant ($P > 0.05$) difference among samples.

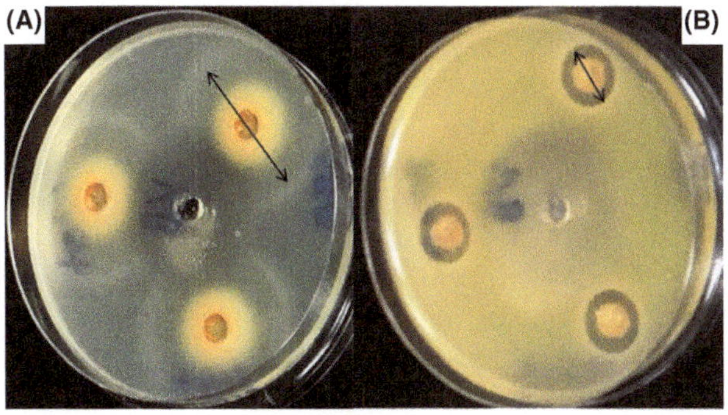

Figure 2. Antibacterial activity (inhibition zone) of Vidal Blanc pomace extract against (A) *L. monocytogenes* ATCC 7644 and (B) *S. aureus* ATCC 29213

Table 6. Minimum inhibitory concentration (MIC) and minimum bactericidal concentration (MBC) of four grape extracts against *Listeria monocytogenes* and *Staphylococcus aureus*.

	Listeria monocytogenes ATCC 7644		*Staphylococcus aureus* ATCC 29213	
Varieties	MIC (mg/mL)	MBC (mg/mL)	MIC (mg/mL)	MBC (mg/mL)
Viognier	5.07^{a}	10.2^{a}	40.6^{a}	162.5^{b}
Vidal Blanc	15.6^{b}	31.3^{b}	250^{c}	>250
Cabernet Franc	4.69^{a}	9.38^{a}	75^{b}	150^{b}
Chambourcin	18.8^{b}	37.5^{b}	75^{b}	75^{a}

Data shown for MICs and MBCs are a result of four replicates of which three values were identical for every organism and every tested sample. Means followed by the same letter within a column indicate no significant ($P > 0.05$) difference among the samples.

pomace extracts had higher antibacterial activity against *L. monocytogenes* than *S. aureus*, which are consistent with the results obtained from agar-well diffusion method.

Conclusion

Significant differences were found among the pomaces from four Virginia-grown grape varieties in relation to the concentrations of total phenolics, total flavonoids, total anthocyanins, tannins, and condensed tannins and to DPPH• and ABTS•+ free radical scavenging assays. Cabernet Franc pomace extract exhibited the highest content of phenolics compounds and ABTS•+ free radical scavenging activity. Total phenolics, total flavonoids, tannins, and condensed tannins were positively correlated with each other and with ABTS•+ scavenging capacity. There was a positive correlation between total anthocyanins and DPPH• -scavenging capacity. All pomace extracts exhibited antibacterial activity against *L. monocytogenes* ATCC 7644 and *S. aureus* ATCC 29213, but not against *E. coli* O157:H7 ATCC 3510 or *S. typhimurium* ATCC 14028. Cabernet Franc and Viognier pomaces appear to have the great potential as source of natural antioxidant and antimicrobial agents. Further research will focus on further identification of phenolic compounds, and the relationship of individual phenolic compounds to antioxidant and antibacterial activities in grape pomaces.

Acknowledgments

We thank Mr. Robert Durst at Oregon State University for HPLC analysis for individual flavonoid compounds. Funding was provided through the USDA Capacity Building Grant (Award number: 2013-38821-21124). The research was conducted at Virginia State University Agricultural Research Station (Journal Series number 322).

Conflict of Interest

None declared.

References

Alipour, D., and Y. Rouzbehan. 2010. Effects of several levels of extracted tannin from grape pomace on intestinal digestibility of soybean meal. Livestock Sci. 128:87–91.

Ben Rodn, J., O. Lamikanra, S. Leong, Y. Owusu, M. Abazinge, and I. Inyang. 1994. Bioconversion of muscadine grape waste into livestock feed. Proc. Florida State Horticult. Soc. 107:291–294.

Cerda-Carrasco, A. D. L., R. López-Solís, H. Nuñez-Kalasic, A. Peña-Neira, and E. Obreque-Slier. 2015. Phenolic composition and antioxidant capacity of pomaces from four grape varieties (*Vitis vinifera* L.). J. Sci. Food Agricult. 95(7):1521–1527.

Darra, N. E., J. Tannous, P. B. Mouncef, J. Palge, J. Yaghi, E. Vorobiev, et al. 2012. A Comparative study on antiradical and antimicrobial properties of red grapes extractsobtained from different *Vitis vinifera* varieties. Food Nutr. Sci. 3:1420–1432.

Doshi, P., P. Adsule, and K. Banerjee. 2006. Phenolic composition and antioxidant activity in grapevine parts and berries (*Vitis vinifera* L.) cv. Kishmish Chornyi (Sharad Seedless) during maturation. Int. J. Food Sci. Technol. 41:1–9.

Elfalleh, W., N. Yahia, and A. Ferchichi. 2012. Main pomegranate phytochemicals and their contribution to the antioxidant potencies of pomegranate juice. Pp. 325–329 *in* P. Melgarejo, D. Valero, ed. II International Symposium on the Pomegranate. CIHEAM/Universidad Miguel Hernández, Zaragoza.

Ferrer, J., G. Paez, Z. Marmol, E. Ramones, C. Chandler, M. Marın, et al. 2001. Agronomic use of biotechnologically processed grape wastes. Bioresour. Technol. 76:39–44.

Fontoin, H., C. Saucier, P. L. Teissedre, and Y. Glories. 2008. Effect of pH, ethanol and acidity on astringency and bitterness of grape seed tannin oligomers in model wine solution. Food Qual. Prefer. 19:286–291.

Giusti, M. M., and R. E. Wrolstad. 2001. Anthocyanins: characterization and measurement with UV-visiblespectroscopy. Pp. F1.2.1–F1.213 *in* R. E. Wrolstad, ed. Current protocols in food analytical chemistry. Wiley, NewYork.

González-Centeno, M. R., M. Jourdes, A. Femenia, S. Simal, C. Rosselló, and P.-L. Teissedre. 2013. Characterization of polyphenols and antioxidant potential of white grape pomace byproducts (*Vitis vinifera L.*). J. Agricult. Food Chem. 61:11579–11587.

Gyawali, R., and S. A. Ibrahim. 2014. Natural products as antimicrobial agents. Food Control 46:412–429.

Hasani, S., and M. Hasani. 2014. Antimicrobial properties of grape extract on common carp (Cyprinus carpio) fillet during storage in 4°C. Int. J. Fish. Aquat. Stud. 1:130–136.

He, F., N.-N. Liang, L. Mu, -H. PanQ, J. Wang, M. J. Reeves, et al. 2012. Anthocyanins and their variation in red wines I. Monomeric anthocyanins and their color expression. Molecules 17:1571–1601.

Hogan, S., L. Zhang, J. Li, B. Zoecklein, and K. Zhou. 2009. Antioxidant properties and bioactive components of Norton (*Vitis aestivalis*) and Cabernet Franc (*Vitis vinifera*) wine grapes. LWT-Food Sci. Technol. 42:1269–1274.

Hogan, S., L. Zhang, J. Li, S. Sun, C. Canning, and K. Zhou. 2010. Antioxidant rich grape pomace extract suppresses postprandial hyperglycemia in diabetic mice by specifically inhibiting alpha-glucosidase. Nut. Metab. 7:71.

Korkiel, L. J., B. J. H. Janse, and M. Viljoen-Bloom. 2002. Utilizing grape pomace for ethanol production. South African J. Enol. Viticult. 23:31–36.

Makkar, H. P. S., M. Bluemmel, N. K. Borowy, and K. Becker. 1993. Gravimetric determination of tannins and their correlations with chemical and protein precipitation methods. J. Sci. Food Agric. 61:161–165.

Mazza, G. 1995. Anthocyanins in grape and grape products. Crit. Rev. Food Sci. Nutr. 35:341–371.

Nile, S. H., S. H. Kim, E. Y. Ko, and S. Park. 2013. Polyphenolic contents and antioxidant properties of different grape (*V. vinifera*, *V. labrusca*, and V. hybrid) cultivars. BioMed Res. Int., 2013, Article ID 718065.

Nittiema, L. W., A. Savadogo, J. Simpore, D. Dianou, and A. S. Traore. 2012. In vitro antimicrobial activity of some phenolic compounds (coumarin and quercetin) against gastroenteritis bacterial strains. Int. J. Microbiol. Res. 3:183–187.

Oliveira, D. A., A. A. Salvadora, A. Jr Smânia, E. F. A. Smâniab, M. Maraschinc, and S. R. S. Ferreiraa. 2013. Antimicrobial activity and composition profile of grape (*Vitis vinifera*) pomace extracts obtained by supercritical fluids. J. Biotechnol. 164:423–432.

Ozkan, G., O. Sagdic, N. G. Baydar, and Z. Kurumahmutoglu. 2004a. Antibacterial activities and total phenolic contents of grape pomace extracts. J. Sci. Food Agric. 84:1807–1811.

Ozkan, G., O. Sagdic, N. G. Baydar, and H. Baydar. 2004b. Antioxidant and antibacterial activities of *Rosa damascena* flower extracts. Food Sci. Technol. Int. 10:277–281.

Parry, J. W., H. Li, J.-R. Liu, K. Zhou, L. Zhang, and S. Ren. 2011. Antioxidant activity, antiproliferation of colon cancer cells, and chemical composition of grape pomace. Food Nut. Sci. 2:530–540.

Petti, S., and C. Scully. 2009. Polyphenols, oral health and disease: A review. J. Dent. 37(6):413–423.

Porter, L. J., L. N. Hrstich, and B. G. Chan. 1986. The conversion of procyanidins and prodelphinidins to cyanidin and delphinidin. Phytochemistry 25:223–230.

Puupponen-Pimia, R., L. Nohynek, C. Meier, M. Kahkonen, M. Heinonen, A. Hopia, et al. 2001. Antimicrobial properties of phenolic compounds from berries. J. Appl. Microbiol. 90:494–507.

Ramirez-Lopez, L. M., and C. A. M. DeWitt. 2014. Analysis of phenolic compounds in commercial dried grape pomace by high-performance liquid chromatography electrospray ionization mass spectrometry. Food Sci. Nut. 2:470–477.

Re, R., N. Pellegrini, A. Proteggente, A. Pannala, M. Yang, and C. Rice-Evans. 1999. Antioxidant activity applying an improved ABTS radical cation decolorization assay. Free Radic. Biol. Med. 26:1231–1237.

Rockenbach, I. I., E. Rodrigues, L. V. Gonzaga, V. Caliari, M. I. Genovese, A. E. de Souza Schmidt Gonçalves, et al. 2011. Phenolic compounds content and antioxidant activity in pomace from selected red grapes (*Vitis vinifera* L. and *Vitis labrusca* L.) widely produced in Brazil. Food Chem. 127:174–179.

Rondeaua, P., F. Gambiera, F. Jolibert, and N. Brossea. 2013. Compositions and chemical variability of grape pomaces from French vineyard. Ind. Crops Prod. 43:251–254.

Ruberto, G., A. Renda, C. Daquino, V. Amico, C. Spatafora, C. Tringali, et al. 2007. Polyphenol constituents and antioxidant activity of grape pomace extracts from five Sicilian red grape cultivars. Food Chem. 100:203–210.

Sagdic, O., I. Ozturk, M. T. Yilmaz, and H. Yetim. 2011. Effect of grape pomace extracts obtained from different grape varieties on microbial quality of beef patty. J. Food Sci. 76:M5 15–M5 21.

Samatha, T., R. Shyamsundarachary, P. Srinivas, and N. R. Swamy. 2012. Quantification of total phenolic and total flavonoid contents in extracts of *Oroxylum Indicum L.* Kurz. Asian J. Pharm. Clin. Res. 5:177–179.

Sánchez-Moreno, C., J. A. Larrauri, and F. Saura-Calixto. 1998. A procedure to measure the antiradical efficiency of polyphenols. J. Sci. Food Agric. 76:270–276.

Smith-Palmer, A., J. Stewart, and L. Fyfe. 1998. Antimicrobial properties of plant essential oils and essences against five important food-borne pathogens. Lett. Appl. Microbiol. 26:118–122.

Tabart, J., C. Kevers, J. Pincemail, J.-O. Defraigne, and J. Dommes. 2009. Comparative antioxidant capacities of phenolic compounds measured by various tests. Food Chem. 113:1226–1233.

Teixeira, A., N. Baenas, R. Dominguez-Perles, A. Barros, E. Rosa, D. A. Moreno, et al. 2014. Natural bioactive compounds from winery by-products as health promoters: a review. Int. J. Mol. Sci. 15:15638–15678.

Vuorinen, H., K. Määtta, and R. Törrönen. 2000. Content of the flavonols myricetin, quercetin, and kaempferol in Finnish berry wines. J. Agricult. Food Chem. 48:2675–2680.

Xia, E.-Q., G.-F. Deng, Y.-J. Guo, and H.-B. Li. 2010. Biological activities of polyphenols from grapes. Int. J. Mol. Sci. 11:622–646.

Yang, J., T. E. Martinson, and R. Liu. 2009. Phytochemical profiles and antioxidant activities of wine grapes. Food Chem. 116:332–339.

Zhou, K., and J. J. Raffoul. 2012. Potential anticancer properties of grape antioxidants. J. Oncol. 2012, Article ID 803294.

17

Sensory quality of soymilk and tofu from soybeans lacking lipoxygenases

Aijun Yang[1], Heather Smyth[2], Mridusmita Chaliha[3] & Andrew James[1]

[1]CSIRO Agriculture, 306 Carmody Road, St Lucia, Queensland 4067, Australia
[2]Queensland Alliance for Agriculture and Food Innovation, The University of Queensland, St Lucia, Queensland 4072, Australia
[3]Department of Agriculture, Fisheries and Forestry, Coopers Plains, Queensland 4108, Australia

Keywords
Lipoxygenase, sensory quality, soy milk, soybean, tofu

Correspondence
Aijun Yang, CSIRO Agriculture, 306 Carmody Road, St Lucia, Queensland 4067, Australia.

E-mail: Aijun.Yang@csiro.au

Funding Information
Grains Research and Development Corporation, Australia.

Abstract

The oxidation of unsaturated lipids by lipoxygenases in soybeans causes undesirable flavors in soy foods. Using a traditional and a nontraditional soy food user group, we examined the cultural difference in perceiving the sensory characteristics of soymilk and tofu produced from soybeans with or without lipoxygenases (Lx123). The two groups described the samples using similar terms. The traditional users preferred the control soy milk and lipoxygenase-free tofu while the nontraditional users preferred the lipoxygenase-free soymilk with no preference for tofu. In a separate study, a trained descriptive taste panel compared the odor of soymilk and tofu from control soybeans or those lacking lipoxygenase-1 and lipoxygenase-2 (Lx12) or all three isomers (Lx123). The rancid/grassy odor was rated the lowest in Lx123 products, followed by Lx12 products with the control products given the highest rating. The Lx12 and Lx123 products were also sweeter and less bitter than the controls. Taken together, our results demonstrated that soybeans lacking lipoxygenases can produce soy foods with less undesirable aromas and are therefore likely more acceptable to the consumers.

Introduction

Soy foods produced from whole soybean seeds such as soymilk and tofu have been part of the traditional foods in East Asia for a long time. Soybean is also an important ingredient in many processed foods. Its production and use has increased rapidly due to its high nutritional value and potential health benefits. Utilization of soybean seeds as food materials, however, has sometimes been limited, particularly in Western societies, because of their "grassy/beany" flavor (Krishna et al. 2003) and certain consumers prefer a bland or neutral flavor in soy products. The consumers from traditional soy food consumption countries, on the other hand, generally favorably associate beany flavor with soy products such as soymilk and tofu. Cross-cultural variations in food preferences are well known and cultural differences in consumption of soy products might account for some differences in perception of sensory attributes. These undesirable flavors, characterized as beany, green, grassy, painty, astringent, and bitter, have been associated with off-flavors from the oxidation of polyunsaturated lipids by lipoxygenases (LOX) present in soybeans.

Soybeans are known to be a rich source of LOX and mature soybean seeds contain three major lipoxygenases: LOX-1 (lipoxygenase-1), LOX-2 (lipoxygenase-2), and LOX-3 (lipoxygenase-3). Soybean also contains high amount of polyunsaturated fatty acids (PUFA), predominantly linoleic acid (C18:2) at around 50% and linolenic acid (C18:3) up to 11% (King et al. 1998; Gerde and White 2008). Both C18:2 and C18:3 contain a *cis,cis*-1,4-pentadiene structure potentially leading to the production of hydroperoxides when oxidized, which in turn are converted into volatile compounds associated with undesirable flavors (Kitamura 1984). Full-fat soy flour is especially prone to such deterioration and has a disagreeable taste that is difficult to mask. Before beans are crushed or ground, LOX and PUFA are separated within the cell, but following soaking and homogenization in the process of making soymilk, they are mixed and begin to react to form the oxidation products and volatile compounds. Among the volatile compounds detectable in soy products, hexanal is primarily responsible for the objectionable flavor or aroma of soy foods and has a very low detection threshold (Wilkens and Lin 1970). The removal of all or some of the LOX present in soybeans through breeding has produced soybean lines lacking LOX and subsequent lower levels of volatiles responsible for the rancid flavor, which could be useful in improving the acceptance of Western consumers. While LOX-free soybean has been shown to produce lower hydroperoxide and hexanal levels than that with LOX or lacking LOX-1, -2, or -3 isozyme (Hildebrand et al. 1991; Kobayashi et al. 1995; Furuta et al. 1996), there have also been mixed results in the literature on the impact of these LOX-free soybean lines on controlling the beany flavor of soy foods produced. For example, using GC-MS, Kobayashi et al. (1995) showed that almost all volatiles in soymilk produced from mutants lacking LOX were markedly lower than those from a normal variety. Wilson (1996) reported that tofu made from LOX-2 null lines of soybeans were less beany than their respective controls as evaluated by a sensory panel. However, while LOX-free soybeans reduced the beany flavor in certain types of soy products such as soymilk and tofu (Wilson 1996; Torres-Penaranda et al. 1998), they showed no effect in oils, breads, and meat patties (King et al. 1998, 2001; Liu et al. 2008). Besides improved flavor and aroma, soybeans null in LOX could be more resistant to adverse storage conditions than the normal soybeans with regard to changes in pH and solid content of the soymilk (Lambrecht et al. 1996), although Torres-Penaranda and Reitmeier (2001) reported significant sensory differences between soymilks from soybeans lacking LOX stored for 3 months and 15 months and no difference for the soymilks from the normal soybeans stored for these times.

The LOX-null lines, including those developed in Australia, have been shown to have similar agronomic traits including yield (Narvel et al. 1998; Reinprecht et al. 2006) (A. James, 2013 unpubl. data). However, the LOX-free lines from Australia have not been evaluated for their effect on storage stability, beany flavor, and other quality attributes in soy foods. There are two types of commercial soymilk in Australia, one made from imported soy protein isolates and one made from domestically sourced whole soybean. The grassy/beany flavor of the whole bean soymilk is reported to be a limitation on the uptake of this type by the market. Therefore, soybean without lipoxygenase may offer an opportunity to expand the market for Australian-grown soybeans. Studies using panels from different cultural backgrounds to evaluate the sample product may give some indication as to whether such differences should be considered. The Australian market for soy products has consumers of many cultural and ethnic backgrounds. The objectives of this study were therefore to compare soymilk and silken tofu from normal and lipoxygenase-free soybeans using a predominantly native Chinese panel ("traditional soy users") and an Anglo-Australian panel ("nontraditional soy users") in Australia and to investigate the impact of LOX-free soybeans developed in Australia on sensory attributes of soy products in order to improve our understanding of the potential utility of these traits for the Australian market.

Materials and Methods

Soybeans, soymilk and tofu

Normal soybeans and soybean lines selected for LOX-null in Australia were used in these studies. All the lines used were grown, harvested, and stored together before use. In the preliminary study, a commercial line and a genotype lacking all three major LOX isozymes (Lx123) were used. In the following sensory study, normal soybeans and lines lacking LOX-1 and LOX-2 (Lx12) or all three isomers (Lx123) were selected. The LOX-1 and LOX-2 genes are tightly linked and inherited together, while the LOX-3 gene is independently inherited (Davies and Nielsen 1986). All the materials were kept at around 22°C until use.

All soybean lines were checked for LOX using a screening method (Suda et al. 1995; Narvel et al. 2000) and SDS-PAGE (sodium dodecyl-polyacrylamide gel electrophoresis) (Yang and James 2013) to confirm the absence of LOX-1 and LOX-2 or all three LOX isomers. A typical SDS-PAGE profile of soybean seed proteins with or without LOX isozymes is presented in Figure 1.

Soymilk and silken tofu were produced according to the procedure optimized by Yang and James (2013) and stored at 4°C overnight before use in sensory and focus group assessments. Briefly, the beans were soaked overnight before they were ground in a domestic blender. The slurry was cooked at 98°C and then filtered using a juice extractor to obtain soymilk. The required amount of the soymilk for assessment was transferred to 4°C. The

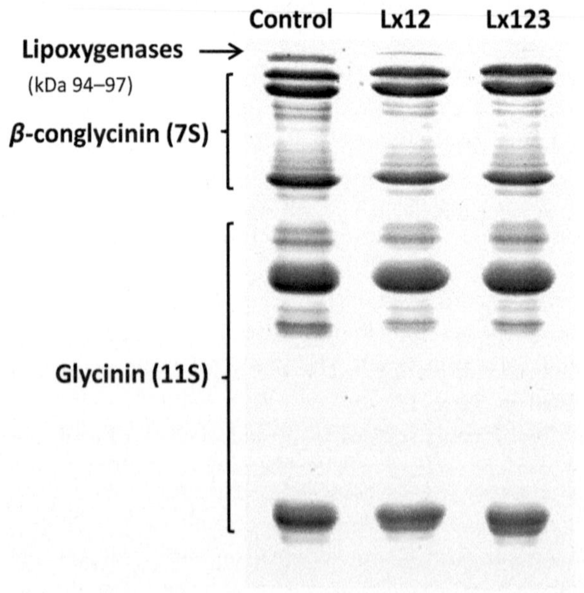

Figure 1. Sodium dodecyl-polyacrylamide gel electrophoresis profile of seed proteins from control, Lx12 or Lx 123 soybeans.

remaining soymilk was made into silken tofu by adding 0.3% coagulant (nigari, mostly magnesium chloride) and allowing the curd to form at 85°C. The soymilk and tofu were kept at 4°C until use.

Preliminary study of soymilk and tofu from control and LOX-free soybeans

Sensory evaluation using panels of "traditional" and "nontraditional" soy users

Two semiformal focus groups were held (each of 1 h duration) involving two target groups namely "nontraditional soy users" (the Australian panel) and "traditional soy users" (the Chinese panel). The profiles of the participants for each group are given in Table 1. The participants in each group were presented samples of soy milk and silken tofu made from commercial beans (control) and lipoxygenase-free soybeans (LOX-free) together with paper questionnaires. Participants were asked to describe the appearance, aroma, texture and mouth feel, flavor, and aftertaste of samples and to rate the overall acceptability of each sample on an unstructured 15-cm hedonic line scale anchored from "dislike extremely" to "like extremely". The individual assessments were made under controlled conditions (light, temperature) and samples were labeled with 3-digit codes. Presentation order of samples was identical across the participants as follows: control soy milk, LOX-free soy milk, control silken tofu, and LOX-free tofu. Samples (15–20 g each) were presented in disposable plastic pots (tofu) and cups (milks). Participants were also asked to complete a short demographic questionnaire and indicate their soy product knowledge and consumption behavior. Following the taste session, a focus group discussion was held in which participants were asked to share and discuss their thoughts on the sensory properties and acceptability of the samples and their past soy product experiences and consumption behavior.

Table 1. Profiles of participants involved in soy focus group study.

		Age range (years)	Ethnicity	Soy product consumption
Nontraditional soy product users	2 male 5 female	20–70	Anglo-Australian	Daily – never
Traditional soy product users	1 male 5 female	40	Chinese	Daily – weekly

Instrumental analysis of volatile compounds by GC-MS

Replicated samples of soy milk and silken tofu (control and LOX-free) after 1 day and 8 days stored at 4°C were sampled and frozen (−19°C) for volatile analysis. Aliquots of 5 mL of soy milk or 5 g of silken tofu were placed in 25 mL glass vials for SPME (solid phase microextraction) and immediately closed with screw caps with PTFE/silicone septa (Supelco, Bellefonte, PA).

The method used for volatile analysis was a modified version of the method reported by Achouri et al. (2006). Samples were analyzed with a 6890N GC (gas chromatograph) equipped with a 5975 MSD (mass spectrometric detector) (Agilent Technologies, Palo Alto, CA). The GC was fitted with a DB-WAX column (J&W Science, i.d. = 0.25 μm, length = 30.0 m, film thickness = 0.25 μm), and helium (BOC gases, ultrahigh purity) was used as a carrier gas at a linear velocity of 56 cm/min and at a flow rate of 2.4 mL/min.

The polydivinylbenzene and carbowax and polydimethylsiloxane (DVB–CAR–PDMS, Gray, 50/30 µm, Supelco) fiber was introduced into the headspace of the sample vial and was allowed to incubate at 45°C for 20 min. After the incubation, the fiber was retracted into a needle and desorbed into the injection port of the GC for 6 min. The fiber remained in the injection port for 6 min to eliminate the possible residues on the fiber. Extraction was supported by magnetic stirring at 250 rpm/s and a fiber blank experiment was performed. The mass spectrometer was operated in the electron impact ion mode with a source temperature of 250°C. The electron energy was 70 eV and the mass range was 35–300 m/z. The GC oven temperature started at 35°C for 3 min, was increased at 6.0°C/min to 220°C, and was held for 10 min.

Data analysis was carried out with MSD ChemStation Data Analysis software (Agilent Technologies) to obtain peak responses of volatiles. Peak identification was achieved by comparison of spectra and retention times with authentic reference standards.

Sensory study on comparing control, Lx12, and Lx123 soy products

Soybean seed characterization

The moisture, oil, and protein content of the soybeans were determined as described by Yang and James (2013). The seeds were analyzed for their fatty acid composition using GC. Briefly, soybean seeds were ground to a fine powder and oil was extracted twice with n-hexane. The combined hexane extractions were evaporated under nitrogen. The oil, 0.1 g, was methylated with 0.5 mol/L sodium methoxide solution at 80°C for 10 min. After cooling to room temperature, 0.05 mL of glacial acetic acid, 2.5 mL of distilled water, and 2.5 mL of petroleum spirit (or hexane) were added. The mixture was vortexed and 0.5 μL of the clear upper phase was used for analysis. The separation and distribution of fatty acid methyl esters were obtained using GC (Perkin Elmer Autosystem Gas Chromatograph, MA, USA) fitted with a FID (flame ionization detector) and a capillary column (SGE BPX70, 25 m × 0.22 mm). The carrier gas was helium at 15 psi. The injector temperature was 240°C and detector temperature was 280°C. The oven temperature started at 150°C before reaching 200°C.

The ground full-fat soybean meal was also stored at 37°C for 1 week and the total volatiles were measured using a SPME-GC-FID procedure.

Sensory evaluation

Three replicates of each silken tofu and soy milk sample were prepared from the composite samples of soybeans the day prior to the commencement of sensory testing and training and formal assessments were completed within a 3 day period to ensure freshness of samples. Sensory descriptive analysis techniques were applied to assess and quantify the major sensory properties of six samples including tofu and soy milk made from commercial soybeans (control), from triple-null soybeans (Lx123), and from double-null soybeans (Lx12). A total of 11 panelists (four male, seven female), who were experienced in descriptive sensory studies and who were staff and students at the Health and Food Sciences Precinct, Coopers Plains, Queensland, participated in the study. Their profiles are listed in Table 1.

Two training sessions were conducted in a board-room style round table suitable for discussions. The first training session involved presentation of all samples to panelists, individual aroma and taste assessments, and vocabulary development through discussion (Table 2). The second training session involved practicing rating attributes for each of the samples and developing a concise list of attributes, scales, and definitions. Attributes selected during training, together with their definitions, are shown in Table 3.

Formal assessments were conducted in the sensory laboratory of the Health and Food Sciences Precinct, Coopers Plains, Queensland. The laboratory consists of individual tasting booths equipped with computers, daylight equivalent lighting, and temperature control. Three replicate sessions were held whereby all six samples were presented and assessed according to a balanced presentation design. Data were collected using sensory software Compusense five (version 5.0, Compusense Inc., Guelph, ON, Canada) and data were exported and analyzed using XLSTAT (version 2014.6.05, Addinsoft 1995–2014, CA, USA). During training and formal sessions, samples of tofu and milk (~10–15 g) were presented to panelists in small plastic cups covered with plastic lids. Milks were freshly stirred and tofu was freshly sliced prior to serving.

Table 2. Sensory descriptors and vocabulary from the training session in the preliminary evaluation of control and LOX-free soymilk and tofu.

LOX-free soymilk	Control soymilk
Yellowish Cooked pasta, floury, evaporated milk, cooked, sour, grassy, raw, less intense/subtle, beany, sweet floral, raw soy Soy, painty, potato, alfalfa sprouts, snow pea, green-sweet, macadamia, savory, soft-nutty sourness, sweeter, less intense	Off-white, lighter color, thicker looking "Typical" Chinese-style, strong, stale-earthy, starchy, raw beans, green, floral, nutty, chalky, rancid, flour and water paste, raw green pea Raw beans, soy, fresh veg, grassy, aged oil/rancid, painty, green astringent, earthy, bitterness, legume, dry milk, more intense
LOX-free tofu	**Control tofu**
Lighter, yellower More subtle, less intense, green bean, fresh bean, grassy, green-floral, rubber tree, sappy, fermented, legume, pleasant Bitter, metallic, nutty, sourness, potato, dairy, buttery, raw bean, sweeter, fresher, clean aftertaste	Creamy, beige More intense, rancid, raw bean, starch, nutty, grain, painty, old rancid wheat bran, floury Rancid, aged oil, sour, low-intensity flavors, bitterness, raw taste, metallic, green, legume, painty, oxidized, potato

Table 3. Sensory attributes and definitions developed and used in the sensory descriptive study of control and LOX-free soymilk and tofu.

Attribute	Definition
Aroma intensity	The overall intensity of the samples aroma from subtle to intense
Fresh pea aroma	A fresh pea, cucumber, melon-like or lettuce aroma
Grassy rancid aroma	A grassy rancid aroma, sappy, sour, raw and painty, like rancid oil
Floury aroma	A floury, starchy, potato-like aroma, reminiscent of clay and earth
Flavor intensity	The overall flavor intensity of the sample when in the mouth
Sweetness	The perceived sweetness of samples experienced in the mouth
Bitterness	The perceived bitterness of samples experienced in the mouth

Statistical analysis

All measurements in this study were replicated three times. The data were subject to analysis of variance to examine the effect of genotypes on each of the sensory attributes examined in soymilk and tofu. The means were separated using least square difference at the 5% significance level.

Results

Preliminary study using panels of "traditional" and "nontraditional" soy users

Typically, the participants from each target group described the samples using similar terms. The control soy milk was paler in color than the LOX-free soy milk. Both groups described the LOX-free milk as being less intense and more subtle with more floury, cooked pasta-type aromas which also came through on the palate together with some sweet green snow pea-like flavors. The LOX-free milk was also described as sweeter than the control and less intense in flavor overall. The control soy milk was stronger in odor with raw green pea/bean, stale-earthy, and rancid-type aromas. The flavor was also stronger, raw, and grassy with some rancid oil, painty, and bitter-type flavors. Similarly for the silken tofu samples, the control was described overall as being more intense in odor and flavor. The LOX-free tofu was described as having fresher/cleaner, more subtle attributes, while the control was described as being rancid (not fresh) and more intense aroma and flavor. Interestingly, the Chinese panel ("traditional soy users") described the control soy milk as "typical" Chinese-style whereas they described the LOX-free milk as unusual. Overall, the Chinese panel preferred the control soymilk and the LOX-free tofu while the Australian panel ("nontraditional soy users") preferred the LOX-free soymilk and did not seem to like either of the tofu products (Fig. 2).

The presence or absence of the three major lipoxygenases was confirmed using SDS-PAGE (Fig. 1) and a screening method. The soymilk from the control and LOX-free soybean had similar solid content in soymilk (~11%). The major volatiles in these products as determined by GC-MS were hexanal with some 1-hexanol and butanol. A GC-MS profile showing the difference in the major volatiles in soymilk stored at 4°C for 1 day is presented in Figure 3. The peak area data (×100,000) revealed that all three volatiles in the control products were much higher than that in the LOX-free products, 1.85, 2.75, and 1.22 for control soymilk and 0.60, 2.05, and 0.42 for LOX-free soymilk for hexanal, 1-hexanol, and butanol, respectively; 4.5, 2.15, and 1.03 for control tofu and 1.25, 1.75, and 0.40 for LOX-free tofu for hexanal, 1-hexanol, and butanol, respectively. The difference in the major volatile, hexanal, between control and LOX-free products seemed to have increased after 8 days of refrigerated storage (Fig. 4).

Sensory study on comparing control and Lx12 and Lx123 soy products

The seed characteristics of the soybeans containing the three major lipoxygenases, lacking LOX-1 and LOX-2 (Lx12) or lacking all three isomers (Lx123) are presented in Table 4. The similar genetic background of the three soybean types, except for lipoxygenases, was expected to yield products with similar characteristics other than the beany aroma/flavor. While the seeds of Lx12 were smaller and, compared with the controls, contained more protein,

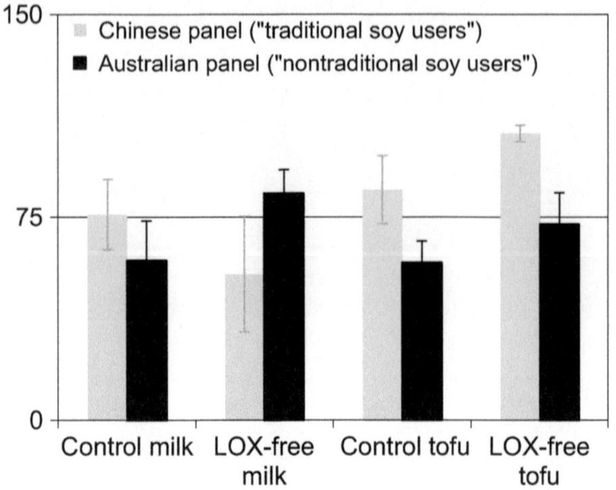

Figure 2. Difference in preference between an Australian (n = 8) and a native Chinese (n = 6) panel for control and LOX-free soymilk and tofu.

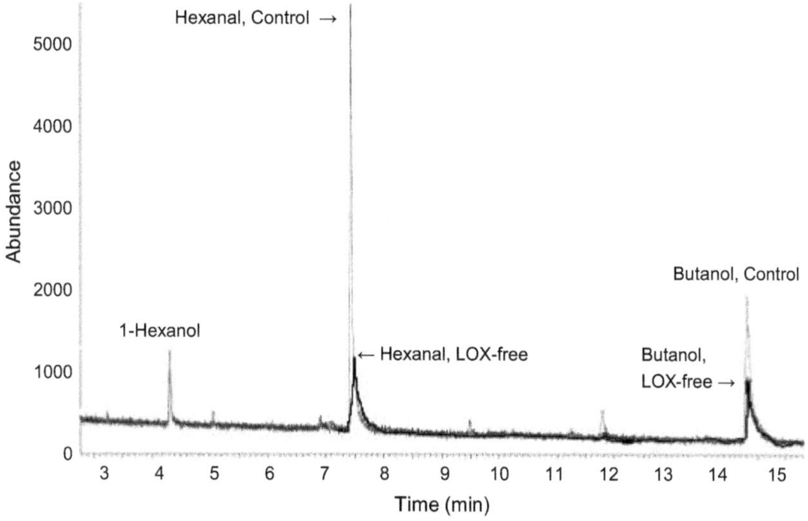

Figure 3. Major volatiles in control soymilk and LOX-free soymilk.

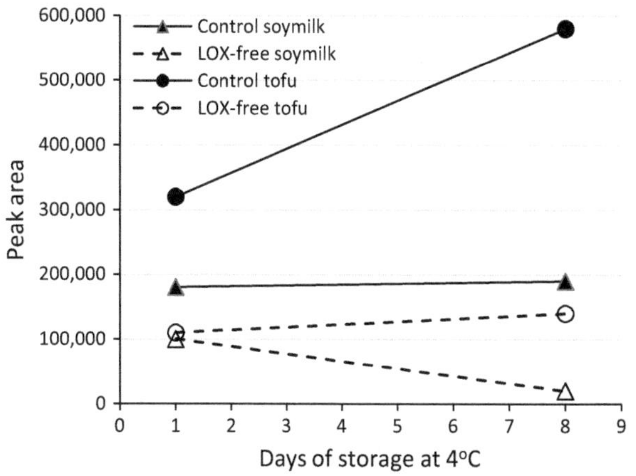

Figure 4. Hexanal peak area for tofu and soymilk after 1 and 8 days of storage at 4°C

Table 4. Seed characteristics of control, Lx1-2 null and Lx1-3 null samples.

	Control	Lx12	Lx123
Seed wt (g/100 seeds)	26.49^{a}*	21.49^{b}	25.34^{a}
Oil (%)	19.80	20.09	19.75
Protein (%)	39.56^{b}	44.33^{a}	42.86^{ab}
Major fatty acids			
C16:0	10.18	9.99	10.33
C18:0	1.53	1.78	1.63
C18:1c	20.03	20.67	23.36
C18:2	53.34	51.50	49.55
C18:3	9.09	9.52	8.82
PUFA ratio (18:2/18:3) (PR)	5.73	5.41	5.62
Total SFA	14.13	14.25	14.26
Total PUFA	61.53	61.02	58.37
Total PUFA/Total SFA (PI)	4.36	4.28	4.09
Total volatile increase in full-fat soy meal after 1 week storage at 37°C	4.10^{a}	1.32^{b}	1.38^{b}

SFA, saturated fatty acids; PUFA, polyunsaturated fatty acids; PR, polyunsaturation ratio; PI, polyunsaturation index.

*Means with the same superscripts within the same row are not statistically different, $P > 0.05$.

the three groups had similar oil content and fatty acids profiles, in particular total saturated fatty acids, total PUFA, and the ratio of linoleic to linolenic fatty acids. As rancidity results from the oxidation of PUFA, the similar fatty acid composition provided an important basis for comparing differences in the sensory attributes or storage stability. After 1 week's storage at 37°C, the total peak area for the major volatiles detected using SPME-GC-FID increased over fourfold for the control full-fat soybean meal while the increase for double-null and triple-null samples was only 1.3-fold ($P < 0.05$).

The sensory analysis of the soy products made from control soybeans or those lacking LOX-1 and LOX-2 (Lx12) or all three isomers (Lx123) showed clear and significant differences in the major aroma notes between these three groups for soymilk (Fig. 5A) or silken tofu (Fig. 5B). The objectionable rancid/grassy odors were rated the lowest by the taste panel in both soymilk and tofu from Lx123 soybeans, followed by Lx12 products with the control products given the highest rancid odor rating. The difference between these three soybeans was statistically significant for both soymilk and tofu ($P < 0.05$). Bitterness, another negative sensory note, was rated significantly lower in the soymilk and tofu made from the soybeans lacking two or three lipoxygenases compared with those made from the soybean containing all three isozymes ($P < 0.05$). Aroma intensity

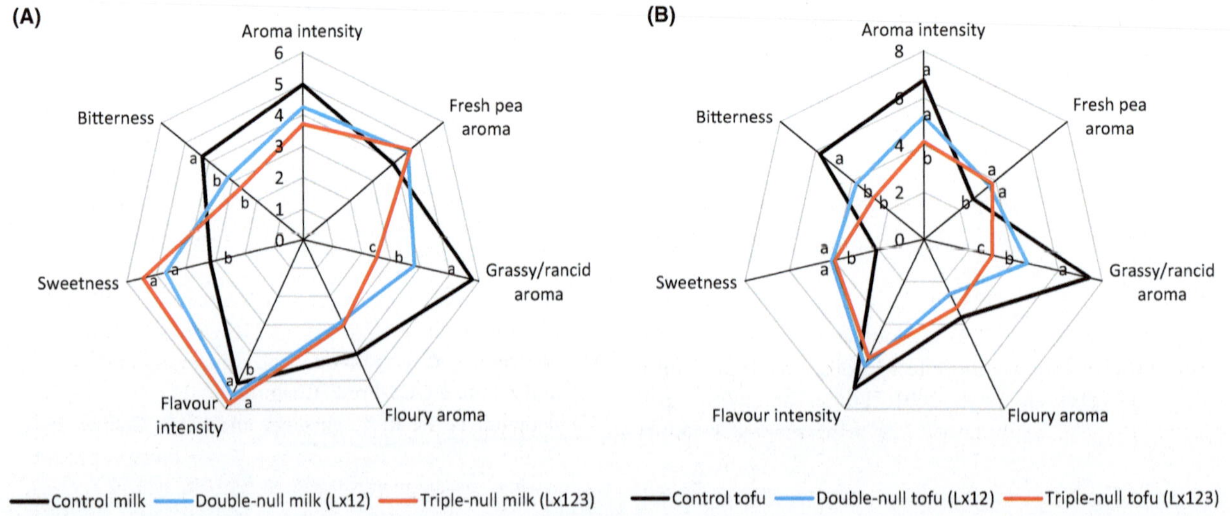

Figure 5. Plot of sensory scores for soymilk (A) and silken tofu (B) samples. $n = 3 \times 11$, for each sensory attribute, the scores with a different letter are significantly different ($P < 0.05$).

was also scored significantly lower for tofu produced from Lx12 and Lx123 soybeans, although this difference was not statistically significant for soymilk. On the other hand, sweetness, a positive sensory note, was rated significantly higher in the Lx12 and Lx123 products than the controls for both soymilk and tofu ($P < 0.05$). Fresh pea aroma was also rated higher in the Lx12 and Lx123 products than the controls, although this difference was only significant for tofu. Flavor intensity was rated differently by the taste panels for soymilk and tofu. It was scored lower for the control soymilk ($P < 0.05$) and higher for the control tofu, although this difference was not statistically different.

Discussion

Cultural difference and preference, as a result of long-term or traditional consumption of soy foods, has been reported in the perception of sensory attributes of soy foods, although the results are not clear-cut (Torres-Penaranda et al. 1998). The preference for control soymilk from an almost-native Chinese panel in this study was therefore expected as "traditional" soy users would associate the "beany" flavor with the typical flavor of soy milk. It is possible that consumers of traditional soy foods such as soymilk and tofu may find the products without lipoxygenases too bland due to the absence of the familiar beany flavor and taste. As a result, while soybean varieties lacking lipoxygenases have been developed in countries of traditional soy food consumption such as Korea and China, these varieties have not been widely taken up (K. Lee 2014 and M. Zhang 2013, pers. comm.). For "nontraditional" soy users, the traditional tofu is usually too bland in flavor and mushy in texture to their liking. They may still prefer the seasoned and harder products irrespective of lipoxygenases.

Among the volatile compounds contributing to the beany/rancid/off-flavor in soy products, hexanal is the major volatile responsible and has been studied most. The lower hexanal level observed in this study in the soymilk and tofu made from the LOX-free soybeans was consistent with the results from many studies which reported that LOX-free soybeans produce lower hydroxyperoxide and hexanal levels than those with LOX or lacking the LOX-1, -2, or -3 isozyme alone (Hildebrand et al. 1991; Kobayashi et al. 1995; Furuta et al. 1996; King et al. 1998; Ma et al. 2002, 2015). There have also been attempts to link soybean oil profile, lipoxygenase status, and off-flavor development in soy foods and a direct relationship between the degree of oil polyunsaturation, volatile compounds, hexanal level in particular, and off-flavor determining parameters has been reported (Furuta et al. 1996; Yuan and Chang 2007; Mandal et al. 2014). The significantly larger increase in the total volatiles in the full-fat soy meal after 1 week's storage at 37°C was similar to those reported by Kobayashi et al. (1995), although King et al. (1998) observed no difference in hexanal level between control and LOX-free oils and an increased hexanal level and peroxide values in LOX-free oil after 2 weeks' storage at 35°C and 50% humidity. The authors attributed these results to the differences in initial fatty acid composition.

The effects of removing lipoxygenases from soybeans on the sensory attributes, in particular on the objectionable beany/grass flavor, of soy products are mixed and seem to be product-dependent. For example, Torres-Penaranda et al. (1998) reported significant less cooked beany aroma and flavor in soy milk made from the LOX-free soybean than that from the normal line, although no difference was observed in tofu in the same study. They also found significant interactions between soybean types and panelist ethnic backgrounds for raw beany aroma and flavor, which was attributed to the low intensity of the raw aroma and flavor making differentiation between soymilk from normal and LOX-free soybeans difficult. Wilson (1996) also reported that tofu made from LOX-2 null lines of soybeans were less beany than their respective controls as evaluated by a sensory panel. LOX-free soybeans, however, showed no effect in oils, breads, and meat patties (King et al. 1998, 2001; Liu et al. 2008). It is possible that the beany flavor was being masked by other stronger sensory notes in these products. In evaluating 70 genotypes including two series of near isogenic lines with or without lipoxygenase isozymes, no effect of lipoxygenase absence was observed on soymilk flavor parameters (Ma et al. 2015). Our results clearly showed that soybeans null in two or three of the major lipoxygenases positively reduced the negative sensory notes including rancidity, bitterness, and aroma intensity and improved the positive sensory notes such as sweetness and fresh pea aroma in soymilk and tofu. Soybeans lacking all three major isomers seemed to have an additive effect on reducing the negative notes in these soy products.

Taken together, our results demonstrated that soybean seeds lacking lipoxygenases can produce whole-bean-based soy foods such as soymilk and tofu with improved flavor and aroma which are likely more acceptable to the consumers, particularly "nontraditional" soy users, and perhaps allow their utilization into other products. The soybean lines lacking lipoxygenases will also provide the Australian food industry with additional ingredients that would broaden and increase the utilization of soybeans and soy proteins in a wide range of food applications.

Acknowledgments

This research was funded in part by the Grains Research and Development Corporation in Australia under the auspices of the National Soybean Breeding Program.

Conflict of Interest

None declared.

References

Achouri, A., J. I. Boye, and Y. Zamani. 2006. Identification of volatile compounds in soymilk using solid-phase microextraction-gas chromatography. Food Chem. 99:759–766.

Davies, C. S., and N. C. Nielsen. 1986. Genetic-analysis of a null-allele for lipoxygenase-2 in soybean. Crop Sci. 26:460–463.

Furuta, S., Y. Nishiba, M. Hajika, K. Igita, and I. Suda. 1996. DETBA value and hexanal production with the combination of unsaturated fatty acids and extracts prepared from soybean seeds lacking two or three lipoxygenase isozymes. J. Agric. Food Chem. 44:236–239.

Gerde, J. A., and P. J. White. 2008. Lipids. Pp. 193–227 *In* L. A. Johnson, P. J. White and R. Galloway, eds. Soybeans: chemistry, production, processing and unilization. AOCS Press, Champaign, IL.

Hildebrand, D. F., R. T. Versluys, and G. B. Collins. 1991. Changes in lipoxygenase isozyme levels during soybean embryo development. Plant Sci. 75:1–8.

King, J. M., L. K. Svendsen, W. R. Fehr, J. M. Narvel, and P. J. White. 1998. Oxidative and flavor stability of oil from lipoxygenase-free soybeans. J. Am. Oil Chemists Soc. 75:1121–1126.

King, J. M., S. M. Chin, L. K. Svendsen, C. A. Reitmeier, L. A. Johnson, and W. R. Fehr. 2001. Processing of lipoxygenase-free soybeans and evaluation in foods. J. Am. Oil Chemists Soc. 78:353–360.

Kitamura, K. 1984. Biochemical-characterization of lipoxygenase lacking mutants, l-1-less, l-2-less, and l-3-less soybeans. Agric. Biol. Chem. 48:2339–2346.

Kobayashi, A., Y. Tsuda, N. Hirata, K. Kubota, and K. Kitamura. 1995. Aroma constituents of soybean glycine-max (l) merril milk lacking lipoxygenase isozymes. J. Agric. Food Chem. 43:2449–2452.

Krishna, A., G. Singh, D. Kumar, and K. Agrawal. 2003. Physico-chemical characteristics of some new varieties of soybean. J. Food Sci. Tech.-Mysore 40:490–492.

Lambrecht, H. S., S. S. Nielsen, B. J. Liska, and N. C. Nielsen. 1996. Effect of soybean storage on tofu and soymilk production. J. Food Quality 19:189–202.

Liu, C., X. Wang, H. Ma, Z. Zhang, W. Gao, and L. Xiao. 2008. Functional properties of protein isolates from soybeans stored under various conditions. Food Chem. 111:29–37.

Ma, H., C. Guan, X. He, G. Zhang, and A. Din. 2002. Effects of lipoxygenase null genes of soybean in controlling beany-flavor of soymilk and soyflour. Agric. Sci. China 1:965–971.

Ma, L., B. Li, F. Han, S. Yan, L. Wang, and J. Sun. 2015. Evaluation of the chemical quality traits of soybean seeds, as related to sensory attributes of soymilk. Food Chem. 173:694–701.

Mandal, S., A. Dahuja, A. Kar, and I. M. Santha. 2014. In vitro kinetics of soybean lipoxygenase with combinatorial fatty substrates and its functional significance in off flavour development. Food Chem. 146:394–403.

Narvel, J. M., W. R. Fehr, and G. A. Welke. 1998. Agronomic and seed traits of soybean lines lacking seed lipoxygenases. Crop Sci. 38:926–928.

Narvel, J. M., W. R. Fehr, and L. C. Weldon. 2000. Analysis of soybean seed lipoxygenases. Crop Sci. 40:838–840.

Reinprecht, Y., V. W. Poysa, I. Rajcan, G. R. Ablett, and K. P. Pauls. 2006. Agronomic performance of soybean with seed lipoxygenase nulls and low linolenic acid content. Can. J. Plant Sci. 86:379–387.

Suda, I., M. Hajika, Y. Nishiba, S. Furuta, and K. Igita. 1995. Simple and rapid method for the selective detection of individual lipoxygenase isozymes in soybean seeds. J. Agric. Food Chem. 43:742–747.

Torres-Penaranda, A. V., and C. A. Reitmeier. 2001. Sensory descriptive analysis of soymilk. J. Food Sci. 66:352–356.

Torres-Penaranda, A. V., C. A. Reitmeier, L. A. Wilson, W. R. Fehr, and J. M. Narvel. 1998. Sensory characteristics of soymilk and tofu made from lipoxygenase-free and normal soybeans. J. Food Sci. 63:1084–1087.

Wilkens, W. F., and F. M. Lin. 1970. Gas chromatographic and mass spectral analyses of soybean milk volatiles. J. Agric. Food Chem. 18:333–336.

Wilson, L. A. 1996. Comparison of lipoxygenase-null and lipoxygenase-containing soybeans for foods. Pp. 209–225 *In* G. Piazza, ed. Lipoxygenase and lipoxygenase pathway enzymes. AOCS Press, Champaign, IL.

Yang, A., and A. T. James. 2013. Effects of soybean protein composition and processing conditions on silken tofu properties. J. Sci. Food Agric. 93:3065–3071.

Yuan, S., and S. K.-C. Chang. 2007. Selected odor compounds in soymilk as affected by chemical composition and lipoxygenases in five soybean materials. J. Agric. Food Chem. 55:426–431.

18

Proximate, mineral, and antinutrient compositions of indigenous Okra (*Abelmoschus esculentus*) pod accessions: implications for mineral bioavailability

Habtamu Fekadu Gemede[1,2], Gulelat Desse Haki[3], Fekadu Beyene[1], Ashagrie Z. Woldegiorgis[2] & Sudip Kumar Rakshit[4]

[1]Department of Food Technology and Process Engineering, Wollega University, P.O. Box 395, Nekemte, Ethiopia
[2]Center for Food Science and Nutrition Program, Addis Ababa University, P.O. Box 1176, Addis Ababa, Ethiopia
[3]Department of Food Science and Technology, Botswana Collage of Agriculture, Botswana University, Gaborone, Botswana
[4]Department of Chemical Engineering, Canada Research Chair (Tier 1), Lakehead University, Thunder Bay, ON, Canada P7B 5E1

Keywords
Accession, antinutrient, bioavailability, mineral, Okra, pod, proximate

Correspondence
Habtamu Fekadu Gemede, Department of Food Technology and Process Engineering, Wollega University, P.O. Box 395, Nekemte, Ethiopia.

E-mail: fekadu_habtamu@yahoo.com

Funding Information
No funding information provided.

Abstract

The promotion and consumption of indigenous vegetables could help to mitigate food insecurity and alleviate malnutrition in developing countries. Nutrient and antinutrient compositions of eight accessions of Okra Pods were investigated. Molar ratios and mineral bioavailability of Okra pod accessions were also calculated and compared to the critical values to predict the implications for mineral bioavailability. Proximate and mineral composition of Okra pod accessions were determined using standard methods of Association of Official Analytical Chemists. The result of the study revealed that the proximate composition (g/100 g) in dry weight basis was significantly ($P < 0.05$) varied and ranged: moisture/dry matter 9.69–13.33, crude protein 10.25–26.16, crude fat 0.56–2.49, crude fiber 11.97–29.93, crude ash 5.37–11.30, utilizable carbohydrate 36.66–50.97, and gross energy 197.26–245.55 kcal/100 g. The mineral concentrations (mg/100 g) were also significantly ($P < 0.05$) varied and ranged: calcium (111.11–311.95), Iron (18.30–36.68), potassium (122.59–318.20), zinc (3.83–6.31), phosphorus (25.62–59.72), and sodium (3.33–8.31) on dry weight bases. The Okra Pods of "OPA#6" accession contained significantly higher amounts of crude protein, total ash, crude fat, calcium, iron, and zinc than all other accessions evaluated in this study. The results of antinutrients analysis showed that, except phytate, tannin, and oxalate contents of all the accessions were significantly ($P < 0.05$) varied. The range of phytate, tannin, and oxalate contents (mg/100 g) for Okra pod accessions studied were as follows: 0.83–0.87, 4.93–9.90, and 0.04–0.53, respectively. The calculated molar ratios of phytate: calcium, phytate: iron, phytate: zinc, oxalate: calcium and [Phytate][Calcium]/[Zinc] were below the critical value and this indicate that the bioavailability of calcium, iron, and zinc in these accessions could be high. The results of the study revealed that Okra pod contain appreciable amount of vital nutrients like protein, fiber, calcium, iron, and zinc and low in antinutrient contents with high mineral bioavailability. Therefore, increase in the production and consumption of these nutrient- rich indigenous Okra pods will help to supplement/formulate the diets and alleviate the problems associated with malnutrition in the country.

Introduction

Traditional vegetables are valuable sources of nutrients (Nesamvuni et al. 2001; Yang and Keding 2009), with some having important medicinal properties (Hilou et al. 2006). Vegetables contribute substantially to food security (Yiridoe and Anchirinah 2005). Overcoming food and nutritional insecurity among women, pregnant and lactating mothers, and children under 5 years of age, remains a challenge in many developing countries in sub-Saharan Africa (Andersen et al. 2003; Tchientche Kamga et al. 2013).

Okra (*Abelmoschus esculentus*) is an important vegetable crop (Oyelade et al. 2003; Andras et al. 2005; Saifullah and Rabbani 2009) originated in Ethiopia (Getachew 2001; Simmone et al. 2004; Dandena 2010; Sathish and Eswar 2013). This crop is one of the most widely known and utilized species of the family Malvaceae (Naveed et al. 2009). Okra is known by many local names in different parts of the world (Nzikou et al. 2006). It is called lady's finger in England, gumbo in the United States of America, guino-gombo in Spanish, guibeiro in Portuguese, and bhindiin India (Ndunguru and Rajabu 2004; Sorapong Benchasr 2012). In its origin of Ethiopia it is also called Kenkase (Berta), Andeha (Gumuz), Bamia (Oromica/Amharic) (Gemede et al. 2015). The name Okra probably derives from one of Niger-Congo group of languages (the name for okra in the Twi language is nkuruma) (Benjawan et al. 2007). The term okra was in the use of English by the late 18th century (Arapitsas 2008).

Okra is a multipurpose crop due to its various uses of the pods, fresh leaves, buds, flowers, stems, and seeds. Okra immature fruits (pods), which are consumed as vegetables, can be used in salads, soups, and stews, fresh or dried, fried or boiled (Habtamu et al., 2014). Despite its nutritional compositions, Okra pod is a powerhouse of valuable nutrients (Adetuyi et al. 2011) and affordable source of protein, carbohydrates, minerals, vitamins, and dietary fiber (Habtamu et al., 2014). Therefore, promoting the consumption of Okra pods could provide cheap sources of nutrients that can improve the nutritional status and reducing the prevalence of malnutrition especially among resource-constrained households and can also used as a means of dietary diversification. On the other hand, the presence of anti-nutritional factors is one of the major drawbacks limiting the nutritional qualities of the food (Kathirvel and Kumudha 2011). Okra pods are not only have beneficial nutrients but might contain traces of antinutritional factors, which may have adverse effects on bioavailability of some minerals like calcium, iron, and zinc. However, okra has been considered as a minor crop and there is no single information or published studies available about nutritional, anti-nutritional, and bioavailability of Okra pods grown in Ethiopia. Therefore, the aim of this study was to evaluate the proximate, mineral, anti-nutrient, and bioavailability of eight indigenous Okra pod accessions grown in Benishangul Gumuz Region, Ethiopia.

Materials and Methods

Sample collection and preparation

Eight Okra pod accessions were harvested from Assosa agricultural research farm in Benishangul Gumiz Region, Ethiopia. Each of the collected accessions were coded, packed in polyethylene bags, kept in an ice box (to prevent moisture loss), and transported to Food Technology and Process Engineering Research laboratory of Wollega University, Ethiopia. Once in the laboratory, each of the Okra pod accessions were washed by distilled water and sliced to uniform thickness 5 mm using a stainless steel knife. The moisture content of each Okra pod accessions was determined immediate after sliced to uniform thickness. The sliced Okra Pod accessions were sun dried, followed by oven drying at 45°C. The dried Okra pod accessions were milled separately into fine powder using electric grinder until to pass through 0.425 mm sieve mesh size, and finally packed into airtight polyethylene plastic bags to minimize heat build-up and stored in the desiccator until required for analysis.

Proximate composition

Moisture content, total ash, crude protein, crude fiber, and crude fat of the Okra pod accessions were determined according to AOAC, (2000) using sub components 925.09, 923.03, 979.09, 962.09, and 920.39, respectively. Utilizable carbohydrate content of Okra pod accessions was calculated by difference (Manzi et al. 2004). The gross energy content of Okra pod accessions was determined by calculation from fat, carbohydrate, and protein contents using the Atwater's conversion factors; 16.7 kJ/g (4 kcal/g) for protein, 37.4 kJ/g (9 kcal/g) for fat and 16.7 kJ/g (4 kcal/g) for carbohydrates and expressed in calories (Guyot et al. 2007).

Determination of mineral contents

Minerals content analysis was determined according to AOAC, (2000). Sodium (Na) and potassium (K) concentrations were determined by using the standard flame emission photometer; phosphorus (P) was determined colorimetrically by vanadomolybdate procedure. Calcium (Ca), iron (Fe), and zinc (Zn) concentrations were measured by atomic absorption spectrophotometer.

Determination of antinutritional factors

Phytate was determined by the method of Vantraub and Lapteva (1988). Oxalate was analyzed using the method originally employed by Ukpabi and Ejidoh (1989) in which the procedures involve three steps: digestion, oxalate precipitation, and permanganate titration. Tannin content was determined by the method of Maxson and Rooney (1972).

Determination of molar ratio of antinutrients to minerals

The molar ratio between antinutrient and mineral was obtained after dividing the mole of antinutrient with the mole of minerals (Woldegiorgis et al. 2015).

Statistical analysis

The completely randomized design was used with two replicates. All the statistical analyses were performed on the results obtained using SPSS version 20.0 (SPSS Institute Inc., Cary, NC) for windows. Data were evaluated by using one way ANOVA (analysis of variance). Means of results for each experiment were separated by the Duncan's multiple range test and reported as mean ± SE (standard error). A P-value of 0.05 or less was considered as statistically significant.

Result and Discussion

Proximate composition

Food analysis is the resolution of the components of food into its proximate or ultimate parts (Onwuka 2005). Proximate analysis involves the determination of the major components of food as moisture, ash, crude fat, crude protein, crude fiber, and carbohydrate (Ekwumemgbo et al. 2014; Aja et al. 2015). The proximate composition of Okra pod accessions is presented in Table 1.

Moisture content determination is an integral part of the proximate composition analysis of food. Moisture content of eight accessions of Okra pods is presented in Table 1. As fresh Okra pods vary considerably in water content, moisture contents were calculated on a dry weight basis, which allows a greater consistency of data. This implies a factor from 1.10 to 1.14 must be multiplied as moisture correction factor for all the other analysis parameters. Okra pod accession "OPA#2" had the highest moisture/dry matter content (13.33 g/100 g) which was significantly ($P < 0.05$) higher than the moisture/dry matter content of all the accessions whereas Okra pod accession "OPA#6" had significantly ($P < 0.05$) lower than the moisture/dry matter content (9.69 g/100 g) of all the accessions except accession "OPA#8" (10.22 g/100 g) and "OPA#7" (10.38 g/100 g). Although fresh Okra pod accessions were ranged from 87.98 to 90.60 g/100 g water and this indicate that the Okra pods have a high moisture content. The high moisture content in okra pods accessions is in agreement with the finding of Adetuyi et al. (2011). Also this is in accordance with the finding of Gopalan et al. (2007) (89 g/100 g) and (Nwachukwu et al. 2014) (88.47 g/100 g). Moisture content of any food is an index of its water activity and is used as a measure of stability and susceptibility to microbial contamination (Uyoh et al. 2013). The high moisture content in vegetables makes them vulnerable to microbial attack, hence spoilage (Nwofia et al., 2012). This high moisture content also implies that dehydration would increase the relative concentrations of other food nutrient and therefore improve the shelf-life and preservation of the fruits (Aruah et al. 2012). There is also need to store the fruit in cool condition if they are to be kept for a long period without spoilage especially in the tropics were wastage of vegetable crops is estimated to be around 50% due to high moisture content (Nwofia, 2012).

The main functions of proteins are growth and replacement of lost tissues in the human body. Table 1 shows the crude protein contents of the eight accessions of Okra pod used in the study. The protein content of the Okra pod accessions was varied significantly ($P < 0.05$) from 10.25 g/100 g in "OPA#2" to 26.16 g/100 g in "OPA#6" on dry weight basis and this variation might be due to genetic factor. The mean value of the accessions obtained in the study is almost comparable with the find of Adetuya et al. (2011) (13.61–16.27 g/100 g) while higher than the

Table 1. Proximate composition of eight Okra pod accessions (dry weight bases).

Accessions	Moisture content (g/100 g)	Crud protein (g/100 g)	Total ash (g/100 g)	Crude fiber (g/100 g)	Crude fat (g/100 g)	Util. carbohy. (g/100 g)	Gross energy (Kcal/100 g)
OPA#1	10.61 ± 0.27^{c,d}	20.75 ± 0.52^{b}	6.05 ± 0.25^{c,d,e}	16.58 ± 0.05^{e}	1.39 ± 0.28^{b,c}	44.62 ± 0.23^{b}	215.24 ± 0.56^{b,c}
OPA#2	13.33 ± 0.28^{a}	10.25 ± 0.69^{e}	6.66 ± 0.03^{c}	17.13 ± 0.39^{e}	1.67 ± 0.02^{b}	50.97 ± 0.00^{a}	245.55 ± 0.05^{a}
OPA#3	12.17 ± 0.16^{b}	13.94 ± 0.02^{d}	10.20 ± 0.28^{b}	21.95 ± 0.03^{d}	1.14 ± 0.01^{c}	40.56 ± 0.49^{c}	213.43 ± 0.82^{c}
OPA#4	11.29 ± 0.26^{c}	17.16 ± 0.65^{c}	5.37 ± 0.01^{e}	24.35 ± 1.17^{c}	1.69 ± 0.01^{b}	40.15 ± 1.55^{c}	197.26 ± 2.21^{d}
OPA#5	10.66 ± 0.24^{c,d}	12.97 ± 0.25^{d}	10.60 ± 0.17^{a,b}	21.69 ± 0.19^{d}	0.56 ± 0.01^{d}	43.52 ± 0.85^{b}	221.52 ± 2.71^{b}
OPA#6	9.69 ± 0.29^{e}	26.16 ± 0.12^{a}	11.30 ± 0.19^{a}	11.97 ± 0.83^{f}	2.49 ± 0.28^{a}	38.41 ± 0.56^{c,d}	221.16 ± 3.9^{b}
OPA#7	10.38 ± 0.26^{d,e}	14.16 ± 0.14^{d}	5.62 ± 0.45^{d,e}	26.42 ± 0.21^{b}	0.58 ± 0.01^{d}	42.87 ± 1.06^{b}	198.98 ± 2.41^{d}
OPA#8	10.22 ± 0.22^{d,e}	16.24 ± 0.94^{c}	6.39 ± 49^{c,d}	29.93 ± 0.09^{a}	0.56 ± 0.01^{d}	36.66 ± 0.85^{d}	214.16 ± 1.38^{e}

Means not followed by the same superscript letters in the same column are significantly different ($P < 0.05$).
Data are expressed as mean ± SE of replicate determinations ($n = 2$).
OPA stands for Okra Pod Accession and # stands for number.

value reported by Nwachukwu et al. (2014) (4.81 g/100 g). Ogungbenle and Omosola (2015) is also reported that the crude protein content of Okra pod is (23.4 g/100 g) which is higher than all the accession in the present study except "OPA#6" (26.16 g/100 g). Okra can be considered a high protein vegetable when compared with *moringa oliefera* (4.2 g/100 g), *Amarantus* (6.1 g/100 g), *Gnetum Africanum* (1.5 g/100 g), and *Pterocarpus* (2.0 g/100 g) (Nzikou et al. 2006) and this implies that Okra pod can serve as a good source of protein. Nwofia et al. (2012) reported that diet is nutritionally satisfactory, if it contains high caloric value and a sufficient amount of protein. It have been shown that any plant foods that provides about 12% of their calorific value from protein are considered good source of protein(Effiong et al. 2009; Ali 2010). The pods of these accessions of Okra meet this requirements and this implies that Okra pod can serve as a good source of protein.

Crude fat content of eight accessions of Okra pods is presented in Table 1. The levels of crude fat varied from 0.56 g/100 g ("OPA #8" and "OPA #5") to 2.49 g/100 g ("OPA #6"). Okra pod accession "OPA#6" had the highest crude fat content (2.49 g/100 g) which was significantly ($P < 0.05$) higher than the crude fat content of all the accessions whereas Okra pod accession "OPA#8" and "OPA#5" had significantly ($P < 0.05$) lower than the crude fat content (0.56 g/100 g) of all the accessions except accession "OPA#7" (0.58 g/100 g). In these finding, the crude fat content is higher than the value reported by Nwachukwu et al. (2014) (0.18 g/100 g) whereas lower than the value reported by Adetuyi et al. (2011) (9.22–10.57 g/100 g). Dietary fats function in the increase of palatability of food by absorbing and retaining flavors (Antia et al. 2006). Excess consumption of fat have been implicated in certain cardiovascular disorders such as atherosclerosis, cancer, and aging, whereas a diet providing 1–2% of its caloric of energy as fat is said to be sufficient to human beings (Aruah et al. 2011), in this regard, the consumption of Okra pod diet should be encouraged to reduce the risk of above diseases in man.

Dietary fiber promotes the growth and protects the beneficial intestinal flora. Moreover, high intake of fiber reduces the risk of colon cancer (Dawczynski et al. 2007). The crude fiber content among the accessions of Okra pod varied from 11.97 g/100 g to 29.93 g/100 g in "OPA#6" and "OPA#8" accessions, respectively. The accession, "OPA#8" had significantly ($P < 0.05$) higher (29.93 g/100 g) in crude fiber content and was followed by "OPA#7" (26.42 g/100 g), "OPA#4" (24.35 g/100 g), "OPA#3" (21.95 g/100 g) in that order, however, the accession "OPA#6" recorded the lowest (11.97 g/100 g) crude fiber content on dry weight basis. Adetuya et al. (2011) reported that the fiber content of Okra pod ranges from 10.15 to 11.63 g/100 g which is lower than the crude fiber obtained in this study. Adetuya et al. (2011) also reported that the fiber content of okra is high when compared with *Amarantus hybridus* (1.6 g/100 g) and *Laurea taraxifolia* (2.0 g/100 g) but very low in comparison with *Gnetumn africanum* (3.0 g/100 g). In this study, the fiber content is relatively high which may suggest that consumption of okra will can improve its digestibility and absorption processes in large intestine, helping to stimulate peristalsis, thereby preventing constipation (Ogungbenle and Omosola 2015). Interest in fiber evaluation has increased due to the recent information on the potential role of dietary fiber in human nutrition (Mensan et al. 2008). Evidences from epidemiological studies suggest that high fiber consumption may contribute to a reduction in the incidence of certain diseases like diabetes, coronary heart disease, colon cancer, high blood pressure, obesity, and various digestive disorders (Ikewuchi and Ikewuchi 2009). Dietary fiber is known to alter the coronary environment in such a way as to protect against colorectal diseases (Ekumankama 2008). It provides protection by increasing fecal bulk, which dilutes the increased colonic bile that occurs with high fat diet (Dillard and German 2000; Zhao et al. 2007). When found in excess, it may bind some essential trace elements leading to deficiency of some minerals such as iron and zinc (Ekwumemgbo et al. 2014). Therefore, okra pod diet is considered as a main source of crude fiber.

The ash content is a measure/reflection of the nutritionally important mineral contents present in the food material (Omotosho 2005; Nnamani et al. 2009). Table 1 shows the crude ash contents of the eight accessions of Okra pod used in the study. The level of ash content was ranged from 5.37 g/100 g (OPA#4) to 11.30 g/100 g (OPA#6). The ash content was significantly ($P < 0.05$) higher in "OPA#6" (11.30 g/100 g) followed by "OPA#3" (10.20 g/100 g), "OPA#2" (6.66 g/100 g), and "OPA#8" (6.39 g/100 g) in that order, whereas accession "OPA#4" had the lowest (5.37 g/100 g) ash content value but this did not differ significantly ($P < 0.05$) from accession "OPA#7" (5.62 g/100 g) and "OPA#1" (6.05 g/100 g) on dry weight basis. The results showed that the sample contains high ash content which indicates that the okra pods would provide essential valuable and useful minerals needed for body development. The mean of ash content in this result agrees with the findings of Adetuya et al. (2011) (7.19–9.63 g/100 g).

Table 1 shows the utilizable carbohydrate contents of the eight accessions of Okra pod used in the study. The utilizable carbohydrate content of Okra pod accessions varied from 36.66 g/100 g to 50.97 g/100 g in "OPA#8" and "OPA#2" accessions, respectively. Utilizable carbohydrate content of pod accession "OPA#2" had higher (50.97 g/100 g), whereas accession "OPA#8" had the lowest

(36.66 g/100 g) but this did not differ significantly from accession "OPA#6" (38.41 g/100 g) utilizable carbohydrate contents. The sample could be considered as potential source of carbohydrate when compared with the content of some conventional sources like cereals with 72–90 g/100 g Carbohydrate (Elinge et al. 2012).

The gross energy was calculated by multiplying the mean values of crude proteins, crude fat, and total carbohydrate by Atwater factors of 4, 9, and 4, respectively. Gross energy content was ranged from 197.26 kcal/100 g in "OPA#4" to 245.55 kcal/100 g in "OPA#2" accessions. Gross energy content of pod accession "OPA#2" had higher (245.55 kcal/100 g), whereas accession "OPA#4" had the lowest (197.26 kcal/100 g) but this did not differ significantly ($P < 0.05$) from accession "OPA#7" (198.98 kcal/100 g) on dry weight basis. This energy value indicates that these accessions can serve as a good source of energy for the body.

Mineral composition

Minerals are considered to be essential in human nutrition (Ibanga and Okon 2009; Valvi and Rathod 2011). These minerals are vital for the overall mental and physical well being and are important constituents of bones, teeth, tissues, muscles, blood, and nerve cells (Soetan et al. 2010). They also help in the maintenance of acid-base balance, response of nerves to physiological stimulation and blood clotting (Hanif et al. 2006). The mineral composition of eight Okra pod accessions is shown in Table 2.

Calcium is the major component of bone and assists in teeth development. Calcium concentrations are also necessary for blood coagulation and for the integrity of intracellular cement substances (Okaka and Okaka 2001). Calcium content in the eight Okra pod accessions is shown in Table 2. The concentration of Calcium in the sample is varied from 111.11 mg/100 g to 311.95 mg/100 g in "OPA#1" and "OPA#3" accessions, respectively. Okra pod accession "OPA#3" had the highest calcium content (311.95 mg/100 g) which was significantly ($P < 0.05$) higher than the Calcium content of all the accessions except accession "OPA#6" (311.35 mg/100 g), whereas Okra pod accession "OPA#1" had the lowest Calcium content (11.11 mg/100 g) on dry weight basis. This result appeared to be far higher than the Calcium contents of Okra variety reported by Adetuya et al. (2011) varying between 58.22 mg/100 g to 58.31 mg/100 g.

Iron is an essential trace element for hemoglobin format on, normal functioning of central nervous system and in the oxidation of carbohydrates, protein, and fats (Kermanshah et al. 2014; Mlitan et al. 2014). It also facilitates carbohydrates, protein, and fat to control body weight, which is very important factor in diabetes (Moses et al. 2012). Iron is necessary for the formation of hemoglobin and also plays an important role in oxygen transfer in human body and low iron content causes gastrointestinal infection, nose bleeding myocardial infection (Ullah et al. 2012). Table 2 shows Iron content of the eight accessions of Okra pod used in the study. The contents of Iron varied from 18.30 mg/100 g in "OPA#7" to 36.68 mg/100 g in "OPA#5". The Iron content of Okra pod accession "OPA#5" had higher (36.68 mg/100 g), but this did not differ significantly ($P < 0.05$) from accession "OPA#6" (32.90 mg/100 g), whereas accession "OPA#7" had the lowest (18.30 mg/100 g) but nonsignificant ($P < 0.05$) from accession "OPA#2" (20.98 mg/100 g) on dry weight basis. The values obtained in this study were far higher than the value reported by Adetuya et al. (2011) which is varied from 0.87 mg/100 g to 0.96 mg/100 g. This indicates that Okra pod is a rich source of Iron.

Zinc is an essential trace element and plays an important role in various cell processes including normal growth, brain development, behavioral response, bone formation, and wound healing (Mlitan et al. 2014). Zinc also plays

Table 2. Mineral concentrations of eight Okra pod accessions (dry weight bases).

	Mineral content (mg/100 g)					
Accessions	Calcium	Iron	Potassium	Zinc	Phosphorous	Sodium
OPA#1	111.11 ± 0.37^{g}	$25.41 \pm 1.36^{c,d}$	169.82 ± 8.25^{c}	$4.13 \pm 0.04^{d,e}$	33.02 ± 0.46^{e}	$5.01 \pm 0.54^{b,c}$
OPA#2	276.29 ± 0.96^{b}	$20.98 \pm 0.75^{d,e}$	318.20 ± 6.67^{a}	4.61 ± 0.01^{c}	42.17 ± 0.78^{c}	8.31 ± 0.51^{a}
OPA#3	311.95 ± 0.57^{a}	31.77 ± 0.37^{b}	177.96 ± 2.89^{c}	6.30 ± 0.09^{a}	27.61 ± 0.91^{f}	$3.97 \pm 0.56^{b,c}$
OPA#4	140.88 ± 1.39^{f}	23.30 ± 0.48^{d}	277.82 ± 9.62^{b}	$4.16 \pm 0.09^{c,d,e}$	54.11 ± 1.62^{b}	$5.61 \pm 1.13^{b,c}$
OPA#5	253.52 ± 4.02^{c}	36.68 ± 0.84^{a}	122.59 ± 11.00^{d}	3.83 ± 0.24^{e}	59.72 ± 0.55^{a}	$3.91 \pm 0.57^{b,c}$
OPA#6	311.35 ± 0.27^{a}	$32.90 \pm 2.65^{a,b}$	263.12 ± 1.06^{b}	6.31 ± 0.19^{a}	36.32 ± 0.68^{d}	$6.06 \pm 0.57^{a,b}$
OPA#7	188.79 ± 3.30^{e}	18.30 ± 0.18^{e}	183.52 ± 7.79^{c}	5.65 ± 0.05^{b}	25.62 ± 0.83^{f}	$4.99 \pm 0.57^{b,c}$
OPA#8	203.89 ± 1.08^{d}	$28.49 \pm 1.77^{b,c}$	174.04 ± 2.75^{c}	$4.35 \pm 0.19^{c,d}$	58.48 ± 1.21^{a}	3.33 ± 1.11^{c}

Means not followed by the same superscript letters in the same column are significantly different ($P < 0.05$).
Data are expressed as mean ± SE of replicate determinations ($n = 2$).
OPA stands for Okra Pod Accession and # stands for number.

a very important role in protein and carbohydrate metabolism and also help in mobilizing vitamin A from its storage site in the liver and facilitates the synthesis of DNA and RNA necessary for cell production (Jabeen et al. 2010). Zinc deficiency is common in people suffering from Chrohn's disease, hypothyroidism, and gum disease, and probably plays a part in susceptibility to viral infections and diabetes mellitus. It can be beneficial in the treatment of viral infections, including those of AIDS, prostate gland enlargement, rheumatoid arthritis, healing of wounds, acne, eczema, and stress (Kermanshah et al. 2014). Zinc content in the eight Okra pod accessions is shown in Table 2. The content of Zinc varied between 3.83 mg/100 g in "OPA#5" and 6.31 mg/100 g in "OPA#6". Zinc content of pod accession "OPA#6" had higher (6.31 mg/100 g) but this did not differ significantly from accession "OPA#3" (6.30 mg/100 g) while accession "OPA#5" had the lowest (3.83 mg/100 g) but this did not differ significantly ($P < 0.05$) from Okra pod accession "OPA#1" (4.13 mg/100 g) and "OPA#4" (4.16 mg/100 g) on dry weight basis. The values obtained in this study are higher than the values reported by Adetuya et al., (2011) (1.29 mg/100 g–1.37 mg/100 g).

Phosphorus content of the accessions of eight Okra pod is shown in Table 2. In this study, the phosphorus content is varied from 25.62 mg/100 g (OPA#7) to 59.72 mg/100 g (OPA#5). The Phosphorus content of pod accession "OPA#5" had higher (59.72 mg/100 g) but did not differ significantly from accession "OPA#8" (58.48 mg/100 g) while accession "OPA#7" had the lowest (25.62 mg/100 g) but did not differ significantly ($P < 0.05$) from Okra pod accession "OPA#3" (27.61 mg/100 g) on dry weight basis. The value of this study is lower than the value reported by Adetuya et al. (2011) which is varied from 60.05 mg/100 g to 62.17 mg/100 g.

Potassium content of the accessions of eight Okra pod is shown in Table 2. The Potassium content of pod accession "OPA#2" had significantly ($P < 0.05$) higher (318.20 mg/100 g), whereas accession "OPA#5" had the lowest (122.59 mg/100 g) on dry weight basis. High amount of potassium in the body was reported to increase iron utilization (Elinge et al. 2012) and beneficial to people taking diuretics to control hypertension and suffer from excessive excretion of potassium through the body fluid (Arinanthan et al. 2003).

Sodium content of the accessions of eight Okra pod is shown in Table 2. In this study, the sodium content is varied from 3.33 mg/100 g (OPA#8) to 8.31 mg/100 g (OPA#2). Sodium content of Okra pod accession "OPA#2" had higher (8.31 mg/100 g) but this did not differ significantly from accession "OPA#6" (6.06 mg/100 g) while accession "OPA#8" had the lowest (3.33 mg/100 g) but this did not differ significantly ($P < 0.05$) from all the five remaining accessions on dry weight basis.

Antinutritional factors

Antinutritional factors are a chemical compounds synthesized in natural food and/or feedstuffs by the normal metabolism of species which exerts effect contrary to optimum nutrition (Gemede and Ratta 2014). Antinutritional factors are also reduce the maximum utilization of nutrients especially proteins, vitamins, and minerals, thus preventing optimal exploitation of the nutrients present in a food and decreasing the nutritive value (Ugwu and Oranye 2006; Fekadu et al. 2013). The antinutritional composition of eight Okra pods accessions are shown in Table 3.

The phytate content of Okra pod accession was highest in "OPA#3" (0.87 mg/100 g) and lowest in "OPA#5" and "OPA#4" (0.83 mg/100 g) whereas value of Okra pod accession "OPA#3" was nonsignificant ($P < 0.05$) from phytate content of the remaining accessions on dry weight bases. The problem with phytate in food is that it can bind some essential mineral nutrients in the digestive tract and can result in mineral deficiencies (Bello et al. 2008). The phytate composition of the sample might not pose any health hazard when compared with a phytate diet of 10–60 mg/100 g which if consumed over a long period of time that has been reported to decrease bioavailability of minerals (Elinge et al. 2012). On the other hand, currently there is evidence that dietary phytate at low level may have beneficial role as an antioxidant, anticarcinogens and likely play an important role in controlling hypercholesterolemia and atherosclerosis (Phillippy et al. 2004). The result of this study is lower than the value reported by Adetuya et al., (2011) (2.64–3.90 mg/100 g). Because Okra pod may provide a substantial portion of phytate, the health benefits of phytate in Okra pod should be investigated.

Tannin content of pod accession "OPA#8" (9.90 mg/100 g) had higher but did not differ significantly

Table 3. Antinutritional factors content of the accessions of eight Okra pod (dry weight bases).

Accessions	Phytate (mg/100 g)	Oxalate (mg/100 g)	Tannin (mg/100 g)
OPA#1	0.85 ± 0.01^{a}	0.04 ± 0.04^{e}	$7.61 \pm 0.55^{b,c}$
OPA#2	0.85 ± 0.01^{a}	0.53 ± 0.53^{a}	$6.75 \pm 0.32^{c,d}$
OPA#3	0.87 ± 0.02^{a}	$0.09 \pm 0.09^{c,d}$	$5.75 \pm 0.38^{d,e}$
OPA#4	0.83 ± 0.02^{a}	0.15 ± 0.15^{c}	8.12 ± 0.38^{b}
OPA#5	0.83 ± 0.01^{a}	0.06 ± 0.06^{e}	$7.48 \pm 0.33^{b,c}$
OPA#6	0.85 ± 0.02^{a}	0.28 ± 0.28^{b}	9.70 ± 0.41^{a}
OPA#7	0.84 ± 0.01^{a}	0.47 ± 0.47^{a}	4.93 ± 0.15^{e}
OPA#8	0.86 ± 0.03^{a}	$0.12 \pm 0.12^{c,d}$	9.90 ± 0.46^{a}

Means not followed by the same superscript letters in the same column are significantly different ($P < 0.05$).
Data are expressed as mean ± SE of replicate determinations ($n = 2$).
OPA stands for Okra Pod Accession and # stands for number.

Table 4. Calculated molar ratio Phy:Ca Phy:Fe, Phy:Zn, Ox:Ca, and [Ca][Phy]/[Zn] molar ratios of Okra pod accessions.

Accessions	Phytate: Ca (Molar ratio)	Phytate: Fe (Molar ratio)	Phytate: Zn (Molar ratio)	Oxalate: Ca (Molar ratio)	Phytate*Ca: Zn (mol/kg)
OPA#1	0.0047 ± 0.050^{a}	0.0028 ± 0.012^{c,d}	0.0204 ± 0.044^{a,b}	0.0016 ± 0.0405^{e,f}	0.0565 ± 0.0014^{c}
OPA#2	0.0019 ± 0.007^{d,e}	0.0034 ± 0.010^{b}	0.0182 ± 0.013^{b}	0.0087 ± 0.0775^{b}	0.1252 ± 0.0013^{a}
OPA#3	0.0017 ± 0.050^{e}	0.0023 ± 0.001^{e,f}	0.0136 ± 0.038^{c}	0.0013 ± 0.0145^{e,f}	0.1059 ± 0.0001^{b}
OPA#4	0.0036 ± 0.170^{b}	0.0030 ± 0.001^{b,c}	0.0198 ± 0.092^{a,b}	0.0049 ± 0.0695^{c}	0.0694 ± 0.0025^{c}
OPA#5	0.0010 ± 0.078^{d}	0.0019 ± 0.007^{f}	0.0216 ± 0.016^{a}	0.0010 ± 0.0255^{f}	0.1363 ± 0.0079^{a}
OPA#6	0.0017 ± 0.057^{e}	0.0022 ± 0.023^{f}	0.0134 ± 0.087^{c}	0.0040 ± 0.0220^{c,d}	0.1037 ± 0.0008^{b}
OPA#7	0.0027 ± 0.021^{c}	0.0039 ± 0.008^{a}	0.0147 ± 0.004^{c}	0.0011 ± 0.0525^{a}	0.0693 ± 0.0014^{c}
OPA#8	0.0026 ± 0.120^{c}	0.0026 ± 0.023^{d,e}	0.0195 ± 0.014^{a,b}	0.0027 ± 0.0460^{d,e}	0.0994 ± 0.0066^{b}

Means not followed by the same superscript letters in the same column are significantly different ($P < 0.05$).

from accession "OPA#6" (9.70 mg/100 g) while accession "OPA#7" (4.93 mg/100 g) had the lowest but did not differ significantly ($P < 0.05$) from Okra pod accession "OPA#3" (5.74 mg/100 g) on dry weight basis. Tannins had been reported to affect protein digestibility, adversely influencing the bioavailability of nonhem iron leading to poor iron and calcium absorption, also carbohydrate is affected leading to reduced energy value of a diet containing tannins (Adeparusi 2001), however, its antinutritional/toxicity effects depend upon their chemical structure and dosage (Fekadu et al. 2013). Therefore, the toxicity effects of the tannin may not be significant since the total acceptable tannic acid daily intake for a man is 560 mg/100 g (Fekadu et al. 2013). Since the tannin content of Okra pod accessions are very low compared to its critical toxicity effect and further reduced during traditional processing, its antinutritional effect may be insignificant in both raw and processed Okra pod.

Oxalate content of pod accession "OPA#2" (0.53 mg/100 g) had higher but this did not differ significantly ($P < 0.05$) from accession "OPA#7" (0.47 mg/100 g) while accession "OPA#1" (0.04 mg/100 g) had the lowest but did not differ significantly ($P < 0.05$) from Okra pod accession "OPA#5" (0.06 mg/100 g), "OPA#3" (0.09 mg/100 g) and "OPA#8" (0.12 mg/100 g) on dry weight basis. The result of this study is comparable with the finding of Adetuya et al., (2011) (0.32–0.506 mg/100 g). Oxalates can have a harmful effect on human nutrition and health, especially by reducing calcium absorption and aiding the formation of kidney stones (Fekadu et al. 2013). High-oxalate diets can increase the risk of renal calcium oxalate formation in certain groups of people (Gemede and Ratta 2014). The majority of urinary stones formed in humans are calcium oxalate stones and currently, patients are advised to limit their intake of foods with a total intake of oxalate not exceeding 50–60 mg per day (Massey et al. 2001). The traditionally processed Anchote tubers analyzed in this study are low compared to the recommendations for patients with calcium oxalate kidney stones. Under these guidelines, processed Anchote tubers analyzed could be recommended not only for normal healthy people but also consumption for patients with a history of calcium oxalate kidney stones, assume about 1 kg of Anchote would be necessary for consumption per day.

Molar ratios and bioavailability of minerals

The molar ratios for oxalate, calcium, zinc, iron, and phytate were calculated to evaluate the effects of elevated levels of oxalate and phytate in the bioavailability of dietary minerals. Bioavailability is the ability of the body to digest and absorb the mineral in the food consumed (Fekadu et al. 2013). The calculated values are also compared with the reported critical toxicity values for these ratios. The calculated Phy:Ca, Ox: Ca, Phy: Zn, Phy: Fe, and [Ca][Phy]/[Zn] molar ratios of Okra pod accessions are shown in Table 4.

Phytic acids markedly decrease Ca bioavailability and the Phy: Ca molar ratio has been proposed as an indicator of Ca bioavailability. The critical molar ratio of [phy]:[Ca] of < 0.24 indicating good calcium bioavailability (Woldegiorgis et al. 2015). The values in this study were lower in all accessions than the reported critical molar ratio of Phytate to Calcium, indicating that absorption of calcium not adversely affected by phytate in all the accessions.

Phytate begins to lose its inhibitory effect on iron absorption when phytate:iron molar ratios are less than 1.0, although even ratios as low as 0.2 exert some negative effect (Hurrell et al., 2003). The phytate:iron molar ratios greater than 0.15 regarded as indicative of poor iron bioavailability (Siegenberg et al. 1991). This result indicated that, the phytate:iron molar ratios of all the accessions are less than the critical value, which implies the absorption of iron all the accessions not inhibited by phytate and as a result the bioavailability of iron is good.

The importance of foodstuffs as a source of dietary zinc depends on both the total zinc content and the level of other constituents in the diet that affect zinc bioavailability. Phytate may reduce the bioavailability of dietary zinc by forming insoluble mineral chelates at a physiological pH (Bhandari and Kawabata 2004) and the formation of the chelates depends on relative levels of both zinc and phytic acid. Hence, the phytate: Zn molar ratio is considered a better indicator of zinc bioavailability than total dietary phytate levels alone (Woldegiorgis et al. 2014). Therefore, the foods with a molar ratio of Phy: Zn less than 10 showed adequate availability of Zn and problems were encountered when the value was >15. Phytate: zinc molar ratios >15, indicative of poor zinc bioavailability (Morris and Ellis 1989). The values of Okra pod accessions were lower than the critical molar ratios of Phy:Zn, which indicates the availability of zinc good.

Oxalic acid and its salts can have deleterious effects on human nutrition and health, particularly by decreasing calcium absorption and aiding the formation of kidney stones (Bhandari and Kawabata 2004). The importance of oxalate contents of an individual plant product in limiting total dietary Ca availability is of significance only when the ratio of Ox:Ca is greater than one (Frontela et al. 2009). From the result, it was observed that, all Okra pod accessions had Ox:Ca values are lower than the reported critical value (1.0), which implies that a low level of oxalate could have no adverse effects on bioavailability of dietary calcium in these accessions.

The potentiating effect of calcium on zinc absorption in the presence of high phytate intakes has led to the suggestion that the [Phy][Ca]/[Zn] millimolar ratio may be a better index of zinc bioavailability than the [Phy]/[Zn] molar ratio alone (Obah and Amusan 2009). High calcium levels in foods can promote the phytate-induced decrease in zinc bioavailability when the [Ca][phytate]/[Zn] millimolar ratio exceeds 0.5 mol/kg (Adetuyi et al. 2011). In this study, the values of [Ca][Phy]/[Zn] millimolar ratios of all the accessions were found less than the critical level.

Conclusions

In conclusion, the study revealed that there is a significant difference ($P < 0.05$) in the proximate and mineral compositions of Okra pod accessions. The most remarkable finding of this study is that Okra pod accessions were found to be a good source of vital nutrients like crude protein, crude fiber, crude ash, calcium, and iron. Specifically, Okra pod of "OPA#6" accession contained significantly higher amounts of crude protein, total ash, crude fat, gross energy, calcium, iron, and zinc than all other accessions and can be recommended as a remedy to alleviate malnutrition in the country. Interestingly, the antinutritional contents of the Okra pods were low and the bioavailability of calcium, iron, and zinc were high and therefore, its cultivation and consumption is encouraged as additional source of minerals to the diet of the indigenous people. Therefore, Okra pods could be employed in fortification, formulation and supplementation of other food materials.

Conflict of Interest

None declared.

References

Adeparusi, E. O. 2001. Effect of processing on the nutrients and antinutrients of lima bean (*Phaseolus lunatus* L.) flour. Nahrung 4:94–96.

Adetuyi, F. O., A. U. Osagie, and A. T. Adekunle. 2011. Nutrient, antinutrient, mineral and bioavailability of okra *Abelmoschus esculentus* (L) Moench. Am. J. Food Nutr. 1:49–54.

Aja, P. M., C. E. Offor, and O. U. Orji. 2015. Proximate and antinutrient compositions of *Parkia biglobosa* fruits in Abakaliki, Ebonyi state, Nigeria. Int. J. Curr. Microbiol. App. Sci 4:394–398.

Ali, A. 2010. A comparative study of nutrients and mineral molar ratios of foods with recommended dietary allowances. J. Food Sci. Technol. 2:104–108.

Andersen, L. T., S. H. Thilsted, B. B. Nielsen, and S. Rangasamy. 2003. Food and nutrient intakes among pregnant women in rural Tamil Nadu, South India. Public Health Nutr. 6:131–137.

Andras, C. D., B. Simandi, F. Orsi, C. Lambrou, D. M. Tatla, C. Panayiotou, et al. 2005. Supercritical carbon dioxide extraction of Okra (*Hibiscus esculentus* L.) seeds. J. Sci. Food Agric. 85:1415–1419.

Antia, B. S., E. J. Akpan, P. A. Okon, and I. U. Umoren. 2006. Nutritive and anti-nutritive evaluation of sweet potatoes (*Ipomoea batatas*) leaves. Pak. J. Nutr. 5:166–168.

AOAC. 2000. Association of Official Analytical Chemists. Official methods of Analysis (Vol. II 17th edition) of AOAC International. Washington, DC, USA. Official methods 925.09, 923.03,979.09, 962.09, 4.5.01 and 923.05.

Arapitsas, P. 2008. Identification and quantification of polyphenolic compounds from okra seeds and skins. Food Chem. 110:1041–1045.

Arinanthan, V., V. R. Mohan, and A. J. Britto. 2003. Chemical composition of certain tribal pulses in South India. Int. J. Food Sci. Nutr. 3:103–107.

Aruah, B. C., M. I. Uguru, and B. C. Oyiga. 2011. Nutritional evaluation of some Nigerian pumpkins (*Cucurbita* spp.). Fruit, Vegetable Cereal Sci. Biotechnol. 5:64–71.

Aruah, B. C., M. I. Uguru, and B. C. Oyiga. 2012. Genetic variability and inter-relationship among some Nigerian pumpkin accessions (Cucurbitaspp). Int. J. Plant Breeding 6:34–41.

Bello, M. O., O. S. Farade, S. R. A. Adewusi, and N. O. Olawore. 2008. Studies of some lesser known Nigerian fruits. Afr. J. Biotechnol. 7:3972–3979.

Benchasr, S.. 2012. Okra (*Abelmoschus esculentus* (L.) Moench) as a valuable vegetable of the world. Ratar. Povrt. 49:105–112.

Benjawan, C., P. Chutichudet, and S. Kaewsit. 2007. Effect of green manures on growth yield and quality of green okra (*Abelmoschus esculentus* L) har lium cultivar. Pak. J. Biological Sci. 10:1028–1035.

Bhandari, M. R., and J. Kawabata. 2004. Assessment of antinutritional factors and bioavailability of calcium and in wild yam(Dioscorea spp.) tubers of Nepal. Food Chem. 85:281–287.

Dandena, G. 2010. Shifting to alternative food source: potential to overcome ethiopias' malnutrition and poverty problems. Emilie Coudel, Hubert Devautour, Christophe-Toussaint Soulard, Bernard Hubert. Cirad-Inra-SupAgro, Montpellier, France, 10 p.

Dawczynski, C., R. Schubert, and G. Jahreis. 2007. Amino acids, fatty acids, and dietary fibre in edible seaweed products. Food Chem. 103:891–899.

Dillard, C. J., and J. B. German. 2000. Photochemical nutraceuticals and human health. J. Sci. Food Agric. 80:1744–1756.

Effiong, G. S., T. O. Ibia, and U. S. Udofia. 2009. Nutritive and energy values of some wild fruit spices in south eastern Nigeria. Electron. J. Environ. Agric. Food Chem. 8:917–923.

Ekumankama, I. O. 2008. Nutrient composition of indigenous vegetables (Pterocarpus soyanxii, pterocarpus santalinoides and *Gnetum africanum*). Nig. J. Nutr. Sci. 29:195–200.

Ekwumemgbo, P. A., M. S. Sallau, K. I. Omoniyi, and S. Y. Zubairu. 2014. Proximate and anti-nutritional constituents of *Abelmoschus esculentus* grown in Fadaman Kubanni, Zaria, Kaduna State, Nigeria. J. Sci. Res. Rep. 3:2015–2027.

Elinge, C. M., A. Muhammad, F. A. Atiku, A. U. Itodo, I. J. Peni, O. M. Sanni, et al. 2012. Proximate, mineral and anti-nutrient composition of pumpkin (*Cucurbitapepo* L) seeds extract. Int. J. Plant Res. 2:146–150.

Fekadu, H., F. Beyene, and G. Desse. 2013. Effect of traditional processing methods on nutritional composition and anti-nutritional factors of anchote (Coccinia Abyssinica(lam.) Cogn) tubers grown in Western Ethiopia. J. Food Process Technol. 4:249.

Frontela, C., M. L. Scarino, S. Ferruzza, G. Ros, and C. Martínez. 2009. Effect of dephytinization on bioavailability of iron, calcium and from infant cereals assessed in the Caco-2 cell model. World J. Gastroenterol. 28:1977–1984.

Gemede, H. F., and N. Ratta. 2014. Antinutritional factors in plant foods: potential health benefits and adverse effects. Int. J. Nutr. Food Sci. 3:284–289.

Gemede, H. F., N. Ratta, G. D. Haki, A. Z. Woldegiorgis, and F. Beyene. 2015. Nutritional quality and health benefits of okra (*Abelmoschus esculentus*): a review. J. Food Process Technol. 6:458.

Getachew, O. 2001. Food source diversification: Potential to ameliorate the chronic food insecurity in Ethiopia. *in* Proceedings of the Potential of Indigenous Wild Foods. Workshop proceedings, 22–26 January 2001. Addis Ababa, Ethiopia.

Gopalan, C., S. B. V. Sastri, and S. Balasubramanian. 2007. Nutritive value of Indian foods. National Institute of Nutrition (NIN), ICMR, India.

Guyot, J. P., I. Rochette, and S. Treche. 2007. Effect of fermentation by amylolytic lactic acid bacteria, in process combinations, on characteristics of rice/soybean slurries: a new method for preparing high energy density complementary foods for young children. Food Chem. 100:623–663.

Habtamu, F., N. Ratta, G. D. Haki, A. Z. Woldegiorgis, and F. Beyene. 2014. Nutritional quality and health benefits of okra (Abelmoschus esculentus): A review. J. Food. Sci. Qual. Manag. 33:87–96.

Hanif, R., Z. Igbal, M. Igbal, S. Hanif, and M. Rasheed. 2006. Use of vegetables as nutritional food: role in human health. J. Agric. Biol. Sci. 1:18–20.

Hilou, A., O. G. Nacoulma, and T. R. Guiguemde. 2006. In vivo antimalarial activities of extract from *Amaranthus spinosus* L., and *Boerhaavia erecta* L. J. Ethnopharmacol. 103:236–240.

Hurrel, R. F., M. B. Reddy, M. A. Juillerat, and J. D. Cook. 2003. Degradation of phytic acid in cereal porridges improves iron absorption by human subjects. Am. J. Clin. Nutr. 77:1213–1219.

Ibanga, O. I., and D. E. Okon. 2009. Minerals and antinutrients in two varieties of African pear (*Dacryodes edulis*). J. Food Technol. 7:106–110.

Ikewuchi, C. C., and J. C. Ikewuchi. 2009. Chemical profile of *Pleurotus tuberregium* (fr) sing's sclerotia pacific. J. Sci. Technol. 10:295–299.

Jabeen, S., M. T. Shah, S. Khan, and M. Q. Hayat. 2010. The typical symptoms of determination of major and trace elements in ten important folk therapeutic plants of Haripur Basin. Pak. J. Med. Plants Res. 4:559–566.

Kathirvel, P., and P. Kumudha. 2011. Chemical composition of prosopis juliflora (SW.) D.C (mosquito bean). Int. J. Appl. Biol. Pharmaceut. Technol. 2:5–14.

Kermanshah, A., P. Ziarati, J. Asgarpanah, and M. Qomi. 2014. Food values of two endemic wild *Almond* species from Iran. Int. J. Plant Anim. Environ. Sci. 4:380–388.

Manzi, P., S. Marconi, A. Aguzzi, and L. Pizzoferrato. 2004. Commercial mushrooms: nutritional quality and effect of cooking. Food Chem. 84:201–206.

Massey, L. K., R. G. Palmer, and H. T. Horner. 2001. Oxalate content of soybean seeds (Glycine max:Leguminosae), Soya foods, and other edible legumes. J. Agric. Food Chem. 49:4262–4266.

Maxson, E. D., and L. W. Rooney. 1972. Evaluation of methods for tannin analysis in sorghum grain. Cereal Chem. 49:719–729.

Mensan, J. K., R. I. Okoli, J. O. Ohaju-Obodo, and K. Eifediyi. 2008. Phytochemical, nutritional and medicinal properties of some leafy vegetables consumed by Edo People of Nigeria. Afr. J. Biotechnol. 7:2304–2309.

Mlitan, A. M., M. S. Sasi, and A. M. Alkherraz. 2014. Proximate and minor mineral content in some selected basil leaves of *Ocimum gratissimum* L, in Libya. Int. J. Chem. Eng. Appl. 5:8–17.

Morris, E. R., and R. Ellis. 1989. Usefulness of the dietary phytic acid/molar ratio as an index of bioavailability to rats and humans. Biol. Trace Elem. Res. 19:107–117.

Moses, A. G., E. G. L. Gitu, and H. Rotich. 2012. Profile of heavy metals in selected medicinal plants used for the treatment of diabetes, malaria and pneumonia in Kisii region, southwest Kenya. Global J. Pharmacol. 6:245–251.

Naveed, A., A. A. Khan, and I. A. Khan. 2009. Generation mean analysis of water stress tolerance in okra (*Abelmoschus esculentus* L.). Pak. J. Bot. 41:195–205.

Ndunguru, J., and A. Rajabu. 2004. Effect of okra mosaic virus disease on the above-ground morphological yield components of okra in Tanzania. Sci. Hortic. 99:225–235.

Nesamvuni, C., N. P. Steyn, and M. J. Potgieter. 2001. Nutritional value of wild, leafy plants consumed by the Vhavenda. S. Afr. J. Sci. 97:51–54.

Nnamani, C. V., H. O. Oselebe, and A. Agbautu. 2009. Assessment of nutritional values of three underutilized indigenous leafy vegetables of Ebonyi state, Nigeria. Afr. J. Biotechnol. 8:2321–2324.

Nwachukwu, E. C., R. Nulit, and R. Go. 2014. Nutritional and biochemical properties of Malaysian okra variety. Adv. Med. Plant Res. 2:16–19.

Nwofia, G. E., N. Nwogu Victoria, and B. K. Nwofia. 2012. Nutritional variation in fruits and seeds of pumpkins (*Cucurbita* Spp) accessions from Nigeria. Pak. J. Nutr. 11:946–956.

Nzikou, J. M., M. Mioula-Tsieri, E. Matouba, J. M. Ouamba, C. Kapser, M. Parmentier, et al. 2006. Study on gumbo seed grown in Congo brazzaville for its food and industrial applications. Afr. J. Biotechnol. 5:2469–2475.

Obah, G., and T. V. Amusan. 2009. Nutritive value and antioxidant properties of cereal gruels produced from fermented maize and sorghum. Food Biotechnol. 23:17–31.

Ogungbenle, H. N., and S. M. Omosola. 2015. The comparative assessment of nutritive values of dry nigerian okra (*Abelmoschus esculentus*) fruit and oil. Int. J. Food Sci. Nutr. Eng. 5:8–14.

Okaka, J. C., and A. N. O. Okaka. 2001. Pp. 54–56 Food composition, spoilage and shelf life extension, ocjarc. Acadamic Publishers, Enugu, Nigeria.

Omotosho, O. T. 2005. Nutritional quality, functional properties and anti-nutrient compositions of the Larva of Cirinda forda (Westwood) (Lepidoptera:saturniidae). J. Zhejiang Univ. Sci. 7:51–55.

Onwuka, G. I.. 2005. Food analysis and instrumentation, proximate composition of food minerals. 1st ed. Naplithali Print, A Division of H.G. Support Nigerian Ltd, Nigeria 64 81, 114 Pp.

Oyelade, O. J., B. I. O. Ade-Omowaye, and V. F. Adeomi. 2003. Influence of variety on protein, fat contents and some physical characteristics of okra seeds. J. Food Eng. 57:111–114.

Phillippy, B. Q., M. Lin, and B. Rasco. 2004. Analysis of phytate in raw and cooked potatoes. J. Food Compos. Anal. 17:217–226.

Saifullah, M., and M. G. Rabbani. 2009. Evaluation and characterization of okra (*Abelmoschus esculentus* L. Moench.) genotypes. SAARC J. Agric. 7:92–99.

Sathish, D., and A. Eswar. 2013. A review on: *Abelmoschus esculentus* (Okra). Int. Res. J. Pharm. App. Sci. 3:129–132.

Siegenberg, D., R. D. Baynes, T. H. Bothwell. 1991. Ascorbic acid prevents the dose-dependent inhibitory effects of polyphenols and phytates on nonheme-iron absorption. Am. J. Clin. Nutr. 53:537–541.

Simmone, E. H., G. J. Hochmuth, D. N. Maynard, C. S. Vavrina, W. M. Stall, T. A. Kucharek, et al. 2004. Okra production in Florida. Horticultural Sciences Department document HS729. Florida Cooperative Extension Service, Institute of Food and Agricultural Sciences, University of Florida.

Soetan, K. O., C. O. Olaiya, and O. E. Oyewole. 2010. The importance of mineral elements for humans, domestic animals and plants: a review. Afr. J. Food Sci. 4:200–222.

Tchientche Kamga, R., C. Kouamé, A. R. Atangana, T. Chagomoka, and R. Ndango. 2013. Nutritional evaluation of five African indigenous vegetables. J. Horticult. Res. 21:99–106.

Ugwu, F. M., and N. A. Oranye. 2006. Effects of some processing methods on the toxic components of African breadfruit *(Treculia africana)*. Afr. J. Biotechnol. 5:2329–2333.

Ukpabi, V. J., and J. I. Ejidoh. 1989. Effect of deep out frying on the oxalate content and the degree of itching of cocoyams. (*Xanthosoma* and *colocassia* spp). Technical paper presented at the 5th annual conference of the Agriculture society of Nigeria. Federal University of Technology Owerri, Nigeria, 3–6 (September).

Ullah, R. J. A., I. Khader, N. M. Hussain, A. M. Talha, and N. Khan. 2012. Investigation of macro and micronutrients in selected medicinal plants". Afr. J. Pharm. Pharmacol. 69:1829–1832.

Uyoh, E. A., E. E. Ita, and G. E. Nwofia. 2013. Evaluation of the chemical composition of *Tetrapleura tetraptera*

(Schum and Thonn.) Tuab. accessions from Cross River State, Nigeria. Int. J. Med. Arom. Plants 3:386–394.

Valvi, S. R., and V. S. Rathod. 2011. Mineral composition of some wild edible fruits from Kolhapur district. Int. J. Appl. Biol. Pharmaceut. Technol. 2:112–119.

Vantraub, I. A., and N. A. Lapteva. 1988. Colorimetric determination of phytate in unpurified extracts of seeds and the products of their processing. Anal. Biochem. 175:227.

Woldegiorgis, A. Z., D. Abate, G. D. Haki, and G. R. Ziegler. 2015. Major, minor and toxic minerals and anti-nutrients composition in edible mushrooms collected from Ethiopia. Food Process. Technol. 6:134–142.

Yang, R. Y., and G. B. Keding. 2009. Nutritional contributions of important African indigenous vegetables. Pp. 105–143 *in* C. M. Shackleton, M. W. Pasquini and A. W. Drescher, eds. African indigenous vegetables in urban agriculture. Earthscan, London.

Yiridoe, E. K., and V. M. Anchirinah. 2005. Garden production systems and food security in Ghana: characteristics of traditional knowledge and management systems. Renew. Agric. Food Syst. 20:168–180.

Zhao, H., J. Lin, H. B. Grossman, L. M. Hernandez, C. P. Dinney, and X. Wu. 2007. Dietary isothiocyanates, GSTMI, NAT2 polymorphisms and bladder cancer risk. Int. J. Cancer 120:2208–2213.

19

Rheological, baking, and sensory properties of composite bread dough with breadfruit (*Artocarpus communis* Forst) and wheat flours

Adegoke H. Bakare[1], Oluwatooyin F. Osundahunsi[2] & Joseph O. Olusanya[3]

[1]Department of Hospitality and Tourism, Federal University of Agriculture, Abeokuta, Nigeria
[2]Department of Food Science and Technology, Federal University of Technology, Akure, Nigeria
[3]Department of Home Economics and Hotel Management, Tai Solarin University of Education, Ijebu Ode, Nigeria

Keywords
Bread, production, rheology, sensory attributes qualities

Correspondence
Adegoke H. Bakare, Department of Hospitality and Tourism Federal University of Agriculture, Abeokuta, Nigeria.

E-mail: bakare65@gmail.com

Funding Information
No funding information provided.

Abstract

The rheological (Pasting, farinograph, and alveograph) properties of wheat flour (WF) replaced with breadfruit four (05–40%) was analyzed. Baking and sensory qualities of the resulting bread were evaluated. Differences in baking properties of loaves produced under laboratory and industrial conditions were analyzed with t-test, whereas ANOVA was used for other analyses. Peak and final viscosities in the composite blends (CB) ranged from 109.20 to 114.06 RVU and 111.86 to 134.40 RVU, respectively. Dough stability decreased from 9.15 to 0.78 min, whereas farinograph water absorption increased 59.7–65.9%. Alveograph curve configuration ratio increased from 1.27 to 7.39, whereas specific volume (Spv) of the loaves decreased from 2.96 to 1.32 cm^3/g. The Spv of WF loaves were not significantly different ($P > 0.05$) from that of the 5% CB, whereas production conditions had no significant effects on absorbed water ($t = 0.532$, df = 18 $P = 0.3005$), weight loss during baking ($t = 0.865$, df = 18, $P = 0.199$), and Spv ($t = 0.828$, df = 14.17, $P = 0.211$). The sensory qualities of the 5% blend were not significantly different from the WF.

Introduction

Bread is a staple food consumed in different parts of the World. Varieties of bread of different sizes, shape, textures, and flavors that contain different ingredients and are baked under different conditions exists across many continents (Zhou and Therdthai 2006). Bread was also described as a fermented confectionery product produced mainly from wheat flour, water, yeast, and salt by a series of process involving mixing, kneading, proofing, shaping, and baking (Dewettinck et al. 2008). Several studies have reported the prospects of composite flour technology as a means of reducing the dependence on wheat for the production of bakery products (Hugo et al. 2000; Doxastakis et al. 2002; Woo and Seib 2002; Hallen et al. 2004; Michiyo et al. 2004; Greene and Bovell-Benjamin 2004; Mepba et al. 2007; Biljan and Bojana 2008; Manuel et al. 2008; Alex et al. 2008; Ade-Omowaye et al. 2008; Lin et al. 2009; Adeleke and Odedeji 2010;. Malomo et al. 2011, 2013).

Consumption of wheat-based products is expected to increase as population and urbanization increases (Bakare 2008; Malomo et al. 2011), and with the exotic lifestyle and food habits adopted by the citizen of most of the nonwheat producing countries. Partial as against the desired complete replacement of wheat flour with available indigenous flours remains the only viable practical option. The challenges with adoption of this technology at industrial scale include minimizing the changes that would occurred in the known quality of the final product, technical issues relating to the use of established manufacturing procedure and availability of flour of suitable quality from various indigenous sources; particularly flour from under utilised crops with less competing uses.

Breadfruit (*Artocarpus communis* Forst) is one of such crops. It is a staple diet in many tropical developing countries of the world. The tree fruits early between May and August, producing 50–200 fruits in a year. The mature fruit is round or ovoid, 15–20 cm in diameter and weighs 2–10 kg on average. The fruit is produced mainly in Malaysia, the South Pacific Island, the Caribbean's and West Africa (Ragone 2009). Total yearly production in Nigerian is about 10 million metric tonnes with potential to exceed 100 million metric tonnes with improved agricultural practice (Adewusi et al. 1995; Amusa et al. 2002). The economic utilization of breadfruit has been limited by its poor storage properties which is about 1–3 days after harvest (Ragone 2009). Conversion of breadfruit to flour would provide a more stable storage form and also enhance its versatility. (Morton 1987; Oladunjoye et al. 2010).

Breadfruit is an underutilized crop in Nigeria, information on its composition, nutritional importance, and the behavior of its flour during cooking had already been studied (Graham and De-Bravo 1981; Oladunjoye et al. 2010; Bakare et al. 2012). This study therefore evaluated the effects of replacing wheat flour with breadfruit flour on the rheological properties of the composite flour blends, the baking and sensory qualities of the resulting bread and also compared some baking qualities of the bread under laboratory and industrial conditions.

Materials and Methods

Source of materials

Seedless variety of breadfruit (*Artocarpus communis* Forst) used for the study was obtained from a farm at Mamu in Ijebu North Local Government area of Ogun State. Wheat flour was obtained from Honey well flour mill, Ltd Apapa, Lagos, whereas other ingredients were purchased in the retail markets.

Preparation of flour

Breadfruit was processed as described by Oladunjoye et al. (2010) with some modifications. Matured breadfruit (Greenish-yellow skin), peel color index - 3 (Ajayi 1997; Ragone 2009) were hand peeled, washed, thinly sliced, and soaked in 5% sodium metabisulfite solution for 30 min to prevent enzymic browning. It was then dried in a cross flow Gallenkamp oven (Model OV-160 size 2 BS, Weiss Technik UK, Loughborough, Leicestershire, UK) at 80°C for 2 h and then, at 35°C for 12 h. The dried chips were milled to flour in a Disk mill (Model FFC-15, Shandong-Jimo Agricultural Machinery, Qingdao City, Shandong Province, China) at 8800 RPM and sieved through a 250 μm mesh sieve (W. S. Tyler, 8570 Tyler Blvd, Mentor, OH, United States).

Analysis of flour

All analyses were performed in triplicates. Protein, moisture, water absorption, and ash contents of wheat flour and blends were analyzed with official methods (AACC, 2000) using a Partens Inframatic analyzer (Model 9140, SE-126 53, Hägersten, Sweden). Alpha-amylase activity was determined with the Hagberg falling numbers instrument (Partens model no 1500, USA), based on (AACC, 2000) approved method. Free sugar and starch in wheat and breadfruit flours samples were determined by the spectrophotometric method of Dubois et al. (1970) and Mcready (1970). Crude fiber content of flour was determined by Trichloroacetic acid method as described by Entwistle and Hunter (1949).

Viscosity characteristics of flour

Pasting characteristic of the four and their blends were determined according to ICC No 162 method. Rapid visco analyzer (RVA) series 4 (RVA; series 4, Newport Scientific P.T.V., Warriewood, Australia) with the aid of thermocline for Windows (version 1.1. Software, 1996) provided by the instrument manufacturer was used for the analysis. The 12-min profile was used for all the analyses. It consists of idle temp of 50°C for 1 min, then 50–95°C in 3 min 45 sec, held at 95°C for 2 min 30 sec, cooled to 50°C over 3 min 45 sec, final, held at 50°C for 2 min. Two paddle speeds of 960 revolutions per minute for the first 10 sec followed by 150 revolutions per minute were employed for the remaining duration of the test cycle. The weight per sample used for each analysis was calculated from the formula:

$$\text{Corrected sample weight for R V A (S)} = \frac{A \times 100}{100 - M},$$

$$(W) = 25 + (A - S),$$

where A = Weight of flour sample: using the $R\ V\ A$ manual as a guide.

S = Corrected sample weight.

M = Actual moisture content of the sample.

W = Volume of water used.

Rheological characteristics of dough

Farinogram characteristics

The farinogram characteristics of dough made from blends of breadfruit/wheat composite Flour samples (10–20%) were determined by approved method (AACC, 2000) using Brabender Farinograph (Model T 150 E, Ohgduisburg, Germany). The instrument provided a means of evaluating the strength of flour, dough consistency, and characteristics (Edmund 1967; Bloksma 1990a;

Abang Zaidel et al. 2010). Inframatic analyzer was used to obtain an estimate of the moisture content of flour sample and hence determine the actual weight of flour samples to be used at the prescribed 14% moisture basis for the farinogram analysis. This was obtained by the expression;

$$\text{Required weight of sample} = \frac{(100 - 14) \times 300\,g}{(100.M)},$$

where M = Percent moisture content of the sample.

Appropriate weight of flour sample was placed in the mixer of the farinogram, which was thermostatically controlled by means of water jacket at a temperature of 30°C. Cold water at 30°C was added to the sample through the attached burette until optimum water absorption content was absorbed by the dough when the farinogram curve was on the 500 line. A fresh sample was taken and the process was repeated using the appropriate water absorption for the mixing and development process. The development of the dough and the resistance offered to mixing were recorded on the farinogram.

Alveogram characteristics

The alveograph (Chopin NG France) was used to measure (AACC, 2010) characteristics that provided insight in to the fermentation tolerance of the dough as may be exhibited during proofing stage of bread making. Characteristics of interest that were measured included the average resistance to expansion indicated by the peak height (mm), extensibility indicated by length (L) of the alveogram curve, energy input (Joules) required for the mechanical deformation of the dough (W), inflation required for maximum development (G), and the elastic resistance (Ie) of the measured dough samples.

Flour sample (250 g) of known moisture content was placed into the mixer, sodium chloride solution (2.5%) was added through a burette (i.e., 129.4 ml for flour with 14% moisture) and mixed for 7 min. The dough was forced through the extrusion gate in the form of a thin strip on to a small oiled steel plate. Five extruded dough pieces of designated length were cut off, rolled with an oiled rolling pin to a uniform thinness, cut into a circular disk, transferred to an oiled steel plate, and subjected to a brief rest period in a tempered compartment of the alveograph for 15 min. Each circular dough test pieces were removed from the compartment and inserted between two metal plates that held it securely in position. The air valve was opened to supply air pressure to the held dough through an orifice. The electrically driven recording manometer was simultaneously activated to record the air pressure inside the dough bubble against time.

Bread production

Bread loaves were produced according to AACC (2010) with slight modification. Formulation included: Breadfruit/Wheat (100:00, 90:10, 80:20, 70:30, and 60:40) composite Flour 100 g (14% moisture), 6.5 g sugar, 1.5 g iodized salt, 3.0 g yeast, 3.9 g fat and 50 ppm of ascorbic acid as dough improver. The water required to form a dough of desired consistency varied between 32.1% and 93.3% of flour using water absorption values obtained from the farinogram as guide.

Bread production was carried out in the laboratory and also in a small-scale industrial bakery (Eucharistic Heart of Jesus, Ibonwon, Lagos state), respectively. Locally fabricated horizontal high speed mixer (Jido Nigeria) and Omega spiral mixer (Model OMJ-25, China Omega Baking Machinery Co. L. No.88, East Taishan Road, Shenzhou City, Hengshui, Hebei, China) were used in the industrial and laboratory mixing, respectively. The dough was fermented (proofed) at initial and final fermentation time of 15 and 28 min and at ambient condition of 28 ± 2°C temperatures and 85 ± 12% relative humidity. Baking trials at laboratory level was done in an oven (Model GP-OV-100-F-SS-DIG, St Helens, Merseyside, Great Britain) at 220°C for 30 min while locally constructed typical clay oven used by local bakeries was used for the industrial production. The bread samples were cooled for 1 h, then placed in low-density polyethylene plastic bags and kept at 24 ± 2 °C.

Determination of physical quality of bread

Weights of bread loaves were measured with a Mettler Toledo (A204) digital weighing scale. Volume of was measured by millet seed displacement method (AACC, 2010) with minor modification.

Weight loss

The weight loss of the bread was determined as described by Kim et al. (2003). The dough was weighed before baking, and the breads were weighed after baking. The percent weight loss of the bread samples was calculated as:

$$\%\text{weight loss} = \frac{A - B \times 100}{A},$$

where, A = weight of dough; B = weight of baked bread.

Sensory analysis

Selection of panelists

Forty people were selected from a pool of volunteers comprising professional bakers, catering officers, lecturers, and students of tertiary institution. The panelists were

Table 1. Attributes, definitions, and references used in the descriptive sensory analysis of bread produced from wheat- breadfruit flour.

Terms	Definitions	References	Quality and score range
Appearances			
Crust color	Light golden brown	100% wheat flour bread	Very pale dark brown to typical yellowish brown: 1–5
Crumb color	Typical white color of bread	100% wheat flour bread	Brown to white: 1–10
Cell size	Cell size of crumb resembling mesh of tiny diameter size	Internal crumb bread from 100% wheat flour.	More cells with small diameter: 1–10
Cell uniformity	Even distribution of the cells throughout the sample	Internal crumb bread from 100% wheat flour.	Extent to which cells are evenly distributed: 1–10
Flavor			
Characteristic taste of Bread	Reminiscent of the characteristic of typical wheat flour bread	Bread made with 100% wheat flour	Foreign to typical: 1–5
Wheaty smell	Reminiscent of the smell of wheat bread	Bread made with 100% wheat flour	Foreign to typical: 1–10
Aroma	Characteristic aroma of freshly baked bread	Bread made with 100% wheat flour	Foreign to typically pleasant: 1–5
Texture			
Mouthfeel	Having chewiness that is associated with freshly baked wheat flour bread	Bread made from 100% wheat flour	Doughy to typical clean easy to breakdown mouth feel: 1–10
Crumb stability and softness	Bread separated slowly when pulled apart	Bread made from 100% wheat flour	Unstable/hard to stable and soft: 1to 10
Nongrittiness	Absence of small coarse particles in the mouth after swallowing	Bread made from 100% wheat flour	Absence of small particles during and after mastication: 1–10
Lightness	Bread loaf has heavy, compact, thick inner structure associated with poorly aerated bread		Denseness to lightness: 1–10

Adapted from Greene and Bovell-Benjamin (2004); Indrani and Rao (2007); Bakare (2008).

selected after an oral interview conducted on the basis of a criteria checklist that included: Good health, non-smoker, nonallergic to wheat/breadfruit, willingness to participate, and passion/likeness for the consumption of bread. They were compensated for their participation. Ten of the selected people were trained as panelists for descriptive analysis aspects of the test, whereas the remaining 30 people were used as untrained panelists for the consumer/preference aspect of the test.

Descriptive sensory analysis

Descriptive sensory analysis was carried out as described by Bakare et al. (2013). Judges rated the intensity of the samples for each attribute using a numerical intensity scale specified in Table 1

Consumer test

Quantitative acceptance test was used to assess consumers liking for the product. Thirty untrained panelists rated their liking or otherwise for cakes produced from the blends on a seven-point hedonic scale (1 = liked very much less as compared to reference sample '*R*', and 7 = liked much more as compared to reference sample '*R*').

Statistical analysis

All experiments and analyses were conducted in triplicates. Data obtained from different aspects of the study were subjected to analysis of variance and the Duncan multiple range test was used to separate the means (Duncan 1955). Independent sample *t*-test was used compare the baking qualities (absorbed water, weight loss, and specific volume) of bread baked under laboratory and industrial conditions. Statistical analysis package software SPSS 17 for windows (IBM, New Orchard Road, Armonk, New York) was used for all the analyses.

Results and Discussion

Composition of the flours and their blends

The breadfruit flour (BF) had relatively lower protein but higher ash and fiber contents than wheat flour (Table 2) and did not have the structural gluten-forming protein found in wheat flour. Protein and gluten contents of the blends decreased as wheat flour (WF) was gradually replaced with BF, whereas ash contents increased in the blends as the proportion of BF increased. Similar trend in protein valued was reported by Olatunji and Akinrele (1978).

Table 2. Composition of breadfruit, wheat flours, and their composite blends.

Flour	Moisture (%)	Protein (%)	Ash (%)	Gluten (%)	Alpha amylase activity (Falling No)	Starch (%)	Damaged starch %	Sugars (%)	Fibers (%)
BF:WF									
00:100	12.5 ± 0.3^{a}	10.9 ± 0.1$_{de}$	0.65 ± .01$_{a}$	12.8 ± 0.1$_{e}$	370.3 ± 2$_{c}$	69.89 ± 8	7.21 ± 0.1	2.63 ± 0.6	2.81 ± 0.7
100:00#	13.7 ± 0.2$_{b}$	2.6 ± 0.1$_{a}$	1.72 ± .01$_{f}$	N.A	N.D	61.30 ± 4	19.3 ± 1.4	3.75 ± 0.7	7.79 ± 0.6
10:90	13.7 ± 0.2$_{b}$	11.1 ± 0.3$_{e}$	0.83 ± .0$_{b}$	11.6 ± 0.1$_{d}$	316.3 ± 0.7$_{b}$				
20:80	12.8 ± 0.1$_{ba}$	10.3 ± 0.3$_{d}$	0.98 ± 0.0$_{c}$	9.8 ± 0.1$_{c}$	302 ± 1.4$_{a}$				
30:60	12.5 ± 0.2$_{a}$	8.59 ± 0.3$_{c}$	1.31 ± .01$_{d}$	7.6 ± 0.2$_{b}$	686 ± 4.2$_{d}$				
60:40	12.5 ± 0.1$_{a}$	6.71 ± 0.1$_{b}$	1.41 ± 01$_{e}$	5.8 ± 0.1$_{a}$	865 ± 2.1$_{e}$				

a–f, Mean in the same column with the same subscripts are not significantly different ($P < 0.05$); N.D, Not determined; N.A, Not available; WF, wheat flour; BF, breadfruit flour; (10–40), composite blends; # = Substitution levels.

Values for protein and ash contents in the blends ranged from 6.71 to 11.1% and 0.83% to 1.41, respectively. Falling number values (which are indicative of the alpha amylase activity) increased from 316.3 to 865 as the proportion of BF was increased in the blends (Table 2). This implied that the extent of liquefaction and diastatic activity of the starches in the blends decreased as the proportion of the BF was increased (Schiller 1984; Watson 1984). The value of damaged starch in WF was within the range specified for bakery flour (Schiller 1984). The BF had a higher value of damaged starch (19.3%) than the WF. It was relatively higher than the value reported for breadfruit starch (Loos et al. 1981). The high fiber content (7.79%) observed in the BF suggested greater tendency to absorb more water during mixing than the WF and this has implication on the quality of bread produced from the blends.

Rheological characteristics

Rheology is the science of the deformation and flow of matter. It is the study of the manner in which materials respond to applied stress or strain (Mirsaeedghazi et al. 2008). The rheological properties of food materials measured or tested by rheometers like rapid visco anlyser, farinograph and alveograph provides empirical information that correlates well with actual results on product's quality. Also, measurements obtained from these instruments have been reported to correlates with result gotten from mixolab (Dapčević et al. 2009) which has been designed to eliminate some of the short comings associated with farinograph and amylograph (Alava et al. 2007; Fustier et al. 2008; Marco and Rosell 2008; Ozturk et al. 2008).

Viscosity characteristic

Pasting temperature gives an indication of temperature required to cook the flour beyond its gelatinization point (BeMiller 2011). It corresponds to the temperature where viscosities first increase by at least 2 RVU over a 20 sec period (Olkku and Rha 1978; Appelqvist and Debet 1997). Changes that may occur when a starch-water system is heated included enormous swelling, increased viscosity, translucency and solubility, and loss of anisotropy (birefringence) (Shimelis et al. 2006). The starch granules of the BF gelatinized at a higher temperature (71.7°C) than that of WF (68.50°C). The starch gelatinization range observed for wheat flour was within the range reported by Hoseney (1994) and Shimelis et al. (2006).

Peak viscosity is the maximum viscosity develops during or soon after the heating phase of the test. It occurred after most of the granule swelling had ceased. Hot starch paste is a mixture of swollen starch granules and granule

Table 3. Pasting characteristics of breadfruit and wheat flours.

Flours	Peak viscosity (RVU)	Holding strength (RVU)	Breakdown viscosity (RVU)	Final viscosity (RVU)	Set back viscosity (RVU)	Peak time (min)	Pasting temperature °C
BF:WF							
00:100	$101.17 \pm 0.7_a$	$64.33 \pm 0.1_a$	$36.83 \pm 0.6_a$	$114.92 \pm 0.7_b$	$50.58 \pm 0.1_e$	$6.20 \pm 0.7_b$	$68.50 \pm 0.4_a$
100:00	$251.90 \pm 0.9_g$	$191.60 \pm 0.7_f$	$60.94 \pm 0.6_c$	$316.00 \pm 0.7_f$	$126.0 \pm 0.7_f$	$4.60 \pm 0.7_a$	$71.74 \pm 0.3_d$
05:95	$109.20 \pm 1.4_b$	$66.14 \pm 0.2_a$	$43.06 \pm 0.4_b$	$111.86 \pm 0.3_a$	$45.70 \pm 0.5_c$	$6.22 \pm 0.1_b$	$68.77 \pm 0.1_{ab}$
10:90	$114.06 \pm 0.7_c$	$77.13 \pm 0.9_b$	$37.03 \pm 0.5_a$	$118.92 \pm 0.7_c$	$42.79 \pm 0.6_{ab}$	$6.19 \pm 0.0_b$	$69.50 \pm 0.4_b$
15:85	$115.8 \pm 1.1_d$	$79.43 \pm 0.2_c$	$36.46 \pm 0.6_a$	$123.44 \pm 0.3_d$	$43.01 \pm 0.2_b$	$6.19 \pm 0.1_b$	$70.12 \pm 0.1_c$
20:80	$119.02 \pm 0.7_e$	$82.15 \pm 0.1_d$	$36.87 \pm 0.6_a$	$124.09 \pm 0.7_d$	$41.94 \pm 0.4_a$	$6.16 \pm 0.1_b$	$70.46 \pm 0.2_c$
40:60	$122.30 \pm 0.6_f$	$85.40 \pm 0.3_e$	$36.93 \pm 0.4_a$	$134.40 \pm 0.3_e$	$48.37 \pm 0.3_d$	$6.07 \pm 0.4_b$	$78.30 \pm 0.2_c$

a–g, Mean in same column with the same subscripts are not significantly different ($P < 0.05$); WF, wheat flour; BF, breadfruit flour; (05–90), composite blends.

fragments, together with colloidal and molecularly dispersed starch molecules. It gelatinizes when heated beyond 50°C. This caused a marked increase in the viscosity and further disintegration of the starch granules. The viscosity of the starch paste dropped at elevated temperature near 95 °C depicting the characteristic peak in the viscosity–temperature curve of the RVA graph (Dengate 1978; Bakare et al. 2012). The peak viscosity also measures the alpha amylase activity and other contributory factors such as the inherent susceptibility of the starch to amylase and the starch gel strength (Watson 1984; Meera 2010). Therefore, a higher value of RVU at the peak of the curve indicated a lower diastatic activity and vice versa (Schiller 1984). The peak viscosity of WF (101.0 RVU) was found to be significantly lower than that of BF (252.0 RVU) (Table 3) indicating a relatively higher diastatic activity and lower gel strength.

Peak viscosities occur at equilibrium between swelling of the granules (that 'increases the viscosity) and the granule rupture and alignment (that reduces viscosity). The relatively high swelling capacity exhibited by the BF may have resulted from a weak internal bonding in the starch granules.

Holding strength indicated the ability of the starch granules to maintain their gelatinized structure when the paste was held at 95°C for 2 min 30 sec under mechanical shearing stress. The BF had a holding strength value that was higher than that of the WF.

Breakdown viscosity is a measure of the degree of starch disintegration. It is an indication of hot paste stability of the starch. The smaller the breakdown viscosity, the higher the paste stability (Hugo et al. 2000; Bakare et al. 2012). The BF had significantly higher (60.9 RVU) breakdown viscosity value than the WF (36.8 RVU) indicating relatively lower hot paste stability.

Final viscosity is the section of the paste gel curve where the gelatinized dispersion of starch becomes viscoelastic on cooling resulting in the formation of a loose paste or gel. The BF had significantly higher final viscosity value (316 RVU) than the WF indicating that it formed a firmer gel after cooking and cooling.

Setback viscosity is the phase of the pasting curve after cooling the starches to 50°C. This stage involved re-association, retrogradation, or reordering of starch molecules. Also, the water previously bounded in the viscoelastic gel are released at this stage in a process referred to as syneresis. The higher the setback viscosity, the greater the tendency toward retrogradation. The BF had relatively higher viscosity value than the WF.

Peak time was the time at which the peak viscosity was attained in minutes. The WF had a significantly higher peak time than the BF.

Farinograph

Mixing, fermentation and baking are the three basic operations involve in bread making. Mixing transforms the flour and water into cohesive viscoelastic dough and also incorporates air in to the dough. The incorporated air provided the gas cells into which the carbon dioxide produced by the yeast fermentation diffuses. Bread dough is a wet mass developed after mixing of wheat flour, water and other ingredients. Development of dough occurs as a result of interactions among flour constituents during mixing operation. Although, these interactions are more complex than what was observed during the farigraph test. The test, however, provided an empirically verifiable insight in to what may be at play during the actual process of dough development. The aim of mixing is to bring about changes in the physical properties of the dough that would improve the ability of the dough to retain the carbon dioxide gas that would be produced during yeast fermentation. Resistance to deformation, extensibility, elasticity, and stickiness are some of the physical properties of dough that are critical for control in bread making process.

The rheological characteristics exhibited by flour during mixing (Table 4) revealed that the WF arrived at the

Table 4. Farinogram of wheat flour and its composite blends with breadfruit flour.

Flours	Arrival time (min)	Departure time (min)	Dough stability (min)	Mixing tolerance index (BU)	Water absorption (%)	Breakdown time (min)	Dough development time (min)
BF:WF							
00:100	$1.86 \pm 0.1_e$	$10.9 \pm 0.1_d$	$9.35 \pm 0.4_e$	$80.5 \pm 0.3_a$	$58.6 \pm 0.4_a$	$10.9 \pm 0.5_c$	$8.25 \pm 0.1_c$
05:90	$1.69 \pm 0.1_d$	$10.6 \pm 0.1_d$	$9.15 \pm 0.2_d$	$82.5 \pm 0.7_a$	$59.7 \pm 0.4_a$	$10.7 \pm 0.4_c$	$8.28 \pm 0.1_c$
10:90	$1.04 \pm 0.1_a$	$3.44 \pm 0.1_c$	$2.25 \pm 0.2_b$	$106.5 \pm 0.9_b$	$64.7 \pm 0.6_b$	$2.56 \pm 0.2_a$	$1.65 \pm 0.3_a$
15:85	$1.06 \pm 0.7_b$	$3.13 \pm 0.4_b$	$2.36 \pm 0.1_c$	$106.80 \pm 1.3_b$	$65.5 \pm 0.4_c$	$2.48 \pm 0.1_a$	$1.63 \pm 0.2_a$
20:80	$1.67 \pm 0.1_c$	$2.54 \pm 0.4_a$	$0.78 \pm 0.1_a$	$161.7 \pm 1.2_c$	$65.9 \pm 0.6_c$	$2.65 \pm 0.1_b$	$2.15 \pm 0.1_b$

d–a, Mean in same column with the same letter are not significantly different ($P < 0.05$); WF, wheat flour; BF, breadfruit flour; (05–20), composite blends.

consistency line in 1.85 min, whereas the blends arrived at relatively short times, indicating faster uptake of water and faster dough development (Lorenz 1990). Arrival time, (AT) was the time to the nearest one-half minutes required for the top of the curve to reach the point of greatest torque after the commencement of mixing (500 BU consistency line). It is a measure of the rate at which water was taken up by the flour (Shuey 1990; Abang Zaidel et al. 2010). Departure time (DT) was the time required for the curve to drop below the 500 BU consistency line. All the blends of BF and WF had shorter DT times compared to the WF.

Dough Stability Time (DST), indicated how much tolerance the flour has to over or under mixing (Schiller 1984). The WF had a DST value of 9.30 min, whereas all the blends have significantly lower DST which decreased as WF was replaced with BF. The DST values of the blends ranged from 0.78 to 9.15 min. This DST trends agreed with the reports of Olatunji and Akinrele (1978) for tropical tuber and breadfruit and Michiyo et al. (2004) for pre-germinated and brown rice.

Water is responsible in hydrating the protein fibrils and facilitating the interactions between the proteins cross-links with the disulfide bonds during dough mixing. An optimum amount of water is needed to develop cohesive, viscoelastic dough with optimum gluten strength. Optimum water level differs from flour to flour depending on the quantity of protein and other dense particles that they contained. Protein content has been known as an important determinant of the extent to which WF would absorbed water during mixing (Sliwinski et al. 2004). In composite flour, the influence of starches, fiber from nonwheat source, and relatively higher damaged starch in the BF on the absorbed water may be more significant than the effect of protein content in the flour blends as substitution of WF for BF progresses.

The water absorption is the amount of water required to develop dough to the point of greatest torque when, for wheat flour, the gluten would have been fully developed. The water absorption values ranged from 58.6 to 65.9% with the WF and the 20% blend having the lowest and highest values, respectively. Earlier studies (Doxastakis et al. 2002; Malomo et al. 2011) have also reported the absorption of more water by composite blends. The increases in water absorption values as the BF replaces WF in the blends may not be unconnected with the higher crude fiber content in the BF (7.8%) compared to the WF (2.81%), respectively (Table 3). Crude fiber have components that are hydrophilic (D'Appolonia and Kim 1976; Hu et al. 2007) and capable forming solution of high viscosity (Yin et al. 2011).

Mixing tolerance index (MTI) values ranged from 80.5 to 161.7 BU with the WF having the lowest values. It also decreased as BF was used to replace WF in the blends. Generally, flours with good tolerance to mixing have low MTI; the higher the MTI value, the weaker the flour (Shuey 1990). Breakdown Time (TBD) like MTI it is also an index of the relative strength of flours. The TBD values ranged from 2.65 to 10.9 min. The WF showed better resilience than the blends of composite flour.

Dough development particularly for the WF begins with addition of water and commencement of mixing operation. Initially all ingredients are hydrated and appeared like a sticky paste. Belton (1999) and Letang et al. (1999) demonstrated that gluten development was mainly brought about by the interactions of glutenin proteins with each other in the loop by disulfide bonds. On further mixing, more protein becomes hydrated and the glutenins tend to align because of the imposed shear and stretching forces (Abang Zaidel et al. 2010). the viscosity also increased, sticky characteristics of dough disappeared and a nonsticky mass was developed at peak consistency of dough typified as the peak of the curve above the 500 BU of the farinogram (Fig. 1A). The interactions between the polymers cross-links was stronger and led to an increase in dough strength, maximum resistance to extension and restoring force after deformation. When the dough was mixed beyond its peak development, the cross-links began to break due to the breaking of disulfide bonds. The glutenins become depolymerized and the dough is overmixed.

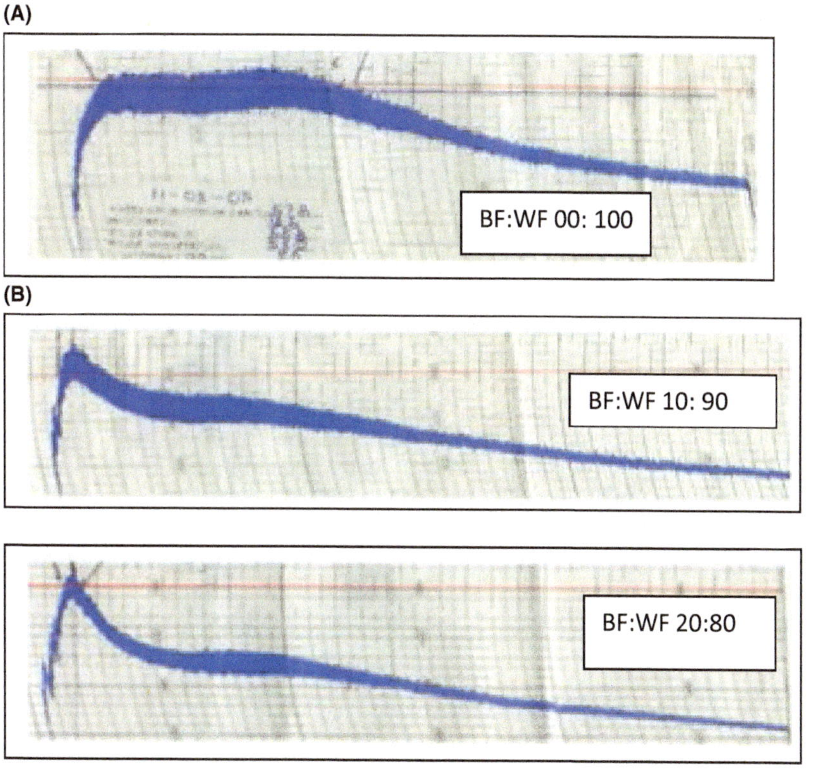

Figure 1. (A) Farinogram of Wheat and Breadfruit-Wheat composite flour. (B) Farinogram of Wheat and Breadfruit-Wheat composite flour.

The monomeric proteins, gliadins form a matrix within the long polymer networks and contribute to resistance to extension by forming viscous dough with reduced elasticity. The presence of smaller chains in the dough makes the dough stickier. In Figure 1B, the ability of the blends to sustain the viscoelastic property of the dough reduced with increasing presence of the BF as shown in the trends in dough stability, breakdown, and dough development time.

Alveograph

The alveograph is an important dough testing instrument use to evaluate the quality of wheat flours for bread and biscuit and cookie making (Bettge et al. 1989; Janssen et al. 1996). It measures the resistance to expansion and the extensibility of a dough by providing the measurement for maximum over pressure, average abscissa at rupture, index of swelling, and deformation energy (Fig. 2) of dough (Indrani and Rao 2007). It impacts strain rates of 0.1–1 sec^{-1}, which are about 100-fold higher than those occurring in actual baking processes (Chin and Campbell 2005).

The Peak height (P) indicated the resistance that the dough offered to deformation and it is related the tensile strength or stability that the dough exhibited during the proofing stage of bread making (Pyler 1988; Mepba et al. 2007). The P values ranged from 90 to 226 mm with the WF and the 10% blend offering the least and highest resistance to expansion, respectively (Table 5). The length (L) indicated the extensibility of the dough. The L values ranged from 33 to 80 mm with the 10% blend and WF having the least and highest extensibility, respectively. The P/L (configuration ratio) ranged from 1.13 to 7.39. The WF and 20% had the highest and lowest values, respectively, and the 5% blend was not significantly ($P < 0.05$) different from the WF.

The energy (W) required for deformation is an indication of the baking strength of the dough. It ranged from 227×10^{-4} J in the 20% blend to 336×10^{-4} J in the 10% blend. Baking strength increased as WF was replaced with BF and peaked at 10% substitution level which was the inflection point in the trend.

The curve configuration ratio (P/L) is an index of gluten behavior. It ranged from 1.13 to 8.04 with the WF and the 15% blend having the lowest and highest values, respectively. Also, there was no significant ($P < 0.05$) difference between the WF and 5% blend. High values of curve configuration ratio may be indicated strong wheat flour as observed by Pyler (1988). However, the strength of composite flour is probably influenced by considerations

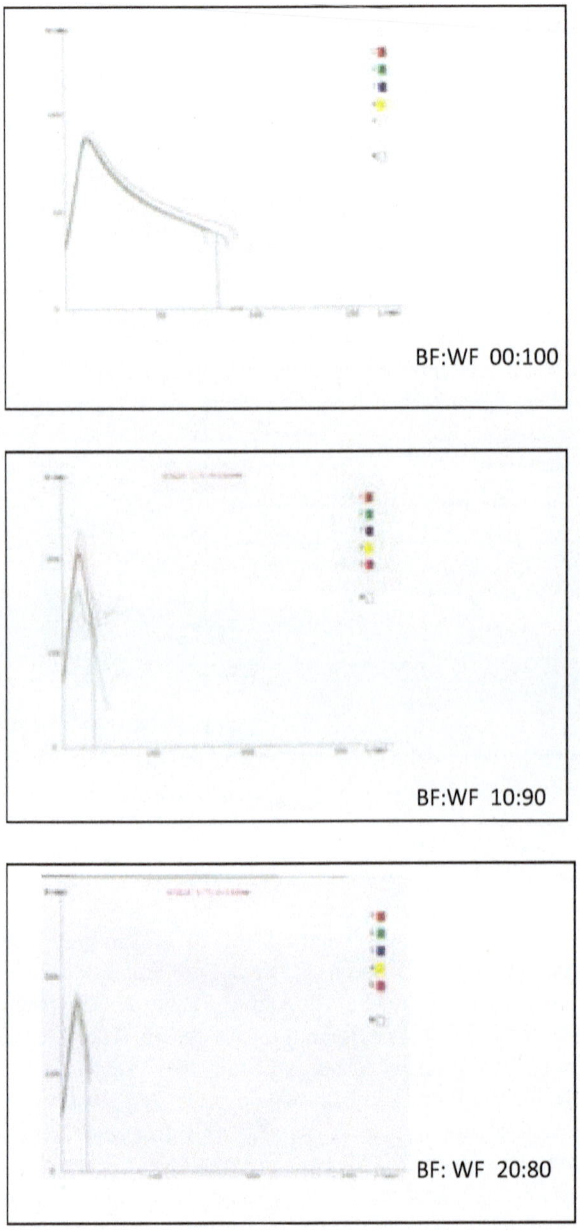

Figure 2. Alveogram of Wheat and Breadfruit-Wheat composite flour.

other than gluten behavior. The significantly higher ratios of the 10–20% blend could not be due their gluten contents alone. This G values (Table 5) depicted the relative abilities of the dough to be inflated for maximum development until they eventually burst. It is a measure of the magnitude of the total response of the dough to the biaxial stress and strain imposed on it by the instrument. It ranged from 11.4 to 19.9, decreased significantly as WF was replaced with BF. The WF and 5% blend had significantly higher values than other blends. Elasticity index (Ie) may be used to characterize the dough on the basis of the elastic resistance that they offer during their bi-axial deformation (Pyler 1988; BaNu et al. 2011). It also decreased with substitution levels and the WF and 5% blend offered significantly better elastic resistance.

The nonlinear viscoelastic behavior of WF dough has been attributed to the continuous gluten matrix and starch granules embedded in it (Collar et al. 2007). It possesses the properties of both solid and liquid bodies, and exhibited the rheological properties that were in between that of the ideal solid and fluid bodies. The inclusion of BF in the blends increased the starch and fiber contents, whereas decreasing the quantity and quality of protein needed to sustain the viscoelastic behavior of their dough. These effects were aptly described by alveograph (Fig. 2) as shown by the significant ($P < 0.05$) decline of important quality indices (Table 5).

Evaluation of bread quality

Absorbed water by dough

The quantity of water used to form dough of consistent quality (Table 6) for baking was significantly (t = 0.540, df = 13.89, P = 0.299) lower than the farinograph water absorption (Table 4). Similar observation was made by El-Dash et al., (1977) and Shuey (1990). This indicated that the presence of other baking ingredients may have been responsible for the reduction in the actual quantity of water used to form the dough.

Table 5. Alveogram of wheat flour and its composite blends with breadfruit flour.

Flours	Peak height (mm) (P)	Length (mm) (L)	Energy (10^{-4}J) (W)	Curve configuration (P/L)	Maximum inflation (G)	Elasticity index (%) (Ie)
BF:WF						
00:100	90 ± 0.4^a	80 ± 1.4^d	304 ± 0.7^c	1.13 ± 0.2^a	19.9 ± 0.6^b	64.6 ± 0.4^e
05:95	96 ± 0.7^a	76 ± 0.7^c	304 ± 1.4^c	1.27 ± 0.4^a	18.4 ± 0.4^b	62.6 ± 0.4^d
10:90	226 ± 0.7^d	33 ± 0.7^b	336 ± 2.8^d	6.79 ± 0.3^b	12.8 ± 0.4^a	59.1 ± 1.4^c
15:85	217 ± 0.6^c	27 ± 0^a	298 ± 1.4^b	8.04 ± 0.2^d	12.1 ± 0.2^a	45.0 ± 0.7^b
20:80	193 ± 0.7^b	26 ± 0.7^a	227 ± 1.4^a	7.39 ± 0.2^c	11.4 ± 0.4^a	0.0^a

d–a, Mean in same column with the same superscripts are not significantly different ($P < 0.05$); WF, wheat flour; BF, breadfruit flour; (05–20), composite blends.

Table 6. Physical quality characteristics of bread.

Flour	Absorbed water (%)	Weight loss (%)	Specific volume (cm^3/g)
BF:WF			
00:100	32.1 ± 0.4^a	2.44 ± 0.3^a	3.00 ± 0.05^d
05:95	37.3 ± 0.3^a	1.58 ± 0.1^a	2.96 ± 0.01^d
10:90	54.3 ± 0.9^b	14.9 ± 0.6^b	2.16 ± 0.04^b
15:85	59.1 ± 0.2^c	14.6 ± 0.6^b	2.17 ± 0.04^b
20:80	67.3 ± 0.1^d	16.4 ± 0.4^c	1.75 ± 0.05^a
30:70	75.3 ± 0.5^e	18.1 ± 0.5^d	1.44 ± 0.03^a
40:60	93.3 ± 0.9^f	15.4 ± 0.5^b	1.32 ± 0.02^a

f–a, Mean in the same column with the same superscripts are not significantly different ($P < 0.05$); WF, wheat flour; BF, breadfruit flour; (05–40), BF/WF composite blends.

Absorbed water ranged from 32.1 to 99.3% with the WF and 40% blend having the highest and lowest values, respectively. The WF was not significantly ($P > 0.05$) different from the 5% blend but the both of them were significantly ($P < 0.05$) different from the rest of the blends. The significantly higher values of absorbed water in the blends when substitution was beyond 10% levels may be due to the relatively higher starch and fiber contents that may be present in the blends as the WF was gradually replaced by the BF.

Specific volume

Loaf volume is used as a criterion to measure the quality of fresh bread in research quality control in industry and by consumers (Penfield and Campbell 1990; Zuwariah and Noor Aziah 2009). Specific volume of loaves of bread provide a uniform basis for comparing results of various studies (Oyeku et al. 2008). It ranged from 1.32 to 3.00 cm^3/g. The WF and 40% blend have the highest and lowest values. The values decreased as BF replaces the WF in the blends but the 5% blend was not significantly ($P > 0.05$) different from the WF.

Specific volume is an indication of the gluten content of the bread (Van Hall 2000; Abang Zaidel et al. 2010) but other constituents such as starch and fiber also contribute to the specific volume of bread. Gluten or more precisely glutenin, is the main structure-forming protein in wheat flour that is responsible for the elastic and extensible properties needed to produce good quality wheat bread (Bloksma 1990b; : Gallagher et al. 2003). Bread made from soft wheat flour usually yield lower loaf volumes. It has also been shown that the difference between weak and strong flours can be explained by differences in the molecular mass distribution of their proteins (MacRitchie 1973). Abundance of glutenin molecules with long chain was observed to have made the protein phase, and consequently the dough, highly extensible (Bloksma 1990a).

Differences in the pasting temperature and peak viscosity of composite starches have been suspected to influence extensibility (Greene and Bovell-Benjamin 2004). Pasting temperature is related to gelatinization temperature because it occurred after gelatinization. It was noted (Table 3) that pasting temperature increased as the WF was replaced with the BF. This implied that peak viscosity of each of the composite blend were attained at different pasting temperatures and may have induced additional tensile stress in dough membranes during baking. This may have over stretched the membranes beyond its capacity, ruptured it and terminating oven rise prematurely.

The differences in specific volume of the composite blend and the WF could therefore be traced to factors (Composition of the flour, their rheological and pasting properties) that directly determines their behavior during processing rather than the behavior of the dough themselves (Bloksma 1990b), because these are factors that influenced the specific volume.

Weight loss

Cut-out dough losses weight during the proofing and baking stages of bread processing. This may be may be due to both fermentation losses brought about by amylases of starch and utilization of soluble sugar by yeast and also by evaporation of moisture during baking. Weight loss decreased as the BF replaces the WF in the blends (Table 6). It ranged from 1.68 to 18.1% with the 5 and 30% blend having the lowest and highest losses, respectively. The weight loss recorded for the 5% blend was not significantly different from the WF. The 20% was significantly different from the 30% blend and both have significantly higher weight loss values than other blends.

Significantly higher weight loss by the blends (except at 5%) could be attributed to their ability to form a viscous dough while imbibing large amount of water (Tables 4 and 6) which were lost during the baking.

Comparison of baking qualities of bread from laboratory and industrial conditions

Relatively more water was absorbed by the dough, greater weight losses were observed and higher specific volumes were recorded in the bread produced under industrial condition (Table 7). This may be due to the high amount of mechanical energy inputted by the locally fabricated horizontal high-speed mixer and humidity condition of the oven. Results of independent t-test for absorbed water (t = 0.532, df = 18, P = 0.3005, one-tailed), weight loss (t = 0.865, df = 18, P = 0.199, one tailed), and specific volume (t = 0.828, df = 14.17, P = 0.211, one-tailed), however, indicated there was no significant ($P > 0.05$) difference (0.601, 0.398, and 0.421 were >0.05) in the mean values of these quality parameters, respectively. These implied that there may be no technical hindrance to successful industrialization of this technology (Table 7).

Descriptive sensory quality

Sensory quality of breads

The summary of the descriptive sensory attributes of the bread samples is presented in Table 8. The mean scores (3.55–6.73) for appearance (crust and crumb color, contour consistency, and grain quality) of the bread samples decreased significantly ($P < 0.05$) as the WF was replaced by the BF. The 5% blend was appreciated better than other blends in terms of appearance. Similar trends were observed for flavor (3.47–7.80) and texture (4.25–8.03). However, the 5% blend was not significantly different from the WF (Fig. 3).

Consumer acceptance

The mean score for consumer acceptance of the bread samples ranged from 3.71 to 8.10 with the 5 and 40% blends having the highest and lowest values, respectively. The panelists felt that bread samples produced when the WF was replaced with the BF up to 15%, was not significantly ($P < 0.05$) different from samples from the WF in terms of acceptance ratings.

Table 7. Comparison of baking qualities of bread produced under laboratory and industrial conditions.

Blends	Absorbed water (%) L	Absorbed water (%) I	Weight loss (%) L	Weight loss (%) I	Specific volume (cm^3/g) L	Specific volume (cm^3/g) I
BF:WF 0:100	32.1	26.1	2.48	3.23	3.00	3.70
BF:WF 05:95	37.3	38.1	1.58	4.71	2.96	3.51
BF:WF 10:90	54.3	42.3	14.9	15.7	2.16	3.31
BF:WF 15:85	59.1	47.4	14.6	15.2	2.17	2.58
BF:WF 20:80	67.3	56.3	16.4	17.2	1.75	2.15
BF:WF 30:70	75.3	81.6	18.1	21.1	1.44	1.12
BF:WF 40:60#	93.3	88.3	15.4	21.6	1.32	1.1

L, laboratory; I, industrial; WF, wheat flour; BF, breadfruit flour; (05–40), BF/WF composite blends; # = Substitution levels.

Table 8. Sensory qualities of bread.

Blends	SCORES	BF:WF/00:100	05:90	10:90	15:85	20:80	30:70	40:60
Attributes								
Appearance								
Crust color	5	3.0	3.5	3.3	3.3	3.3	2.5	1.5
Crumb color	10	7.0	7.3	5.5	6.0	5.0	5.5	3.7
Cell size	10	8.0	8.0	5.0	5.6	4.8	4.3	4.7
Cell uniformity	10	8.0	8.1	5.2	5.1	4.8	5.0	4.3
Mean		6.5 ± 2.4^d	6.73 ± 2.2^d	4.75 ± 1.0^c	5.0 ± 1.2^c	4.48 ± 0.8^{ab}	4.33 ± 1.3^{ab}	3.55 ± 1.4^a
Flavor								
Taste	5	5.0	4.7	3.5	3.5	2.8	2.8	2.7
Wheaty smell	10	10.0	9.6	5.0	5.1	4.7	4.3	4.2
Aroma	10	8.0	8.5	4.5	4.7	3.5	4.5	3.5
Mean		7.67 ± 2.5^b	7.80 ± 2.6^b	4.33 ± 0.8^a	4.4 ± 0.8^a	3.67 ± 1.0^a	3.87 ± 0.9^a	3.47 ± 0.8^a
Texture								
Mouthfeel	10	8.0	8.4	6.5	6.5	5.8	4.7	4.5
Crumb stability and softness	10	8.0	8.0	6.0	5.2	5.2	5.2	4.5
Grittiness	10	7.0	7.2	6.0	5.0	5.2	4.3	3.5
Lightness	10	8.0	8.5	6.0	5.5	5.2	5.2	4.5
Mean		7.75 ± 0.5^d	8.03 ± 0.6^d	6.12 ± 0.3^c	5.55 ± 0.7^{bc}	5.35 ± 0.3^b	4.85 ± 0.4^{ab}	4.25 ± 1.9^a
General acceptance								
		7.85^c	8.1^c	7.04^c	7.01^c	5.83^b	5.20^b	3.71^a

d–a, Mean in same column with the same alphabets are not significantly different ($P < 0.05$); WF, wheat flour; BF, breadfruit flour; (05–40), BF/WF composite blends.

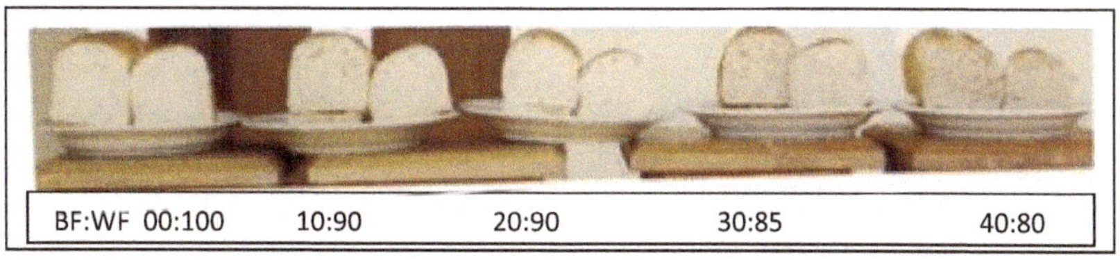

Figure 3. Samples of Wheat and Breadfruit-Wheat composite flour.

Conclusion

In this study, attempt was made to evaluate the extent to which WF can be replaced with BF in the production of bread and to assess whether such efforts could be replicated at industrial scale. This was done by analyzing the rheological properties of the flour and dough, as well as baking qualities of the resulting bread. Nigeria bakers have often complained about the gaps between research results obtained in the laboratory and the practicality of such results at industrial level. Attempt was made in this study to bridge such gap by comparing laboratory baking test result with that at industrial level.

The study concluded that the foam structure of bread crumbs was determined by the network of gelatinized dispersion of starch interwoven with strands of gluten. Gluten, the main structure-forming protein in WF that was responsible for the elastic and extensible properties needed to produce good quality bread decreased as the WF was replaced with the BF. Interactions between gluten (specifically gliadin), starch, and other components of the flour were responsible for the viscosity properties that contributed to the aeration of the dough. Ability of the dough to sustain this aeration particularly during oven rise under baking condition was determined in the blends, by their relative viscosity properties.

The BF that was used to replace the WF had lower starch but higher fiber contents. These therefore altered the pasting characteristics and other rheological (farinograph and alveograph) properties of the blends especially at substitution levels beyond 5% and made them to be significantly different from that of WF. These also resulted in adverse changes in baking qualities. Bread sample whose specific volume was not statistically different from that of WF was only obtained at 5% level of replacement of the WF with BF. The objectivity of these was further reinforced as panelists were unable to significantly detect differences in sensory attributes between the samples from the 5% blend and those from WF. Although, panelist felt that bread of acceptable sensory quality similar to that produced from the WF was obtained within 15% substitution levels. In order to prevent serious deviation from the widely accepted quality attributes of bread and also for ease of adapting the technology to industrial level, it is recommended that substitution should be limited to a range from 5 to 10%. More so, when results have showed that this effort can be replicated at industrial level without significant alteration in baking quality indices.

Conflict of Interest

None declared.

References

AACC 2000. American Association of Cereal Chemists Approved methods of Analysis. St. AACC International, St. Paul, MN. http://dx.doi.org/10.1094/AACCIntMethod.

AACC 2010. American Association of Cereal Chemists International. Approved Methods of Analysis, 11th Ed. Method 54-30.02. Physical Dough Tests: Alveograph Method for Soft and Hard Wheat Flour. AACC International, St. Paul, MN. http://dx.doi.org/10.1094/AACCIntMethod.

Abang Zaidel, D. N., N. L. Chin, and Y. A. Yusof. 2010. A review on rheological properties and measurements of dough and gluten. J. Appl. Sci. 10:2478–2490.

Adeleke, R. O., and J. O. Odedeji. 2010. Functional properties of wheat sweet potato flour blend. PJN 9:535–538.

Ade-Omowaye, B. I. O., B. A. Bolarinwa, and A. O. Adebiyi. 2008. Evaluation of Tigernut (*Cyperus esculentus*) - wheat composite flour and bread. AJES 2:87–89.

Adewusi, S. R. A., J. U. Akpobome, and B. A. Osuntogun. 1995. Studies on the carbohydrate content of Breadfruit (*Artocarpus communis Forst*) from Southwestern Nigeria. Starch/Starke 47:289–294.

Ajayi, O. P. 1997. Studies on some Physico-chemical and enzymatic changes in breadfruit (*Artocarpus atilis*) during storage. M.Sc. Research Thesis. Food technology dept. University of Ibadan. VI + 33.

Alava, J. M., S. S. Sahi, J. Garcia-Alvarez, A. Turo, J. A. Chavez, M. J. Garcia, et al. 2007. Use of Ultrasound for the determination of flour quality. Ultrasonics 46:270–276.

Alex, A. A., A. R. Kelly, M. L. Odean, R. G. Fulcher, and D. A. Susan. 2008. Influence of added bean flour (*Phaseolus vulgaris* L.) on some physical and nutritional properties of wheat flour tortillas. Food Chem. 109:33–41.

Amusa, N. A., L. A. Kehinde, and O. A. Ashaye. 2002. Biodeterioration of breadfruit (*Artocarpus communis*) in storage and its effect on the nutrient composition. Afr. J. Biotechnol. 1(2):57–60.

Appelqvist, I. A. M., and M. R. M. Debet. 1997. Starch – biopolymer interactions – A review. Food Rev. Int. 13:163–224.

Bakare, H. A. 2008. Evaluation of the rheological properties and baking performance of wheat composite flour produced from lye-peeled breadfruit *(Artocarpus communis* Forst) and cassava *(Manihot esculenta* crantz). PhD Thesis in Food Science and Technology. Department, University of Ibadan, Ibadan.

Bakare, H. A., M. O. Adegunwa, O. F. Osundahunsi, and J. O. Olusanya. 2012. Composition and Pasting properties of Breadfruit (*Artocarpus communis* Forst) From South West States of Nigeria. Negerian Food Journal 30:11–17.

Bakare, H. A., O. F. Osundahunsi, M. O. Adegunwa, and J. O. Olusanya. 2013. Batter rheology, baking, and sensory qualities of cake from blends of breadfruit and wheat flours. J. Cul. Sci. Technol. 11:203–221.

BaNu, J., G. StoeNeSCu, V. IoNeSCu, and J. Aprodu. 2011. Estimation of the baking quality of wheat flours based on rheological parameters of the mixolab curve. Czech J. Food Sci. 29:35–44.

Belton, P. S. 1999. On the elasticity of wheat gluten. J. Cereal Sci. 29:103–107.

BeMiller, J. N. 2011. Pasting, paste, and gel properties of starch-hydrocolloid combinations. Carbohydr. Polym. 86:386–423.

Bettge, A., G. L. Rubenthaler, and Y. Pomeranz. 1989. Alveograph algorithms to predict functional properties of in bread and cookie baking. Cereal Chem. 66:81–86.

Biljan, S., and F. Bojana. 2008. Nutritional and sensory evaluation of wheat bread supplemented with oleic-rich sunflower seed. Food Chem. 108:119–129.

Bloksma, A. H. 1990a. Rheology of the bread making process. CFW 35:232–236.

Bloksma, A. H. 1990b. Dough structure, dough rheology and baking quality. CFW 35:237–243.

Chin, N. L., and G. M. Campbell. 2005. Dough aeration and rheology: part 2. Effects of flour type, mixing speed and total work input on aeration and rheology of bread dough. J. Sci. Food Agric. 85:2194–2202.

Collar, C., C. Bollain, and C. M. Rosell. 2007. Rheological behaviour of formulated bread doughs during mixing and heating. Food Sci. Technol. Int. 13:99–106.

Dapčević, T., M. Hadnadev, and M. Pojić. 2009. Evaluation of the possibility to replace conventional rheological whaet flour Quality control Instruments with the New Measurement Tool-Mixolab. Agriculturae Conspectus Scientificus 74:169–174.

D'Appolonia, B. L. 1978. Use of untreated and roasted navy beans in bread baking. Cereal Chem. 55:88–907.

D'Appolonia, B. L., and S. K. Kim. 1976. Bread Stalin studies 1: effect of protein content on stalin rate and bread crumb pasting properties. Cereal Chem. 54:207.

Dengate, H. N. 1978. Swelling, pasting and gelling of wheat starch. Pp. 49–82 *in* Y. Pomeranz, ed. Advances in cereal science and technology. Vol VI. Am Assoc. Cereal Chem, Inc., St. Paul, MN.

Dewettinck, K., F. Van Bockstaele, B. Kühne, D. Van de Walle, T. M. Courtens, and X. Gellynck. 2008. Nutritional value of bread: influence of processing, food interaction and consumer perception- Review. J. Cereal Sci. 48:243–257.

Doxastakis, G., I. Zafiriadis, M. Irakil, H. Marlani, and C. Tananaki. 2002. Lupin, soya and triticale addition to wheat flour dough and their effect on rheological properties. Food Chem. 77:219–227.

Dubois, M., K. A. Giles, J. K. Hamilton, P. A. Rebers, and F. L. Smith. 1970. Colorimetric method for determination of sugars and related substances. Anal. Chem. 28:350–356.

Duncan, D. B. 1955. Multiple range and multiple F-tests. Biometrics 11:1–5. doi:10.2307/3001478. CrossRef, Web of Science® Times Cited: 13957.

Edmund, B. B. 1967. Breadmaking in principle and practice. Oxford Univ. Press, New York, NY. Pp. 313–381.

El-Dash, A. A., A. Tosello, and G. Roa. 1977. Pregelatinized Cara (water yam) flour: Effect on dough and bread quality. Cereal chem 55(6):799–808.

Eliason, A. C. 1983. Rheological properties of concentrated wheat starch gels. J. Cereal Sci. I:199–205.

Entwistle, P. V., and W. L. Hunter. 1949. Report on crude fiber. J. AOAC 32:65–656.

Fustier, P., F. Csataigne, S. L. Turgeon, and C. G. Biladeris. 2008. Flour constituents interactions and their influence on dough rheology and quality of semi-sweet biscuits: a mixture design approach with reconstituted blends of gluten, water solubles and starch fractions. J. Cereal Sci. 48:144–158.

Gallagher, E., T. R. Gormley, and E. M. Arendt. 2003. Crust and Crumb characteristics of gluten free breads. J. Food Eng. 56:153–161.

Graham, H. D., and E. N. De-Bravo. 1981. Composition of the breadfruit. J. Food Sci. 46:535–539.

Greene, J. L., and A. C. Bovell-Benjamin. 2004. Macroscopic and sensory evaluation of bread supplemented with sweet potato flour. J. Food Sci. 69:167–173.

Hallen, E., S. Ibanoglu, and P. Ainsworth. 2004. Effect of fermented/germinated cowpea flour addition on the rheological and baking properties of wheat flour. J. Food Eng. 63:177–184.

Hoseney, R. C. 1994. Gas retention in bread doughs. CFW 29:305–306.

Hu, G. H., F. Yang, Z. Ma, and Q. Zhou. 2007. Development of research and application of rice bran dietary fibre. Chin. Food Addit. 84:80–85.

Hugo, L. F., L. W. Rooney, and J. R. N. Taylor. 2000. Malted Sorghum as a functional ingredient in composite bread. Cereal Chem. 77:428–432.

ICC. 1996. International Association for Cereal Science and Technology Standard (1996). Approved method No 162 Rapid Pasting Method using the Newport Rapid Visco Analyser. Rapid Pasting Method using the Newport Rapid Visco Analyser. ICC standard Methods-Principles. Mht

Indrani, D., and G. V. Rao. 2007. Rheological characteristics of wheat flour dough as influenced by ingredients of parotta. J. Food Eng. 79:100–105.

Janssen, A. M., T. van Vliet, and J. M. Vereijken. 1996. Fundamental and empirical rheological behaviour of wheat flour doughs and comparison with bread making performance. J. Cereal Sci. 23:43–54.

Kim, H. J., N. Morita, S. H. Lee, and K. D. Moon. 2003. Scanning electron microscopic observations of dough and bread supplemented with *Gastrodia elata* blume powder. Food Res. Int. 36:387–389.

Letang, C., M. Piau, and C. Nerdier. 1999. Characterization of wheat flour-water doughs. Part I: rheometry and microstructure. J. Food Eng. 41:121–132.

Lin, L., H. Liu, Y. Yu, S. Lin, and J. Mau. 2009. Quality and antioxidant property of buckwheat enhanced wheat bread. Food Chem. 37:461–467.

Loos, P. J., L. F. Hood, and H. D. Graham. 1981. Isolation and characterization of Starch of breadfruit. Cereal Chem. 58:282–286.

Lorenz, K. 1990. Special uses and techniques of the farinograph. Farinograph manual 1:3–5.

MacRitchie, F. 1973. Conversion of a weal flour to a strong one by increasing the proportion of its high molecular weight gluten protein. J. Sci. Food Agr. 24:1325.

Malomo, S. A., A. F. Eleyinmi, and J. B. Fashakin. 2011. Chemical composition, rheological properties and bread making potentials of composite flours from breadfruit, breadnut and wheat. Afr. J. Food Sci. 5:400–410.

Malomo, O., M. O. Jimoh, O. O. Adekoyeni, O. E. Soyebi, and E. A. Alamu. 2013. Effect of blanching and unblanching on rheological properties of sweet-potato bread. Acad. Res. J. 1:24–41.

Manuel, G., O. Bonastre, M. R. Cristina, P. Valentin, and F. Encarnacion. 2008. Studies on cake quality made of wheat- chickpea flour blends. LWT Food Sci. Technol. 41:1701–1709.

Marco, C., and C. M. Rosell. 2008. Breadmaking performance of protein enriched, gluten-free breads. Eur. Food Res. Technol. 227:1205–1213.

Mcready, R. M. 1970. Determination of Starch dextrins. Pp. 552–557 *in* Methods in food analysis. A series of monograph, 2nd ed. A. M. Joslyn, ed. Academic Press, New York, NY.

Meera, K. 2010. Falling number in wheat-how is it calculated and what does it mean to Producers? USA: USDA, ARS, Soft wheat Quality Lab. Alpha amylase mkweon-FN-012810 [1], pdf. (Accessed 19 May 2011).

Mepba, H. D., L. Eboh, and S. U. Nwaojigwa. 2007. Chemical composition, functional and baking properties of wheat- plantain composite flours. Afr. J. Food Nutr. Dev. 7:1–22.

Michiyo, W., M. Tomoko, T. Kikuchi, K. Hiroshi, and M. Naofumi. 2004. Application of pregerminated brown rice for breadmaking. Cereal Chem. 81:450–455.

Mirsaeedghazi, H., Z. Emam-Djomeh, and S. M. A. Mousavi. 2008. Rheometric measurement of dough rheological characteristics and factors affecting it. Int. J. Agri. Biol. 10:112–119.

Morton, J. 1987. Breadfruit: *Artocarpus altilis*. In J. F. Morton (ed.), Fruits of Warm Climates. Miami, FL: Florida Flair Books. Pp. 50–58.

Oladunjoye, I. O., A. D. Ologhobo, and C. O. Olaniyi. 2010. Nutrient composition, energy value and residual anti- nutritional factors in differently processed breadfruit (*Artocarpus altilis*) meal. Afr. J. Biotechnol. 9:4259–4263.

Olatunji, O., and I. A. Akinrele. 1978. Comparative rheological properties and bread qualities of wheat flour diluted with tropical tuber and breadfruit flour. Cereal Chem. 55:1–6.

Olkku, T., and C. Rha. 1978. Gelatinisation of starch and wheat flour starch – A review. Food Chem. 3:293–317.

Oyeku, M. O., C. F. Kupoluyi, H. A. Osibanjo, C. U. Orji, F. N. Ajuebor, I. O. Ajiboshin, et al. 2008. An economic assessment of commercial production of 10% cassava-wheat composite flour bread. J. Indust. Res. Tech. 2:13–20.

Ozturk, S., K. Kahraman, B. Tiftik, and H. Koksel. 2008. Predicting the cookie quality of fl ours by using Mixolab. Eur. Food Res. Technol. 227:1549–1554.

Penfield, M. P., and A. M. Campbell. 1990. Experimental food science, 3rd ed. San Diego, California, USA: Academic Press.

Pyler, E. J. 1988. Baking science and technology, 3rd ed. 1 and II. Sosland Publishing Company, Reno, NV, USA. P. 345.

Ragone, D. 2009. Farm and Forestry production and marketing profile for breadfruit (*Artocarpus altilis*) Pp. 2–21 *in* C. R. Elvitch, ed. Specialty crops for pacific Island Agro-forestry. Permanent Agricultural Resources (PAR), Holualoa, Hawai'i. Available at http://agroforestry.net/scps.

Schiller, G. W. 1984. Bakery flour specifications. CFW 29:647–651.

Shimelis, E., M. Meaza, and S. Raskshit. 2006. Physico-chemical properties, pasting behaviour and functional

characteristics of flour and starches from improved Bean (*Phaseoulus vulgaris* L.) varieties grown in East Africa. Agricult. Eng. Int. Viii:05–015.
Shuey, W. C. 1990. Interpretation of the farinogram. Farinograph Manual 1:31–36.
Sliwinski, E. L., P. Kolster, and T. Van Vliet. 2004. On the relationship between large-deformation properties of wheat flour dough and baking quality. J. Cereal Sci. 39:231–245.
Stone, H., and J. L. Sidel. 2004. Sensory evaluation practices. Elsevier Academic Press, San Diego, CA. Pp. 201–244.
Van Hall, M. V. 2000. Quality of sweet potato flour during processing and storage. Food Rev. Int. 16:1–37.
Watson, C. A. 1984. An instrument for determining alpha – amylase activity. CFW 29:507–509.
Woo, K. S., and P. A. Seib. 2002. Cross linked resistant starch: preparation and properties. Cereal Chem. 79:819–825.
Yin, S. W., Q. Y. Lu, and X. G. Yang. 2011. Study on the effect of damaged starch on cooking quality of noodles. Food Sci. Technol. 10:68–70.
Zhou, W., and N. Therdthai. 2006. Bread manufacture. Pp 301–316 *in* Bakery products: science and technology. Y. H. Hui, eds. Blackwell Publishing Professional, Iowa.
Zuwariah, I., and A. A. Noor Aziah. 2009. Physicochemical properties of wheat breads substituted with banana flour and modified banana flour. J. Trop. Agric. Fd. Sc. 37:33–42.

20

Methyl jasmonate effectively enhanced some defense enzymes activity and Total Antioxidant content in harvested "Sabrosa" strawberry fruit

Mohammadreza Asghari & Ali Rashid Hasanlooe

Department of Horticulture, Faculty of Agriculture, Urmia University, Urmia, Iran

Keywords
Catalase, methyl jasmonate, peroxidase, polyphenol oxidase, strawberry, total antioxidant content

Correspondence
Mohammadreza Asghari, Department of Horticulture, Faculty of Agriculture, Urmia University, Urmia, Iran.

E-mail: mhamadreza@yahoo.com

Funding Information
Urmia University

Abstract

The use of chemicals in postharvest technology of horticultural crops is highly restricted and it is necessary to introduce safe food preserving methods. Straw-berry is very susceptible to postharvest losses and more than 50% of harvested fruit is lost in Iran. Effect of postharvest treatment with methyl jasmonate (at 0, 8, and 16 μmol L^{-1}) on some quality attributes of Sabrosa strawberry fruit during storage at 1 ± 0.5°C with 90–95% RH for 14 days followed by 24 h at 20°C was studied. Methyl jasmonate, at both concentrations, decreased weight loss and retained marketability of fruits. Catalase activity of treated fruits was decreased during the first days, but showed a substantial increase during the second week. Methyl jasmonate, in a concentration- dependent manner, enhanced peroxidase activity. Fruit total antioxidant capacity was enhanced by methyl jasmonate treatment. The results indicated that methyl jasmonate plays a key role in establishing resistance against stresses, enhancing fruit defense systems, antioxidant capacity, and storage life leading to decreased postharvest losses. This phytochemical has a good potential to be used in postharvest technology of Sabrosa strawberry fruit and enhance the fruit postharvest life.

Introduction

Active oxygen species (AOS) and free radicals are the major players in aging and diseases like inflammation, arthritis, immune system impairment, different cancers, and heart disease, and much more focus has been given to the involvement of antioxidants in free radical scavenging and related senescence, and diseases prevention (Cai et al. 2004; Kaefer and Milner 2008; Huang et al. 2010). Similar to human cells, the aging and senescence process in plant cells is highly related to free radicals and AOS, and several antioxidants are responsible for detoxifying the plant cells from these dangerous agents. The antioxidant systems in plants and harvested crops include antioxidant enzymes such as superoxide dismutase (SOD, EC 1.15.1.1), ascorbate peroxidase (APX, EC 1.11.1.11), peroxidase (POD, EC 1.11.1.7), catalase (CAT, EC 1.11.1.6)) as well as nonenzymatic compounds with antioxidant activity such as ascorbic acid, glutathione, phenolic compounds, flavonoids, catkin, carotenoid, and α-tocopherols (Asghari and Soleimani Aghdam 2010). Since natural antioxidants are more readily acceptable than the synthetic ones, fruits containing high antioxidants are of more commercial importance. Strawberry fruit is a rich source of natural antioxidants and phytochemicals, particularly anthocyanins, flavonoids, phenolic acids, and ellagic acid, which have potent antioxidant and anti-inflammatory functions and also essential minerals making it as one of the most commercial horticultural crops (Rice-Evans and Miller 1996; Heinonen et al. 1998). Fresh juice of strawberries has high oxygen radical absorbance activity against peroxyl radicals (ROO*), superoxide radicals ($O^{*}{}_2{}^-$), hydrogen peroxide (H_2O_2), hydroxyl radicals (OH*), and singlet oxygen ($^{*}O_2$), and it is well demonstrated that the antioxidant activity is different among varieties (Wang and Jiao 2000).

With progress in aging and senescence of harvested crops, they become more susceptible to postharvest losses. Because of the consumption during free radical scavenging process, the antioxidant content of the harvested crops is decreased during postharvest stages leading to accelerated senescence. Strawberries are perishable fruits and more than 50% of produced strawberries are lost in Iran during postharvest handling, and because of using improper postharvest technologies, the remaining part received by the consumers has a very low nutritional quality. Then, the use of proper postharvest technologies is essential to decrease the adverse effects of stress conditions, rate of aging process, keeping nutritional quality, and enhancing storage life of strawberries.

Recently, because of the food safety issues and environmental concerns, use of synthetic chemicals in postharvest technology of horticultural crops is highly restricted and much more researches have been focused on generally regarded as safe compounds (GRASC). Jasmonic acid (JA) and it's methyl ester (methyl jasmonate (MeJA)) are important natural GRAS compounds playing key roles in several plant cell communication and signaling processes including ethylene production, defense responses against different biotic and abiotic stresses, anthocyanin, and other phytochemicals synthesis (Demole et al. 1962; Creelman and Mullet 1995). MeJA treatments have been shown to decrease the changes in physical attributes such as color, weight, firmness, and the amount of bioactive compounds (phenolic content, antioxidants), and enhance storage life in some fruits (Karaman et al. 2012; Concha et al. 2013). Strawberry fruits treated with MeJA has been reported to have higher total phenolics, anthocyanins, and total antioxidant capacity (TAC) after 12 days of cold storage (Ayala-Zavala et al. 2005). Exogenous MeJA has been shown to enhance SOD, CAT, and APX activity in harvested loquat fruits leading to reduced O_2^- and H_2O_2 content (Cao et al. 2009). Furthermore, increase in SOD activity in peaches and CAT activity in tomatoes has been reported as the result of postharvest MeJA treatment (Ding et al. 2002; Jin et al. 2009).

Enzymatic browning mainly caused by polyphenol oxidase (PPO, EC 1.10.3.2) is a main cause of postharvest losses in different fruits as well as strawberries. As a result of accelerated senescence and damaged cell membranes, PPO oxidizes the phenolics to dark brown colored polyphenols leading to a substantial decrease in overall quality and marketability (Gao et al. 2013; Zhou et al. 2015). Different biotic and abiotic stresses such as pathogens and chilling injury are responsible for oxidative burst in the cells of harvested fruits leading to increased membrane damage and subsequent PPO activity. Exogenous MeJA have been reported to activate some heat shock proteins (HSPs), which are preservative agents of plant cells against different stresses (Soleimani Aghdama et al. 2013). Decreased susceptibility to chilling injury and prevention of PPO activity has been reported as the result of treatment with MeJA in peach Fruit (Jin et al. 2009).

The effect of MeJA on antioxidant content and some physiological traits in some crops has been studied, but the exact mechanism of the effects has not been well demonstrated. The purpose of this study was to examine the effect of postharvest treatment with different concentrations of MeJA on TAC and some defense and antioxidative enzymes, and also postharvest life of "Sabrosa" strawberry fruit during cold storage to see if whole antioxidative system is affected or not, and also to determine the response of fruit during short- and long-term storage.

Materials and Methods

Sample preparation

"Sabrosa" strawberry fruits (*Fragaria* × *ananassa* Duch. cv. Sabrosa) were harvested at commercial maturity from a commercial production greenhouse in Urmia (Iran) and transported to postharvest laboratory at Urmia University. Fruit were selected for uniformity of color and size, and any fruit with apparent injuries, disease, or infections were removed.

Treatments with MeJA

MeJA was purchased from Sigma Co. (Sigma Aldrich, Germany). Treatments were performed at 20°C in five replicates by placing the strawberry in a 120 L container, in which the appropriated volume of MeJA to reach the desired concentration (8 and/or 16 μmol L^{-1}) was deposited on filter paper at the bottom of the container and then immediately hermetically sealed. Duration of the treatment was 16 h, after which the fruits from each replicate were randomized and sorted into five fruit lots. Control fruit received no treatment. Both control and treated fruits were put in 100 mL plastic jars and stored at 1 ± 0.5°C with 90–95% RH. for 14 days followed by 24 h at 20°C. Fruit quality attributes were measured after 7 days of cold storage plus 24 h at 20°C and the end of storage.

Weight loss

Fruit weight was recorded several times during the storage period and expressed as percentage of water loss in comparison to initial weight.

Determination of fruit firmness

Universal testing machine (TA.XT Plus; Texture Analyzer, Stable Micro Systems, UK) equipped with a

6 mmol cylinder probe (P/6) and a 5 kg load cell was used to determine the fruit firmness. Test condition consisted of a 10 mm probe displacement distance (constant strain), 2 mm sec^{-1} pretest speed, 1 mm sec^{-1} test speed, and 10 mm sec^{-1} posttest speed. Penetration force was calculated in each case on the force–time curve.

Marketability (overall quality)

Overall quality (percentage of fruit surface area decayed, shrunken and adversely affected) was considered as fruit marketability index and evaluated by 10 trained panelists using a 1–5 scale, where 1 = unacceptable (>50% surface affected), 2 = bad (20–50% surface affected), 3 = acceptable (5–20% surface affected), 4 = good (up to 5% surface affected), and 5 = excellent (no decay, shrinkage, or any other adverse effects on fruit surface were seen). Results were expressed as an overall quality index.

Determination of total antioxidant content (TAC)

Fruit juice TAC was determined by ferric ions reducing antioxidant power assay (FRAP) according to Benzie and Strain (1996) with slight modifications. The stock solutions included 5 mL of a 10 mmol L^{-1} TPTZ (2, 4,6-tripyridyl- s- triazine) with 40 mmol L^{-1} HCL plus 5.41 mL of $FeCl_3$ (20 mmol L^{-1}) and 50 mL of phosphate buffer, (0.3 mol L^{-1}, pH = 3.6), and was prepared freshly and warmed at 37°C. Fruit extracts (150 mL) were allowed to react with 2.85 mL FRAP solution and the absorbance of reaction mixture at 593 nm was measured spectrophotometrically after incubation at 37°C for 10 min. For construction of calibration curve, five concentrations of $FeSO_47H_2O$ (1000, 750, 500, 250, 125 μmol L^{-1}) were used to obtain the calibration curves. The values were expressed as the concentration of antioxidants having a ferric reducing ability equivalent to that of 1 mmol L^{-1} $FeSO_4$. ($y = 0.0009x - 0.0275$, $R^2 = 0.995$).

Determination of CAT enzyme activity

All enzyme extract procedures were conducted at 4°C. CAT activity was measured according to the Beers and Sizer (1952) with slight modifications. The reaction mixture consisted of 2.5 mL sodium phosphate buffer (50 mmol L^{-1}, pH 7.0), 0.2 mL H_2O_2 (1%), and 0.3 mL enzyme. The decomposition of H_2O_2 was measured by the decline in absorbance at 240 nm. The specific activity was expressed as U mg^{-1} protein, where one unit of catalase converts one mol of H_2O_2 per min.

Determination of POD enzyme activity

In order to determine the POD activity, the reaction mixture contained 2.5 mL of 50 mmol L^{-1} phosphate buffer (PH 6.1), 1 mL of 1% hydrogen peroxide, 1 mL of 1% guaiacol, and the enzyme extract. The increase in absorbance at 490 nm was followed up for 1 min (Updhayaya et al. 1985).

Determination of PPO enzyme activity

The PPO activity was assayed by determining the rate of increase in absorbance at 420 nm and 25°C. The reaction mixture contained 0.5 mL of enzyme extract to 2.5 mL of buffered substrate (100 m mol L^{-1} sodium phosphate, pH 6.4, and 50 mmol L^{-1} Catechol). The linear section of the activity curve as a function of time was used to determine the PPO activity (U mg^{-1} protein min^{-1}). The unit for the PPO activity was defined as a change of 0.001 in absorbance at the conditions of the assay (Pizzocaro et al. 1993).

Statistical analysis

The experiment was designed as a completely randomized design with 3 (MeJA concentration) × 2 (storage time) = 6 factors with 5 replicates (each replication was included 10 fruits). ANOVA was performed for the experiment using SAS. Means of data were compared by Duncan's Multiple Range Test. Differences at $P \leq 0.05$ were considered significant. A summary of the statistical results is shown in Table 1.

Results

Weight loss

As shown in Table 1, the weight of control fruit was rapidly decreased during storage, but MeJA, at both concentrations, effectively decreased the rate of weight loss. There was no significant difference between the two levels of MeJA in retaining fruit weight.

Firmness

After 14 days of storage at 1 ± 0.5°C followed by 24 h at 20°C, the firmness was decreased in all fruits, but the control fruits showed a substantially increased firmness value due to water loss and lignification.

Fruit marketability index

Since overall quality is the most important factor determining the marketability, it was considered as the

Table 1. Effect of postharvest MeJA treatment on weight loss, firmness, and marketability index of "Sabrosa" strawberry fruit.

Treatments		Quality attributes		
MeJA (μmol L^{-1})	Storage time (days)	Weight loss (%)	Firmness (N cm^{-2})	Marketability
0	–	0.87^a	0.41^a	2.82^b
8	–	0.65^b	0.36^b	3.52^a
16	–	0.67^b	0.32^b	3.42^a
		**	**	**
–	8	0.51^b	0.41^a	3.75^a
–	15	0.95^a	0.31^b	2.75^b
		**	**	**
0	8	0.59^a	0.49^a	3.42^a
0	15	1.16^a	0.32^c	2.22^a
8	8	0.42^a	0.39^b	3.96^a
8	15	0.89^a	0.32^c	3.08^a
16	8	0.53^a	0.34^{bc}	3.88^a
16	15	0.81^a	0.29^c	2.96^a
		ns	*	ns

Means followed by different letters within a group are significantly different at 5% level.

** and * represent significance at the 0.01, and 0.05 levels, respectively, and NS represents nonsignificance at $P < 0.05$.

marketability index. As shown in Table 1, fruit treated with MeJA showed higher marketability than control fruits and there was no significant difference between the two levels of MeJA in retaining fruit marketability index.

TAC

Fruit TAC was significantly affected by exogenous MeJA treatment. As shown in Table 2, fruit treated with 8 μmol L^{-1} MeJA had the highest TAC after storage for 8 and 15 days. The difference between the two MeJA levels was significant after 8 days, but there was no significant difference between them after 15 days.

CAT enzyme activity

During the first week the activity of CAT enzyme, as an important antioxidant and also the key enzyme in systemic resistance network, was decreased in treated fruits, but it was increased in all fruits during the second week (Table 2). Although MeJA at both concentrations was effective in enhancing CAT activity, it was more significantly enhanced by 8 μmol L^{-1} MeJA.

POD enzyme activity

As shown in Table 2 and Figure 1, control fruit showed a decrease in POD activity but MeJA, in a concentration-dependent manner, effectively enhanced the enzyme activity during the storage period. The activity of POD in both treated and control fruit was significantly decreased during the second week of cold storage.

PPO enzyme activity

After 14 days of storage at 1 ± 0.5°C followed by 24 h at 20°C, PPO enzyme activity declined in all fruits. According to Figure 1, at the end of first week, fruit treated with 8 μmol L^{-1} MeJA showed an increase in PPO enzyme activity, but at the end of storage, there was no significant difference between the treated and control fruit.

Discussion

Fresh fruit and vegetables are living tissues which continue to lose weight due to water loss and respiration after harvest, which is a serious problem in harvested crops (Hung et al. 2011). Fruit flesh firmness is one of the most important indicators for shelf life, preservation potential, consumer acceptance, and market value of horticultural crops (Valero et al. 2003). Ethylene is known as the ripening hormone promoting pectin degradation leading to crop flesh softening together with increase in the rate of various other ripening processes such as discoloration, weight loss, general senescence, and respiration (Singh and Khan 2010). There are conflicting data in different literature about the effects of jasmonates on ethylene production and action in different horticultural crops. It seems that jasmonates may enhance ethylene production in some fruits while blocking its effects. Under different stress conditions, including postharvest storage and transport situations, plant and harvested crop cells may produce jasmonates via membrane lipids breakage. In fact, under these conditions, plant cells undergo jasmonates production as an important defense mechanism. While exogenous MeJA treatment my act as a downregulating factor for internal jasmonates production leading to decreased internal jasmonates production and membrane lipid preservation. As an important result, the retention of membrane lipids is the major reason for blocking ethylene effects, preventing water loss, and decreasing respiration and other senescence-related processes rates such as softening (Creelman and Mullet 1995).

Antioxidant content is a good indicator of internal cell situation. Fruit with high antioxidant content are in a good condition of health and are considered as marketable. Free radicals and AOS are produced during normal cell metabolism and also in response to biotic and abiotic stresses, and antioxidants are consumed for scavenging free radicals and AOS. With progress in senescence and increase in metabolic activities, the rate of free radicals and AOS production is increased. In comparison to whole plant systems, the capacity of harvested fruit to produce antioxidants is limited, and

Table 2. Effect of postharvest MeJA treatment on TAC and CAT, POD and PPO enzymes activity of "Sabrosa" strawberry fruit.

Treatments		Quality attributes			
MeJA (μmol L^{-1})	Storage time (days)	TAC (mmol Fe^{+2} 100 g^{-1} FW)	CAT (U mg^{-1} protein)	POD (U mg^{-1} protein)	PPO (U mg^{-1} protein)
0	–	379.33^b	122.805^a	165.90^b	7791.20^b
8	–	579.78^a	115.872^a	249.62^a	10132.00^a
16	–	385.22^b	114.046^a	269.53^a	8464.00^b
		**	ns	**	**
–	8	498.85^a	104.93^b	243.61^a	9050.10^a
–	15	397.37^b	130.20^a	213.09^a	8541.30^a
		**	**	ns	ns
0	8	406.78^{bc}	118.25^b	168.66^a	7374.40^b
0	15	351.89^c	127.35^{ab}	163.12^a	8208.00^b
8	8	695.22^a	96.33^c	263.77^a	11464.00^a
8	15	464.33^b	135.40^a	235.47^a	8800.00^b
16	8	394.56^{bc}	100.22^c	298.39^a	8312.00^b
16	15	375.89^{bc}	127.86^{ab}	240.66^a	8616.00^b
		**	**	ns	*

Means followed by different letters within a group are significantly different at 5% level.
** and * represent significance at the 0.01, and 0.05 levels, respectively, and NS represents nonsignificance at $P < 0.05$.

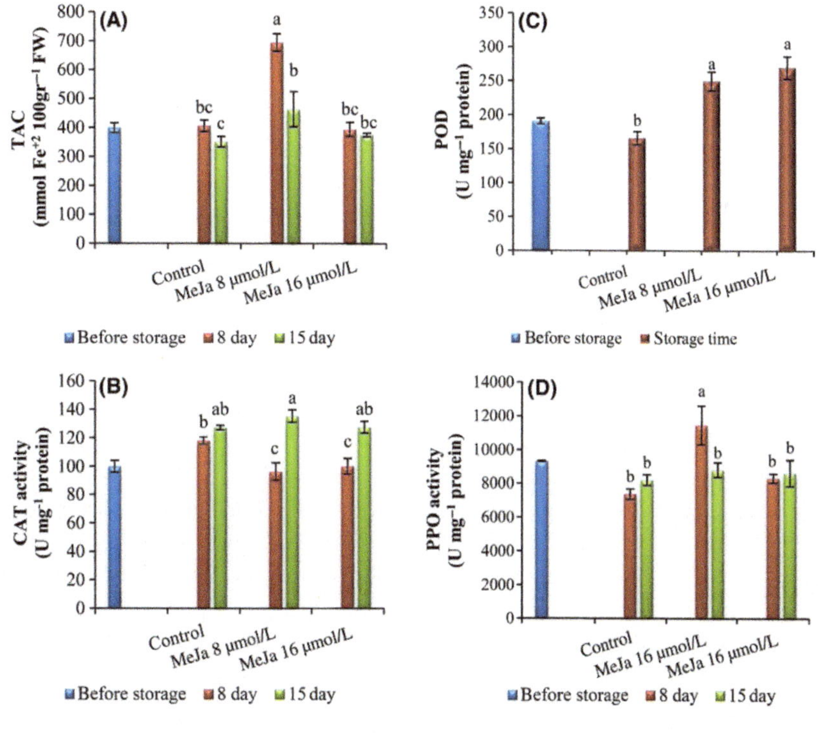

Figure 1. Effects of postharvest MeJA treatment on total antioxidant capacity (A), catalase (B), peroxidase (C), and polyphenol oxidase (D) enzymes activity of "Sabrosa" strawberry fruit after 8 and 15 days of cold storage followed by 1 day at 20°C. Means followed by different letters are significantly different at 5% level.

with progress in ripening and senescence, the rate of free radical and AOS production precedes the antioxidant systems leading to cell damage and subsequent postharvest losses. Then any factor decreasing cell metabolic activities and contributing in defense systems against different stresses will decrease the rate of free radical production and senescence leading to antioxidant preservation. It has been demonstrated that exogenous treatment with MeJA enhances the antioxidant capacity of different harvested fruits and horticultural crops (Wang and Zheng 2005; Chanjirakul et al. 2006; Wang et al. 2008; Sayyari et al. 2011). In this study, MeJA not only enhanced strawberry fruit TAC, but also increased the activity of CAT and POD as two important antioxidant and defense enzymes. Similar results were also observed in peaches (Yao and Tian 2005; Jin et al. 2009), cherrie (Yao and Tian 2005) and loquat fruits (Cao et al. 2008). It is well-known that during the local and systemic acquired resistance in disease and stress-resistant crops, CAT activity decreases in first steps allowing the H_2O_2 to increase as a second messenger, and also as the major player in hypersensitive response, and after the establishment of a resistance system, increase in the activity of CAT is necessary to eliminate the elevated dangerous H_2O_2 molecules (Asghari and Soleimani Aghdam 2010). It has been proposed that JA may play a direct or indirect role in systemic resistance network. Also it is well-known that JA activates phenylalanine amonia-lyase (PAL, EC 4.3.1.24) as the key enzyme in phenolics and salicylic acid biosynthesis, the later considered as the main activator of local and systemic acquired resistance in different plants. Our data indicates that MeJA directly affects the systemic resistance due to the decreasing CAT activity. According to our findings, postharvest MeJA treatment decreased CAT enzyme activity during the first 8 days of storage but enhanced it later, coinciding with the mentioned acquired resistance pattern. POD and PPO are enzymes with important roles in enhancing antioxidant capacity and triggering some resistance systems against biotic and abiotic stresses in plants and harvested crops. Both catalyzing the formation of different antimicrobial phenolic substances such as quinones which are toxic to pathogens (Mohammadi and Kazemi 2002). In addition, POD and PPO activities have been considered as important biochemical markers for crop resistance against different stresses specially the pathogens (Mohammadi and Kazemi 2002). Significant increase in PPO activity also may negatively affect the color of strawberries due to formation of dark brown pigments. According to our data, after an increase during the first week of storage, PPO activity was decreased in the second week indicating that MeJA treatment will not result in a loss in fruit color during long-term storage.

The results of this study indicated that MeJA enhances fruit postharvest life due to enhanced total antioxidant capacity, decreased weight loss, and senescence rate. It is proposed that MeJA may effectively contribute in systemic acquired resistance establishment via decreasing CAT activity during first week and then increasing it during the second week. In addition, the useful effects of MeJA in enhancing fruit postharvest life and decreasing senescence rate by phenolics, and some HSPs, as main cell protecting agents, should be considered.

Conclusion

The results of this study indicate that MeJA directly plays key roles in enhancing fruit storage life, antioxidant and defense systems, and treatment of harvested fruits with MeJA, as a safe phytochemical, may significantly enhance "Sabrosa" strawberry fruit storage life, quality attributes, and nutritional quality by enhancing the fruit's whole antioxidant capacity and defense enzymes activity. The suitable concentration of MeJA for enhancing TAC and antioxidant enzymes activity in Sabrosa strawberry was 8 μmol L^{-1}.

Conflict of Interest

None declared.

References

Asghari, M., and M. S. Soleimani Aghdam. 2010. Impact of salicylic acid on postharvest physiology of horticulture crop. Trends Food Sci. Tech. 21:502–509.

Ayala-Zavala, J. F., C. Y. Wang, and G. A. Gonzalez-Aguilar. 2005. Methyl jasmonate in conjunction with ethanol treatment increases antioxidant capacity, volatile compounds and postharvest life of strawberry fruit. Eur. Food Res. Technol. 221:1438–1443.

Beers, J., and I. W. A. Sizer. 1952. Spectrophotometric method for measuring the breakdown of hydrogen peroxide b catalase. J. Biol. Chem. 95:133–140.

Benzie, I. F. F., and J. J. Strain. 1996. The ferric reducing ability of plasma (FRAP) as a measure of 'antioxidant power': the FRAP assay. Anal. Biochem. 239:70–76.

Cai, Y., Q. Luo, M. Sun, and H. Corke. 2004. Antioxidant activity and phenolic compounds of 112 traditional Chinese medicinal plants associated with anticancer. Life Sci. 74:2157–2184.

Cao, S., Y. Zheng, Z. Yang, S. Tang, P. Jin, K. Wang, et al. 2008. Effect of methyl jasmonate on inhibition of *Colletotrichum acutatum* infection in loquat fruit and the possible mechanisms. Postharvest Biol. Technol. 49:301–307.

Cao, S., Y. Zheng, K. Wang, P. Jin, and H. Rui. 2009. Methyl jasmonate reduces chilling injury and enhances antioxidant enzyme activity in postharvest loquat fruit. Food Chem. 115:1458–1463.

Chanjirakul, K., S. Y. Wang, C. Y. Wang, and J. Siriphanich. 2006. Effect of natural volatile compounds on antioxidant capacity and antioxidant enzymes in raspberries. Postharvest Biol. Technol. 40:106–115.

Concha, C. M., N. E. Figueroa, L. A. Poblete, F. A. Oñate, W. Schwab, and C. R. Figueroa. 2013. Methyl jasmonate treatment induces changes in fruit ripening by modifying the expression of several ripening genes in *Fragaria chiloensis* fruit. Plant Physiol. Biochem. 70:433–444.

Creelman, R. A., and J. E. Mullet. 1995. Jasmonic acid distribution and action in plants: regulation during development and response to biotic and abiotic stress. Proc. Natl Acad. Sci. USA 92:4114–4119.

Demole, E., E. Lederer, and D. Mercier. 1962. Isolement et determination de la structure du jasmonate de methyle, constitutuant odorant characteristique de l'essence de jasmin. Helv. Chim. Acta 45:675–685.

Ding, C. K., C. Y. Wang, K. C. Gross, and D. L. Smith. 2002. Jasmonate and salicylate induce the expression of pathogenesis-related protein genes and increase resistance to chilling injury in tomato fruit. Planta 214:895–901.

Gao, M., L. Feng, and T. Jiang. 2013. Browning inhibition and quality preservation of button mushroom (*Agaricus bisporus*) by essential oils fumigation treatment. Food Chem. 149:107–113.

Heinonen, I. M., A. S. Meyer, and E. N. Frankel. 1998. Antioxidant activity of berry phenolics on human low-density lipoprotein and liposome oxidation. J. Agric. Food Chem. 46:4107–4112.

Huang, W. Y., Y. Z. Cai, and Y. Zhang. 2010. Natural phenolic compounds from medicinal herbs and dietary plants: potential use for cancer prevention. Nutr. Cancer 62:1–20.

Hung, D. V., S. Tong, F. Tanaka, E. Yasunaga, D. Hamanaka, N. Hiruma, et al. 2011. Controlling the weight loss of fresh produce during postharvest storage under a nano-size mist environment. J. Food Eng. 106:325–330.

Jin, P., Y. Zheng, S. Tang, H. Rui, and C. Y. Wang. 2009. A combination of hot air and methyl jasmonate vapor treatment alleviates chilling injury of peach fruit. Postharvest Biol. Technol. 52:24–29.

Kaefer, C. M., and J. A. Milner. 2008. The role of herbs and spices in cancer prevention. J. Nutr. Biochem. 19:347–361.

Karaman, S., B. Ozturk, N. Genc, and S. M. Celik. 2012. Effect of preharvest application of methyl jasmonate on fruit quality of plum (*Prunus salicina* Lindell cv. 'Fortune') at harvest and during cold storage. J. Food Process. Preserv. 37:1049–1059.

Mohammadi, M., and H. Kazemi. 2002. Changes in peroxidase and polyphenol oxidase activities in susceptible and resistant wheat heads inoculated with *Fusarium graminearum* and induced resistance. Plant Sci. 162:491–498.

Pizzocaro, F., D. Torreggiani, and G. Gilardi. 1993. Inhibition of apple polyphenoloxidase (PPO) by ascorbic acid, citric acid and sodium chloride. J. Food Process. Preserv. 17:21–30.

Rice-Evans, C. A., and N. J. Miller. 1996. Antioxidant activities of flavonoids as bioactive components of food. Biochem. Soc. Trans. 24:790–795.

Sayyari, M., M. Babalar, S. Kalantari, D. Martinez-Romero, F. Guillen, M. Serrano, et al. 2011. Vapour treatments with methyl salicylate or methyl jasmonate alleviated chilling injury and enhanced antioxidant potential during postharvest storage of pomegranates. Food Chem. 124:964–970.

Singh, Z., and A. S. Khan. 2010. Physiology of plum fruit ripening. Stewart Postharvest Rev. 2:3.

Soleimani Aghdama, M., L. Sevillano, F. B. Flores, and S. Bodbodak. 2013. Heat shock proteins as biochemical markers for postharvest chilling stress in fruits and vegetables. Sci. Hortic. 160:54–64.

Updhayaya, A., D. Sankhla, T. D. Davis, N. Sankhla, and B. N. Smidth. 1985. Effect of paclobutrazol on the activities of some enzymes of activated oxygen metabolism and lipid peroxidation in senescing soybean leaves. J. Plant Physiol. 121:453–461.

Valero, D., A. D. Martinez-Romero, J. M. Valverde, F. Guillen, and M. Serrano. 2003. Quality improvement and extension of shelf life by 1-methylcyclopropene in plumas affected by ripening stage at harvest. Innov. Food Sci. Emerg. Technol. 4:339–348.

Wang, S. Y., and H. Jiao. 2000. Scavenging capacity of berry crops on superoxide radicals, hydrogen peroxide, hydroxyl radicals, and singlet oxygen. J. Agric. Food Chem. 48:5677–5684.

Wang, S. Y., and W. Zheng. 2005. Preharvest application of methyl jasmonate increases fruit quality and antioxidant capacity in raspberries. Int. J. Food Sci. Technol. 40:187–195.

Wang, S. Y., L. Bowman, and M. Ding. 2008. Methyl jasmonate enhances antioxidant activity and flavonoid content in blackberries (Rubus *spp.*) and promotes anti proliferation of human cancer cells. Food Chem. 107:1261–1269.

Yao, H. J., and S. P. Tian. 2005. Effects of a biocontrol agent and methyl jasmonate on postharvest disease of peach fruit and the possible mechanism involved. J. Appl. Microbiol. 98:941–950.

Zhou, D., L. Li, Y. Wu, J. Fan, and J. Ouyang. 2015. Salicylic acid inhibits enzymatic browning of fresh-cut Chinese chestnut (*Castanea mollissima*) by competitively inhibiting polyphenol oxidase. Food Chem. 171:19–25.

21

Impact of type of child growth intervention program on caregivers' child feeding knowledge and practices: a comparative study in Ga West Municipality, Ghana

Faith Agbozo[1], Esi Colecraft[2] & Basma Ellahi[3]

[1]Department of Family and community Health, School of Public Health, University of Health and Allied Sciences, Ho (Hohoe campus), Ghana
[2]Department of Nutrition and Food Science, University of Ghana, P. O. Box LG 134, Legon, Ghana
[3]Faculty of Health and Social Care, University of Chester, Chester, CH1 4BJ, United Kingdom

Keywords
Caregiving, community-based growth promotion, growth monitoring and promotion, infant and young child feeding

Correspondence
Faith Agbozo, University of Health and Allied Sciences, School of Public Health, PMB 31, Ho, Volta region, Ghana.
E-mail: faagbozo@uhas.edu.gh

Funding Information
No funding information provided.

Abstract

Community-based growth promotion (CBGP) delivered by community volunteers aims at enhancing the traditional growth monitoring and promotion (GMP) program delivered by community health nurses through the promotion of optimum infant and young child feeding (IYCF) leading to improved child growth. This study compared IYCF knowledge and practices among caregiver–child pairs (0–24 months) receiving child welfare services from CBGP (n = 124) and GMP (n = 108) programs. Semistructured questionnaires were used to interview caregivers on IYCF knowledge/practices and validated food frequency questionnaire used to record infants' food intakes. Group differences were determined using Chi-square and independent samples t-tests ($P < 0.05$; 95% confidence interval [CI]). Mean IYCF knowledge scores were similar (CBGP: 10.84 ± 1.69 vs. GMP: 10.23 ± 1.38, $P = 0.062$). However, more CBGP caregivers (17%) were highly knowledgeable than their GMP counterparts (5%) ($P = 0.011$). Early breastfeeding initiation (CBGP: 54% vs. GMP: 28%, $P < 0.0001$), exclusive breastfeeding (CBGP: 73% vs. GMP: 56%, $P = 0.001$), and timely complementary feeding (CBGP: 72% vs. GMP: 49%, $P = 0.014$) were reportedly higher among CBGP caregivers. Underweight was 11% (CBGP: 8% vs. GMP: 14%, $P = 0.154$). Mean dietary diversity scores (10 food groups) were similar (CBGP: 4.49 ± 1.89 vs. GMP: 3.87 ± 1.89, $P = 0.057$) but more CBGP caregivers (77%) achieved minimum dietary diversity than their GMP counterparts (61%) ($P = 0.035$). Few caregivers achieved minimum meal frequency (CBGP: 31% vs. GMP: 29%, $P = 0.486$) and minimum acceptable diet (CBGP: 23% vs. GMP: 21%, $P = 0.464$) indicators. Number of children under 5 years owned by caregiver (adjusted odds ratio [AOR]: 0.405; 95% CI: 1.13–78.53, $P = 0.038$), her educational level (AOR: 0.112; 95% CI: 0.02–0.90, $P = 0.040$), and IYCF knowledge (AOR: 0.140; 95% CI: 0.03–0.79, $P = 0.026$) significantly predicted optimum child feeding. Nutrition education on optimum complementary feeding and birth spacing strategies should intensify.

Introduction

Childhood malnutrition is a serious public health problem associated with adverse health and socioeconomic consequences. Globally, an estimated 26% of children below 5 years of age were stunted, 16% were underweight and 8% were wasted in 2011 (UNICEF-WHO-The World Bank, 2012). The vast majority of undernourished children are in south-central Asia and sub-Saharan Africa. In Ghana, 28% of children under-five years are stunted, 14% are underweight, and 9% are wasted (Ghana Statistical Service, 2008). Child growth monitoring and promotion (GMP) programs have long been identified and recommended as an effective approach to preventing child malnutrition (UNICEF, 2006).

The GMP program was introduced by UNICEF and implemented in Ghana in the 1970s with the main objective of reducing the prevalence of malnutrition (UNICEF, 1990). The earlier growth monitoring program instituted by the WHO in the 1950s was limited to weighing and plotting children's weights to detect abnormal growth (WHO, 1962). Inclusion of a promotion component in the GMP program, intended to foster communication between health workers and caregivers concerning child health and nutrition, was expected to enhance caregivers' child caring and feeding behaviors leading to improved child growth (Pearson 1995).

However, a systematic review of studies on the program revealed that the "promotion" component of "GMP" which encompassed child-centered caregiver counseling was poorly implemented (Pearson 1995). Also, poor attendance and low coverage were reported in UNICEF supported programs in China, Ecuador, Indonesia, Malawi, Thailand, Zaire, and Zambia (Ashworth et al. 2008). In Burkina Faso, Niger and Mozambique, fewer than 30% of mothers were counseled (Hampshire et al. 2004). Reasons cited included lack of health personnel to provide the service, inaccessible child health services and poor attendance by caregivers. However, in Ghana and other developing countries, it is has been shown that adequate caregiver counseling and longer effective participation in child growth programs is associated with improved knowledge of caregivers on infant feeding and positive anthropometric outcomes of children (Owusu and Lartey 1992; Colecraft et al. 2004; Alderman 2007).

Thus, the community-based growth promotion (CBGP) concept was an attempt to address some of the shortcomings of the GMP program and improve coverage, delivery of services and effective participation by caregivers. The program was pioneered by the Manoff Group and promoted by UNICEF during the 1980s as a child survival strategy to engender the caregiver–health worker interaction believed to be crucial for program success (UNICEF, 1990; Mason et al. 2006). Prior to its implementation, the CBGP concept was successfully piloted in Indonesia in 1977 where caloric intake of participating children improved by 200–300 calories per day and consumption of green leafy vegetables doubled with subsequent reduction in malnutrition from 25% to 14% (Griffiths and Nobbe 1985; Griffiths et al. 1996). Following the piloting success, the CBGP concept was adopted and implemented in several countries with outcomes that suggested that the program had positive effects on knowledge, attitudes, and practices of participating families which led to improved growth of children (Van Roekel et al. 2002; Hossain et al. 2005; Galasso and Umapthi 2007; Muyeti-Stevens 2007).

Modalities for rolling out the CBGP program in Ghana have been documented by the Ghana Health Service (Ghana Health Service, 2010). In Ghana, major differences between the CBGP and the GMP programs centers on "where," "who," and "how" the services are delivered. Typically, the GMP program is delivered at child welfare clinics (CWC) situated at health centers or outreach health posts and the services are provided by trained health professionals, mostly community health nurses who are sometimes supported by nutrition extension workers and auxiliary health aides. In contrast, the CBGP program is delivered at the community-level in selected rural and deprived urban communities where the GMP program is readily unavailable and is intended to be owned by the community. Here, services are provided by community volunteers called child growth promoters who have been trained by the Ghana Health Service to carry out growth monitoring of infants and counseling of caregivers on infant and young child feeding (IYCF). The volunteers are supervised by community health nurses who carry out specialized activities such as immunizations. Another difference between the two program types is that whereas the GMP program targets children under 5 years, the CBGP program focuses on children from birth to 24 months. In both programs, monthly attendance by caregiver–child pairs is required where infant growth monitoring is carried out and caregivers are counseled on optimum IYCF practices. However, in the GMP program, the counseling is typically group-based and prescriptive. Conversely, the counseling delivered in the CBGP program is usually individualized and participatory and the community volunteer is expected to negotiate with the caregiver and motivate her to adopt optimum IYCF practices.

After over a decade of implementation, there is little documented information on whether the CBGP program is achieving the intended impact and if it is an improvement over the traditional GMP program. This study evaluated differences in the effects of a CBGP and a GMP program on caregivers' IYCF knowledge and practices in two rural communities in the Ga West municipality, Greater Accra region, Ghana.

Materials and Methods

The study was a cross-sectional survey conducted at Nsakina and Dom Sampaman, both rural communities in the Ga West municipality of the Greater Accra region, Ghana. The study targeted all caregiver–child pairs enrolled in the CBGP and GMP programs in Nsakina and Dom Sampaman communities, respectively. All caregivers who received child welfare services in either the CBGP (N = 124) or GMP (N = 108) programs in the two study locations between January and March 2012 were invited to participate and interviewed after completing an informed consent document.

Socio-demographic, economic, and health characteristics of caregiver–child pairs

A semistructured questionnaire was used to collect data on background characteristics of caregivers. This included questions on socio-demographic characteristics (e.g., age, marital status, educational level, employment, household possessions, etc.) and some maternal experiences such as use of antenatal services during pregnancy, education on IYCF at antenatal and CWCs, home visits by program implementers). Additionally, data on the child's age, age at program enrollment, birth weight, and current body weight were abstracted from the child health record booklets.

Knowledge of caregivers on IYCF

Questions intended to assess caregivers' IYCF knowledge were designed based on IYCF counseling topics documented in the Ghana Health Service revised child health record booklet (Ghana Health Service, 2010) which ought to be communicated to caregivers during child welfare sessions. Caregivers responded to 13 knowledge questions on age-specific IYCF practices regarding breastfeeding and complementary feeding.

IYCF practices

A sample of the food frequency questionnaire used during the 2008 Ghana demographic and health survey was used to collect a 3-day information on habitual dietary intakes of the children on complementary feeding (Ghana Statistical Service, 2008). The food groupings in the 3-day questionnaire were as follows: light cereal porridges; stiff cereal-based meals; roots/tubers/plantain; fruits/vegetables rich in vitamin A; other fruits/vegetables; animal products; milk/dairy products; legumes/nuts/oil seeds; fats/oils; and commercial baby products. The WHO core indicators that were used to assess IYCF practices were early initiation of breastfeeding; exclusive breastfeeding under 6 months; introduction of solid, semi-solid or soft foods (timely initiation of complementary foods); minimum dietary diversity; minimum meal frequency, and minimum acceptable diet (WHO and UNICEF, 2010).

Child anthropometry

Birth weight categorizations and nutritional status of the children was determined using the birth weight and current body weight measurements recorded in the child health record booklets.

Data analyses

Data were analyzed using SPSS (version 20.0; Incorporated, Chicago, IL). Differences between the CBGP and GMP programs were determined using Chi-squared test for categorical variables (e.g., sex, proportions of underweight children) and independent samples *t*-test for continuous variables (e.g., age, difference in children's mean weight-for-age *Z*-scores [WAZ]) at $P < 0.05$ (95% confidence interval [CI]). Infant body weight measurements were converted to WAZ using WHO Anthro software (version 3.2.2) (World Health Organization, Geneva, Switzerland). Underweight was defined as WAZ-score <-2. Similarly, their birth weights were classified as normal ($\geq$2.5 kg) and low ($<$2.5 kg). Univariate binary logistic regression model was developed for both known and unknown caregiver–child pair determining factors for child feeding according to WHO minimum IYCF standards and significant independent association (unadjusted odds ratios, UOR) determined. Variables were selected into the final model by considering independent variables with a significance of $\leq$0.500. In the final model, a multivariate binary logistic regression analysis was done to identify the effects of interaction of the explanatory variables (adjusted odds ratio, AOR) on the outcome variable (optimum child feeding).

Measurement of socioeconomic status (SES) index

Variables used in the determination of socioeconomic status (SES) index were education, occupation, income, source of water supply, toilet facilities, fuel for cooking, and household possessions. Each variable was scored based on a method described by Caro and Cortes (Caro and Cortés 2012). The total possible score ranged from 26 to 88 (Table 1). The predetermined SES constituent indicators were analyzed using principal component analysis (factor analysis). The Kaiser-Meyer-Olkin measure of sampling adequacy statistic and Bartlett's test of sphericity tests were applied to determine the usefulness of the data for SES index rating. Based on the possible minimum and maximum values, SES index was determined by providing arbitrary cut-offs for the cumulative scores. Total score >65 indicated high SES; 40–65, average SES and <40, low SES.

Evaluation of caregivers IYCF knowledge

Every knowledge-based question was given a score of either zero or one for questions that demanded a "Yes" or "No" response (e.g., should colostrum be fed to newborns?) and on a 0–2 scale for questions that required caregivers to give specific examples (e.g., give examples of foods rich in vitamin A). Cumulative scores, ranging from 0 to 15 points were computed for each caregiver. Using the Ghana

Table 1. Indicators and associated scores used to measure SES.

SES indicator	Variable	Score
Education[1]	None or primary	1
	Junior high school	2
	Technical/vocational or senior high school	3
Occupation[1]	Housewife	22
	Trading or artisan	31
	Farming	37
Household possessions[1]	House	7
	Land	5
	Vehicle	4
	Milling machine, livestock, or motor	3 each
	Bicycle, refrigerator, sewing machine, television or farm produce	2 each
	Radio, fan or mobile phone	1 each
Income (Ghana cedis) spent on food per week[2]	<20[3]	1
	20–50	2
	>50	3
Sources of water supply[2]	Borehole or well	2
	Rainwater/river	1
Fuel for cooking[2]	Gas	3
	Charcoal	2
	Firewood	1
Household access to toilet facilities[2]	Private toilet	2
	Public latrine	1
	Open defecation	0

[1]These indicators were described by Caro and Cortés (2012).
[2]These were extra indicators added by the authors.
[3]Exchange rate at data collection was 1 dollar to 1.8 Ghana cedis.

Health Service counseling topics as a guide, an interquartile range was determined for the knowledge scores obtained. Relying on distribution of the scores, knowledge rating cut-offs were assigned as follows: low knowledge (0–8); fair knowledge (9–12); and high knowledge (13–15).

Assessment of complementary feeding

The WHO core indicators used to assess complementary feeding are introduction of solid, semisolid or soft foods (timely complementary feeding); minimum dietary diversity; minimum meal frequency and minimum acceptable diet (optimum feeding) (WHO and UNICEF, 2010). The minimum dietary diversity indicator was calculated based on the proportion of children 6–24 months who received foods from four or more food groups during the previous day. The minimum meal frequency indicator was calculated as a proportion of breastfed infants 6–8 months who received at least two meals and 9–24 months who received at least three meals the previous day. The infant or young child met the minimum acceptable diet indicator if the minimum dietary diversity and minimum meal frequency indicators were both met. Based on this, the feeding was classified as either optimum or suboptimum.

Ethical considerations

Ethical clearance was obtained from the Institutional Review Board of the Noguchi Memorial Institute for Medical Research, University of Ghana, Legon (040/11-12). Permission was granted from the Ga West Municipal Health Management Team before commencement of study. Written informed consent was obtained from the caregivers with signature (if literate) or thumbprint (if illiterate).

Results

Socio-demographic, economic, and health characteristics of caregiver–child pairs enrolled in the CBGP and GMP programs

Children in the two programs were similar in age and the average age was about 8 months (Table 2). Based on age at program enrollment, children in the GMP and CBGP programs were enrolled at average ages of 6 and 8 weeks, respectively ($P = 0.04$). Mean birth weights of children were similar. Compared to caregivers in the GMP program, the CBGP caregivers were older and more likely to have completed higher than primary level education, be married or cohabiting and had higher parity. While borehole was the main source of water for nearly 90% of the GMP caregivers' households, over 30% of the CBGP caregivers said their households relied on wells or rainfall as their main water supply ($P < 0001$). The CBGP caregivers were significantly more likely than the GMP caregivers to use charcoal and gas rather than firewood as their main fuel source. There were no significant group differences in the other socio-demographic variables assessed.

Healthcare services received by caregivers

Prior to enrolling in the child growth programs, about 91% of caregivers in the CBGP program received antenatal care services during their last pregnancy compared to 71% of GMP caregivers ($P < 0.0001$). In both programs, about 90% of caregivers had received education on IYCF during their visits to antenatal and or CWCs. Compared to caregivers enrolled in the CBGP program (31%), more GMP caregivers (57%) reported having received home visits from the community health nurses ($P < 0.001$).

IYCF knowledge of caregivers

Generally, there were no significant group differences in caregivers' knowledge on breastfeeding initiation, frequency of breastfeeding in 24 h, duration of exclusive breastfeeding, timely complementary feeding initiation, duration of complementary feeding, minimum meal frequency and

Table 2. Socio-demographic characteristics of caregivers–child pairs.

Characteristics	CBGP (*n* = 124)	GMP (*n* = 108)	*P*-value[1]
Children's age (months)	8.3 ± 5.5	7.5 ± 4.2	0.207
Sex			
Males	61 (49.2)	52 (48.1)	0.489
Females	63 (50.8)	56 (51.9)	
Child's age at program enrollment (weeks)	8.3 ± 0.81	6.3 ± 0.63	0.042
Child's birth weight (kg)	3.08 ± 0.55	2.97 ± 0.51	0.286
Caregivers' age (years)	27.9 ± 5.8	23.9 ± 5.1	<0.0001
Educational level			
None	19 (15.3)	21 (19.4)	0.023
Primary	25 (20.2)	34 (31.5)	
Junior high school	46 (37.1)	41 (38.0)	
Technical/vocational school	27 (21.8)	9 (8.3)	
Senior high school	7 (5.6)	3 (2.8)	
Marital status			
Married	77 (62.1)	51 (47.2)	0.007
Cohabiting	36 (29.0)	38 (35.2)	
Single	11 (8.9)	19 (17.6)	
Parity	2.8 ± 1.6	2.1 ± 1.4	0.001
Number of children under 5 years	1.6 ± 0.7	1.6 ± 0.9	0.741
Household size	4.8 ± 1.7	4.9 ± 2.0	0.860
Occupation			
Trading	69 (55.7)	45 (41.7)	0.173
Vocational[2]	29 (23.4)	30 (27.8)	
Housewife	23 (18.5)	28 (25.9)	
Farming	3 (2.4)	5 (4.6)	
Water supply			
Borehole	82 (66.2)	93 (86.1)	<0.0001
Well	37 (29.8)	6 (5.6)	
Rainwater/river	5 (4.0)	9 (8.3)	
Toilet facilities			
Private toilet	104 (83.8)	77 (71.5)	0.113
Public latrine	15 (12.2)	23 (21.3)	
Open defecation	5 (4.0)	8 (7.2)	
Cooking fuel			
Charcoal	103 (83.1)	72 (66.7)	<0.0001
Firewood	7 (5.6)	30 (27.7)	
Gas	14 (11.3)	6 (5.6)	
Weekly expenditure on food (GH¢)			
<20	6 (4.8)	13 (12.1)	0.080
20–50	23 (18.5)	24 (22.2)	
>50	95 (76.6)	71 (65.7)	
SES index			
Low	66 (53.2)	63 (58.3)	0.337
Average	58 (46.8)	45 (41.7)	

[1]Independent sample *t*-test or Chi-square test, significance ($P < 0.05$).
[2]Hairdressing and dressmaking.

Table 3. Infant and young child feeding knowledge of study caregivers in the CBGP and GMP programs.

Knowledge assessment	CBGP (*n* = 124)	GMP (*n* = 108)	*P*-value[1]
Breastfeeding initiation			
Within an hour after birth	66 (53.2)	45 (41.7)	0.099
Breastfeeding frequency in 24 h			
On demand	106 (85.5)	82 (75.9)	0.113
Duration of exclusive breastfeeding			
Six months	92 (74.2)	65 (60.2)	0.074
Timing of complementary feeding			
Six months	92 (74.2)	66 (61.1)	0.097
Duration of complementary feeding			
6–24 months	79 (63.7)	65 (60.2)	0.270
Minimum meal frequency per day			
6–8 months (≥2 times daily)	108 (87.1)	87 (80.6)	0.175
9–11 months (≥3 times daily)	93 (75.0)	82 (75.9)	0.870
12–24 months (≥4 times daily)	30 (24.2)	36 (33.3)	0.124
Minimum dietary diversity per day			
6–8 months (≥3 food groups)	101 (89.4)	70 (90.9)	0.730
9–11 months (≥3 food groups)	112 (90.3)	95 (88.0)	0.563
12–24 months (≥4 food groups)	114 (91.9)	93 (86.1)	0.112
Knowledge of vitamin A-rich foods			
>2 foods mentioned	17 (13.7)	2 (1.9)	0.004
1–2 foods mentioned	24 (19.4)	20 (17.9)	
None mentioned	83 (66.9)	86 (80.2)	
Knowledge of iron-rich foods			
>2 foods mentioned	11 (8.9)	18 (16.7)	0.099
1–2 foods mentioned	66 (53.2)	45 (41.7)	
None mentioned	47 (37.9)	45 (41.6)	
Knowledge score[2]	10.84 ± 1.69	10.23 ± 1.38	0.062
Knowledge rating			
Low	7 (5.6)	9 (8.3)	0.011
Fair	96 (77.4)	94 (87.0)	
High	21 (16.9)	5 (4.6)	

[1]Independent sample *t*-test or Chi-square test, significance ($P < 0.05$).
[2]The maximum score is 15.

minimum dietary diversity for infants and young children (Table 3). In both groups, with the exception of timely breastfeeding initiation where approximately 50% caregivers (CBGP: 53.2% vs. GMP: 41.7%, $P = 0.099$) were aware of it being within an hour after delivery, in most cases, more than 60% of caregivers in both programs gave correct responses to the other IYCF knowledge questions asked. However, CBGP caregivers were significantly more likely to correctly mention foods rich in vitamin A and tended to have a higher mean knowledge score (CBGP: 10.84 ± 1.69 vs. GMP: 10.23 ± 1.38, $P = 0.062$). Also, significantly more CBGP caregivers were rated as having high IYCF knowledge (CBGP: 17% vs. GMP: 5%, $P = 0.011$).

IYCF practices of caregivers

Breastfeeding practices of caregivers

With the exception of feeding colostrum to newborns, where there was no group difference in caregivers

Table 4. Breastfeeding practices of caregivers in the CBGP and GMP programs.

Breastfeeding practices	CBGP (*n* = 124)	GMP (*n* = 108)	*P*-value[1]
Breastfeeding initiation			
<1 h	67 (54.0)	30 (27.8)	<0.0001
1–24 h	26 (21.0)	36 (33.3)	
>24 h	31 (25.0)	42 (38.9)	
Feeding colostrum to newborns	103 (83.1)	79 (74.5)	0.112
Exclusive breastfeeding for 6 months	91 (73.4)	60 (55.6)	0.001
Pre-lacteal feeds given to newborns			
Coconut juice	8 (6.5)	20 (18.4)	0.022
Formula	12 (9.6)	4 (3.7)	
Fluids given <6 months infants			
Water	11 (8.9)	30 (27.8)	0.002
Gripe water	19 (15.3)	14 (13.0)	
Water and gripe water	3 (2.4)	4 (3.8)	
Timely complementary feeding	57 (72.2)	32 (48.5)	0.014
First complementary food served			
Fermented corn dough porridge	55 (69.6)	33 (50.8)	0.078
Commercial products[2]	23 (29.1)	28 (43.1)	
Sugar solution	1 (1.3)	4 (6.2)	

[1]Chi-square test, significance ($P < 0.05$).
[2]Include formula milk and cereal blends.

breastfeeding practices, significantly more caregivers in the CBGP program followed recommended IYCF practices (Table 4). The CBGP caregivers were significantly more likely to report initiating breastfeeding within one hour of birth (54% vs. 28%; $P < 0.0001$), practicing exclusive breastfeeding for 6 months (73% vs. 56%; $P = 0.001$) and timely initiation of complementary feeding (72% vs. 49%; $P = 0.014$). Fermented corn dough porridge was the most common first complementary food given to infants in both groups but use of commercial products for complementary feeding tended ($P = 0.078$) to be higher among the GMP caregivers.

Types and frequency of consumption of complementary foods by study children aged 6–24 months

Figure 1 shows the types of foods consumed by the children age 6–24 months over the 3-day assessment period. The most commonly consumed food groups (at least 50% consumption rate) among children in both groups were cereal-based meals, cereal porridges, fats and oils, and nonvitamin A-rich fruits and vegetables. Conversely, the least consumed foods (less that 30% consumption rate) were milk and dairy products, vitamin A-rich fruits and vegetables, roots and tubers, commercial foods and legumes, and nuts. The mean dietary diversity scores of children in the CBGP program tended to be higher than those in the GMP program (CBGP: 4.49 ± 1.89 vs. GMP: 3.87 ± 1.89; $P = 0.057$).

Children aged 6–24 months who were fed according to the minimum IYCF guidelines

Of the 232 study children, 141 participants were aged 6–24 months and were on complementary feeding. However, only 31 (22.0%) were optimally fed. Overall, higher proportions of CBGP children were fed according to minimum IYCF guidelines (Table 5). Minimum dietary

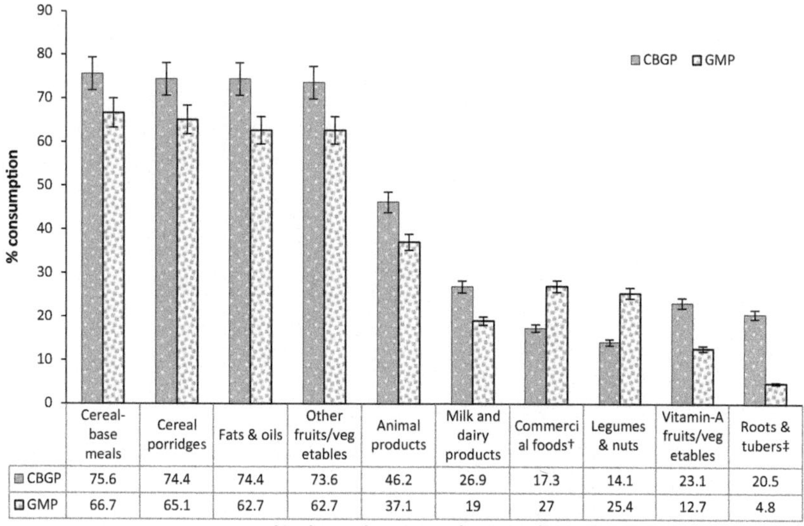

	Cereal-base meals	Cereal porridges	Fats & oils	Other fruits/vegetables	Animal products	Milk and dairy products	Commercial foods†	Legumes & nuts	Vitamin-A fruits/vegetables	Roots & tubers‡
CBGP	75.6	74.4	74.4	73.6	46.2	26.9	17.3	14.1	23.1	20.5
GMP	66.7	65.1	62.7	62.7	37.1	19	27	25.4	12.7	4.8

†Cerelac was the main item. ‡Signigicant (*P*=0.006)

Figure 1. Types of complementary foods consumed by study children aged 6–24 months enrolled in the CBGP and GMP programs.

Table 5. Study children between 6 and 24 months who were fed according to minimum IYCF guidelines.

Minimum IYCF indicator	CBGP (n = 78)	GMP (n = 63)	P-value[1]
Minimum dietary diversity			
6–8 months	10 (45.5)	8 (42.1)	>0.999
9–24 months	50 (89.3)	30 (69.8)	0.020
Cumulative: 6–24 months	60 (76.9)	38 (61.3)	0.035
Minimum meal frequency			
6–8 months: ≥2 daily	13 (59.1)	9 (47.4)	0.538
9–24 months: ≥3 daily	11 (19.6)	9 (20.9)	>0.999
Cumulative: 6–24 months	24 (30.8)	18 (29.0)	0.486
Minimum acceptable diet			
6–8 months	7 (31.8)	5 (20.3)	0.744
9–24 months	11 (19.6)	8 (18.6)	>0.999
Cumulative: 6–24 months	18 (23.1)	13 (21.0)	0.464

[1]Chi-square test, significance ($P < 0.05$).

diversity (CBGP: 77% vs. GMP: 61%; $P = 0.035$) was the only IYCF indicator that over half of the caregivers were able to meet. In both programs, about a third of the caregivers met the minimum meal frequency indicator (CBGP: 31% vs. GMP: 29%; $P = 0.486$) with only a quarter meeting the minimum acceptable diet indicator to achieve optimum child feeding. (CBGP: 23% vs. GMP: 21%; $P = 0.464$).

Anthropometric measurements of study children

Anthropometric data showed no significant difference among children participating in the two programs. Mean WAZ-scores for children in the CBGP (−0.49 ± 1.41) and GMP (−0.65 ± 1.19) programs were low ($P = 0.372$). Although the prevalence of underweight was low among children in the CBGP program (8.1%) and medium in the GMP group (13.9%), the difference was insignificant ($P = 0.154$). Of 141 children on complementary feeding, 11.8% (CBGP: 7.7% vs. GMP: 16.1%, $P = 0.119$) were underweight.

Predictors of child feeding according to minimum IYCF guidelines

In the full model, among caregivers who achieved optimum child feeding according to WHO minimum IYCF standards for their infants aged 6–24 months, the number of children less than 5 years owned by the caregiver was the only significant predictor among the known determining factors of optimum child feeding (UOR: 4.90; 95% CI: 138–17.34, $P = 0.014$). Caregivers who had not more than two children under the age of 5 years were almost five times more likely to optimally feed their 6–24 months old infants than caregivers who had above two children under 5 years. However, caregivers who enrolled their newborns within the postnatal period had 2.5 increased odds of optimally feeding their infants though it was insignificant (UOR: 2.51; 95% CI: 0.97–6.48, $P = 0.057$). The full univariate binary logistic regression model is presented in Table 6.

In the final model, presented in Table 7, again, number of children <5 years owned by the caregiver, educational level of the caregiver, and her IYCF knowledge rating were the explanatory variables in which significant associations were observed. The odds of caregivers with ≤2 children under 5 years optimally feeding their infants increased by additional 4.5 points in the final model (AOR: 0.405; 95% CI: 1.13–78.53, $P = 0.038$). Caregivers who were educated to only the junior the high school level had a significant 0.11 reducing odds of optimally feeding their infants on complementary feeding compared to those who were educated to at least the senior high school level (AOR: 0.112; 95% CI: 0.02–0.90, $P = 0.040$). Similarly, caregivers with fair knowledge on IYCF had a significant 0.14 reducing odds of optimally feeding their infants on complementary feeding compared to those with high IYCF knowledge (AOR: 0.140; 95% CI: 0.03–0.79, $P = 0.026$). Compared to the full model, increasing odds for optimal infant feeding were observed in two variables in the final model: caregiver's SES and when infant was enrolled on the child growth promotion program.

Discussion

Some differences were observed in the socio-demographic variables of caregivers enrolled on the CBGP and GMP programs (age, educational level, marital status, parity, source of water, and type of fuel used for cooking). However, these did not translate into differences in the SES of the two groups. Caregivers participating on the CBGP programs were 4 years older than their GMP counterparts. Usually, persons who are relatively older tend to be in a marriage relationship, have higher parity, and attain higher level of education. The lower education of the GMP caregivers could probably be due to their relatively younger age. If age of caregivers in both groups were similar, it is possible their educational status would also be similar. However, the influence of educational status on caregivers child care giving and seeking behaviors cannot be over-emphasized. After adjusting for caregiver–child pairs' socio-demographic factors, educational level was a significant determinant of optimum child feeding. This finding has been confirmed in other studies (Abuya et al. 2012; Bornstein et al. 2015). Mothers with at least secondary education have decreased likelihood of their infants being stunted (UOR: 1.28; CI: 1.096–1.498, $P = 0.002$) (Abuya et al. 2012).

Table 6. Full univariate binary logistic regression model showing predictors of child feeding according to WHO IYCF indicators.

Explanatory variables	OR_{unadj}	95% CI	*P*-value
Type of child growth promotion program			
CBGP	REF		
GMP	0.922	0.41–2.07	0.844
Age of caregiver			
>20 years	REF		
≤20 years	0.516	0.19–1.42	0.200
Educational level			
Senior high school & above	REF		
Junior high school & below	0.486	0.16–1.52	0.215
Marital status[1]			
Married	REF		
Single	0.657	0.18–2.44	0.530
Parity			
≤4 children	REF		
>4 children	0.751	0.15–3.67	0.724
No. of children <5 years owned by caregiver			
>2 children	REF		
≤2 children	4.896	1.38–17.34	0.014
Household size			
≤6 members	REF		
>6 members	0.712	0.19–2.66	0.613
Weekly food expenditure[2]			
>50 cedis	REF		
≤50 cedis	1.043	0.43–2.51	0.925
Socioeconomic status			
Low SES	REF		
High SES	0.627	0.27–1.44	0.269
Caregiver educated on IYCF at antenatal clinic[3]	1.650	0.34–7.96	0.533
Educated on IYCF at child welfare clinic[3]	1.661	0.35–7.93	0.524
Ever visited at home by program worker[3]	1.414	0.64–3.15	0.397
Caregiver's IYCF knowledge rating			
High knowledge	REF		
Fair knowledge	1.000	0.17–5.77	1.000
Poor knowledge	0.505	0.16–1.62	0.252
Age of child			
≥12 months	REF		
<12 months	0.970	0.39–2.42	0.949
Sex of child			
Female	REF		
Male	0.763	0.34–1.70	0.507
Child's birth weight			
≥2.5 kg	REF		
<2.5 kg	0.509	0.14–1.92	0.319
Underweight			
WAZ ≥2	REF		
WAZ <–2	1.173	0.35–3.93	0.796
When child was enrolled on the program			
Postnatal period	REF		
After postnatal period	2.509	0.97–6.48	0.057

[1]All caregivers who were living with their partners were regarded married.
[2]The exchange rate then was 1 US dollar = 1.8 Ghana cedi.
[3]The reference (OR = 1.00) is a "yes" response.

Table 7. Final multivariate binary logistic regression model showing interaction of the explanatory variables on achievement of optimum infant feeding.

Explanatory variables	OR_{adj}	95% CI	*P*-value
Age of caregiver			
>20 years	REF		
≤20 years	0.283	0.03–2.46	0.253
Educational level			
Senior high school & above	REF		
Junior high school & below	0.112	0.02–0.90	0.040
No. of <5 year children owned by caregiver			
>2 children	REF		
≤2 children	9.405	1.13–78.53	0.038
Socioeconomic status			
Low SES	REF		
High SES	1.489	0.38–5.82	0.567
Home visit by a program worker	0.735	0.16–3.33	0.689
Caregiver's IYCF knowledge rating			
High knowledge	REF		
Fair knowledge	0.140	0.03–0.79	0.026
Poor knowledge	0.896	0.04–20.01	0.945
Child's birth weight			
≥2.5 kg	REF		
<2.5 kg	0.393	0.08–1.83	0.235
When child was enrolled on the program			
Postnatal period	REF		
After postnatal period	3.308	0.66–16.58	0.146

Hosmer–Lemeshow goodness of fit: Chi-square = 10.820, $P = 0.212$.

Knowledge of study participants on appropriate breastfeeding and complementary feeding practices was generally good with minimal differences between the two groups. Although mean knowledge scores were similar for both groups, on the knowledge ranking scale, some interesting differences were observed; 87% of GMP caregivers were moderately informed on IYCF practices but this was 10 points less in the CBGP group. However, 17% of the CPGP caregivers were highly knowledgeable compared to only 5% in GMP group. Since both child growth promotion programs focus on improving the nutrition knowledge of caregivers, it is disappointing to report low IYCF knowledge among the caregivers as this influenced their IYCF practices. In a similar study in Honduras where the community nutrition program was assessed, mean knowledge scores of caregivers participating in the program was higher (6.02 out of 9 points) than that for the control communities (4.91; $P = 0.001$) (Van Roekel et al. 2002). However, it is worth noting that in this study, disparity between the mean knowledge scores and the knowledge rankings may be a result of the cut-offs used.

Assessment of IYCF practices of caregivers revealed some differences. A significant proportion of CBGP caregivers translated their breastfeeding knowledge into practice having reported practicing early initiation of breastfeeding, exclusive breastfeeding and timely introduction of complementary diets. Effective caregiver counseling has been shown to increase breastfeeding rates (Bhutta et al. 2008; Arabi et al. 2012; Negash et al. 2014). Findings from this study also indicated that caregivers in the CBGP program fed their 6–24 months infants with varied food resources than their GMP counterparts but in both groups, the mean dietary diversity score was less than half of the 10 food groups investigated. Since the CBGP caregivers spend relatively more of their income on food per week, coupled with a higher number being married, employed and better educated, it appears these factors might have positively influenced the number of foods they fed their infants with. Consequently, a significant difference existed in the proportion of CBGP and GMP caregivers who met the IYCF guideline relating to minimum dietary diversity. But in both groups, just a quarter met the minimum meal frequency indicator. Therefore, over almost 80% caregivers did not achieve the minimum acceptable diet (optimum child feeding). This finding did not come as a surprise because in both groups, caregivers' knowledge on minimum meal frequency was poor. They believed that young children should be fed three times, just like adults. Suboptimum complementary feeding has become a public health problem globally (Onyango et al. 2014). In Haiti, minimum dietary diversity, minimum meal frequency and minimum acceptable diet were achieved in 29.2%, 45.3%, and 17.1% of children aged 6–23 months, respectively (Heidkamp et al. 2013).

The child growth promoters were observed to render client-centered counseling using counseling cards and often negotiated and agreed with the caregivers on the exact IYCF actions to take (data not reported in this paper). Literature attest that the success of child growth programs rely heavily on the crucial one-to-one counseling contact which caregivers and their family members receive from community workers (Hossain et al. 2005; Muyeti-Stevens 2007; Imdad et al. 2011). Although this study did not prove that the type of growth promotion program that caregiver–child pairs participate in affect the IYCF practices, the caregivers IYCF knowledge has been shown to be a crucial predictor for optimum child feeding. Contrary to findings from Waswa et al. (2015), this study and others have shown that nutrition knowledge of caregivers positively predicts adequate dietary intakes of infants (Dewey and Adu-Afarwuah 2008; Inayati et al. 2012). In Honduras, caregivers' knowledge gained from counseling messages received in the community nutrition program was translated into practice evidenced by their higher child feeding scores (Van Roekel et al. 2002). In Senegal also, caregivers participating in a similar program exhibited significant gains in IYCF practices (Alderman et al. 2009). A year into its implementation, caregivers who practiced adequate complementary feeding increased from 35% to 72%.

Prevalence of underweight among children in the GMP program was similar to the 14% national prevalence recorded in the 2008 Ghana demographic and health survey (Ghana Statistical Service, 2008). However, there was 6 point decrease in the CBGP group. Breastfeeding practices of over half of the caregivers was appropriate but complementary feeding practices of over two-thirds were suboptimum. Most studies have documented widespread growth faltering during the complementary feeding period where infant feeding practices become suboptimum (Heidkamp et al. 2013; Mishra et al. 2014). In both the unadjusted and adjusted binomial regression models, the number of children under 5 years owned by the caregiver was the significant predictor of optimum child feeding. Children under 5 years are vulnerable and require special care. Therefore, having more than two children <5 years would imply a reduction in the caregiving and care-seeking attention rendered to each of them while the limited family food and other resources would have to be shared among these vulnerable ones. The result will be regular suboptimum feeding which will predispose such children to growth faltering. This is a significant finding with little literature from other studies to back it. However, maternal parity in general have been found to correlate with both child feeding practices and nutritional status (Abuya et al. 2012; Radwan 2013).

Poor nutrition knowledge of community health workers and volunteers could adversely affect program outcomes. This was the case with the community-based growth monitoring program in South Africa (Faber et al. 2009). In developing countries, one of the current challenges to child nutrition is the considerable global and national efforts being devoted to breastfeeding promotion to the neglect of complementary feeding practices (Dewey and Adu-Afarwuah 2008; Lartey 2008). From this study, however, it remains unclear whether the IYCF knowledge and practices of the caregivers was a result of the counseling received from the program facilitators. Also, whether the counseling yielded the intended impact of behavior change is an issue worth exploring. Another limitation of the study is the lack of information on nutrition knowledge of the community volunteers and health workers giving education to the caregivers thus making it difficult to assume a relationship between the nutrition knowledge and counseling provided.

Lesson learned and recommendations

Findings from this study provide a firm basis for strengthening and expansion of the CBGP program to augment the traditional GMP program in Ghana as it addresses

Key messages

- Caregivers in the CBGP program were more knowledgeable on IYCF. Most caregivers in both programs practiced appropriate breastfeeding but could not meet the complementary feeding indicators.
- Underweight prevalence was lower in the CBGP program which suggests that the program has the potential to make significant contribution to child health in Ghana.
- Caregivers with fewer children <5 years, high IYCF knowledge and higher education had increased odds for optimum infant feeding.
- Counseling of caregivers and their families on adequate complementary feeding and birth spacing should intensify and should be integrated into all maternal and child health interventions.
- Both programs should be strengthened to enhance their outcomes

some short-falls in the traditional GMP program such as high prevalence of underweight and poor IYCF knowledge. Addressing some operational challenges in the CBGP and GMP programs would help make both programs more effective. Capacity of child growth promoters (community volunteers), community health nurses and other categories of health workers who provide child welfare services should be built through regular training on evidenced-based contemporary IYCF recommendations. They should also be equipped with modern behavior change communication skills to appropriately deliver these messages to the target audience. In filling the knowledge deficit gap, special attention should be given to dietary diversification, food consistency, quantity of meals and feeding frequency. Since infants are particularly vulnerable during the transition period, counseling on child feeding should provide core information on timeliness, adequacy, safety and proper preparation of complementary diets. Emphasis should be placed on involvement of caregivers to understand their challenges to meeting complementary feeding recommendations and where possible, solutions offered to suit their child(ren) and family needs. Finally, since the CBGP program is not meant to replace the traditional GMP program, the Ghana Health Service should take pragmatic steps to strengthen the institutional systems within the GMP program to make it relevant to the needs of caregivers, families and communities.

Acknowledgments

The authors would like to acknowledge the contributions of the management team of the Ga West Municipal Health Directorate and all the community health nurses, health assistants, and child growth promoters (community volunteers) of Nsakina and Dom Sampaman in the Ga West Municipality of the Greater Accra region, Accra for their diverse contributions toward the success of the study.

Conflict of Interest

None declared.

References

Abuya, B. A., J. Ciera, and E. Kimani-Murage. 2012. Effect of mother's education on child's nutritional status in the slums of Nairobi. BMC Pediatr. 12:80.

Alderman, H. 2007. Improving nutrition through community growth promotion: longitudinal study of the nutrition and early child development program in Uganda. World Dev. 35:1376–1389.

Alderman, H., B. Ndiaye, S. Linnemayr, A. Ka, C. Rokx, K. Dieng, et al. 2009. Effectiveness of a community-based intervention to improve nutrition in young children in Senegal: a difference in difference analysis. Public Health Nutr. 12:667–673.

Arabi, M., E. A. Frongillo, R. Avula, and N. Mangasaryan. 2012. Infant and young child feeding in developing countries. Child Dev. 83:32–45.

Ashworth, A., R. Shrimpton, and K. Jamil. 2008. Growth monitoring and promotion: review of evidence of impact. Matern. Child Nutr. 4:86–117.

Bhutta, Z. A., T. Ahmed, R. E. Black, S. Cousens, K. Dewey, E. Giugliani, et al. 2008. What works? Interventions for maternal and child undernutrition and survival. Lancet 371:417–440.

Bornstein, M. H., D. L. Putnick, R. H. Bradley, J. E. Lansford, and K. Deater-Deckard. 2015. Pathways among caregiver education, household resources, and infant growth in 39 low-and middle-income countries. Infancy 20(4):353–376.

Caro, D. H., and D. Cortés. 2012. Measuring family socioeconomic status: an illustration using data from PIRLS 2006. IERI Monogr. Series Issues Methodol. Large-Scale Assessments 5:9–33.

Colecraft, E. K., G. S. Marquis, A. A. Bartolucci, L. Pulley, W. B. Owusu, and H. M. Maetz. 2004. A longitudinal assessment of the diet and growth of malnourished children participating in nutrition rehabilitation centres in Accra, Ghana. Public Health Nutr. 7:487–494.

Dewey, K. G., and S. Adu-Afarwuah. 2008. Systematic review of the efficacy and effectiveness of complementary feeding interventions in developing countries. Matern. Child Nutr. 4:24–85.

Faber, M., S. Schoeman, C. M. Smuts, V. Adams, and T. Ngomane. 2009. Evaluation of community-based growth monitoring in rural districts of the Eastern Cape and KwaZulu-Natal provinces of South Africa. South Afr. J. Clini. Nutr. 22(4):185–194.

Galasso, E., and N. Umapthi. 2007. Improving nutritional status through behavioral change: Lessons from Madagascar. Policy Research Working Paper 4424; Impact Evaluation Series No. 19. The World Bank Development Research Group Poverty Team; Washington, D.C., United States.

Mason, J.B., D. Sanders, P. Musgrove, and G.R. Soekirman. 2006. Community Health and Nutrition Programs, In: Disease Control Priorities in Developing Countries. 2nd edition, chapter 56, 37–58. World Bank; Washington D.C. United States.

Ghana Health Service. 2010. Growth monitoring and promotion for child survival. Trainers guide for training the trainers of community child growth promoters. Nutrition Department, Ghana Health Service, Accra.

Ghana Statistical Service. 2008. Ghana Demographic and Health Survey 2008. Ghana Health Service, ICF Macro Calverton, Ghana Statistical Services, Maryland, Accra, Ghana.

Griffiths, M., and E. Nobbe. 1985. A communication strategy to improve nutrition in Indonesia. Dev. Commun. Rep. Autumn; 51(5):14–19.

Griffiths, M., K. Dickin, and M. Favin. 1996. Promoting the growth of children: what works. World Bank Nutrition Toolkit Tool, 4 p.

Hampshire, R. D., V. M. Aguayo, H. Harouna, J. A. Roley, A. Tarini, and S. K. Baker. 2004. Delivery of nutrition services in health systems in sub-Saharan Africa: opportunities in Burkina Faso, Mozambique and Niger. Public Health Nutr. 7:1047–1053.

Heidkamp, R. A., M. A. Ayoya, I. N. Teta, R. J. Stoltzfus, and J. P. Marhone. 2013. Complementary feeding practices and child growth outcomes in Haiti: an analysis of data from Demographic and Health Surveys. Matern. Child Nutr. 11(4):815–828.

Hossain, S. M., A. Duffield, and A. Taylor. 2005. An evaluation of the impact of a US $60 million nutrition programme in Bangladesh. Health Policy Plann. 20:35–40.

Imdad, A., M. Y. Yakoob, and Z. A. Bhutta. 2011. Impact of maternal education about complementary feeding and provision of complementary foods on child growth in developing countries. BMC Public Health 11:S25.

Inayati, D. A., V. Scherbaum, R. C. Purwestri, N. N. Wirawan, J. Suryantan, S. Hartono, et al. 2012. Improved nutrition knowledge and practice through intensive nutrition education: a study among caregivers of mildly wasted children on Nias Island, Indonesia. Food Nutr. Bull. 33:117–127.

Lartey, A. 2008. Maternal and child nutrition in Sub-Saharan Africa: challenges and interventions. Proc. Nutr. Soc. 67:105–108.

Mishra, K., P. Kumar, S. Basu, K. Rai, and S. Aneja. 2014. Risk factors for severe acute malnutrition in children below 5 y of age in India: a case-control study. Indian J. Pediatr. 81:762–765.

Muyeti-Stevens, R. A. D. R. J.. 2007. Uganda Community Based Growth Promotion: Program Review. JSI Research & Training Institute Inc (Kampala; Uganda), the Manoff Group and USAID (Washington, DC).

Negash, C., T. Belachew, C. J. Henry, A. Kebebu, K. Abegaz, and S. J. Whiting. 2014. Nutrition education and introduction of broad bean–based complementary food improves knowledge and dietary practices of caregivers and nutritional status of their young children in Hula, Ethiopia. Food Nutr. Bull. 35:480–486.

Onyango, A. W., E. Borghi, M. de Onis, Md C Casanovas, and C. Garza. 2014. Complementary feeding and attained linear growth among 6–23-month-old children. Public Health Nutr. 17:1975–1983.

Owusu, W. B., and A. Lartey. 1992. Growth monitoring: experience from Ghana. Food Nutr Bull; 14:97–100.

Pearson, R. 1995. Thematic evaluation of UNICEF support to growth monitoring. Unicef.

Radwan, H. 2013. Patterns and determinants of breastfeeding and complementary feeding practices of Emirati Mothers in the United Arab Emirates. BMC Public Health 13:171.

UNICEF. 1990. Strategy for improved nutrition of children and women in developing countries. A UNICEF policy review. United Nations Children's Fund, New York.

UNICEF. 2006. Progress for children: a report card on nutrition. United Nations Children's Fund, New York, NY.

UNICEF-WHO-The World Bank. 2012. UNICEF-WHO-World Bank Joint Child Malnutrition Estimates. Levels & Trends in Child Malnutrition United Nations Children's Fund, World Health Organization and The World Bank, UNICEF, New York; WHO, Geneva; and The World Bank, Washington, DC.

Van Roekel, K., B. Plowman, M. Griffiths, Vivas de Alvarado V., and J. Matute. 2002. BASICS II midterm evaluation of the AIN program in Honduras 2000. Survey report.

Waswa, L. M., I. Jordan, J. Herrmann, M. B. Krawinkel, and G. B. Keding. 2015. Community-based educational intervention improved the diversity of complementary diets in western Kenya: results from a randomized controlled trial. Public Health Nutr. 10:1–14.

WHO. 1962. Joint FAO/WHO Expert Committee on Nutrition, Sixth Report. WHO Technical Report Series 245. World Health Organization, Geneva.

WHO and UNICEF. 2010. Indicators for assessing infant and young child feeding practices. Part 3: country profiles. World Health Organization, Geneva, Switzerland.

PERMISSIONS

All chapters in this book were first published in FSN, by John Wiley & Sons Ltd.; hereby published with permission under the Creative Commons Attribution License or equivalent. Every chapter published in this book has been scrutinized by our experts. Their significance has been extensively debated. The topics covered herein carry significant findings which will fuel the growth of the discipline. They may even be implemented as practical applications or may be referred to as a beginning point for another development.

The contributors of this book come from diverse backgrounds, making this book a truly international effort. This book will bring forth new frontiers with its revolutionizing research information and detailed analysis of the nascent developments around the world.

We would like to thank all the contributing authors for lending their expertise to make the book truly unique. They have played a crucial role in the development of this book. Without their invaluable contributions this book wouldn't have been possible. They have made vital efforts to compile up to date information on the varied aspects of this subject to make this book a valuable addition to the collection of many professionals and students.

This book was conceptualized with the vision of imparting up-to-date information and advanced data in this field. To ensure the same, a matchless editorial board was set up. Every individual on the board went through rigorous rounds of assessment to prove their worth. After which they invested a large part of their time researching and compiling the most relevant data for our readers.

The editorial board has been involved in producing this book since its inception. They have spent rigorous hours researching and exploring the diverse topics which have resulted in the successful publishing of this book. They have passed on their knowledge of decades through this book. To expedite this challenging task, the publisher supported the team at every step. A small team of assistant editors was also appointed to further simplify the editing procedure and attain best results for the readers.

Apart from the editorial board, the designing team has also invested a significant amount of their time in understanding the subject and creating the most relevant covers. They scrutinized every image to scout for the most suitable representation of the subject and create an appropriate cover for the book.

The publishing team has been an ardent support to the editorial, designing and production team. Their endless efforts to recruit the best for this project, has resulted in the accomplishment of this book. They are a veteran in the field of academics and their pool of knowledge is as vast as their experience in printing. Their expertise and guidance has proved useful at every step. Their uncompromising quality standards have made this book an exceptional effort. Their encouragement from time to time has been an inspiration for everyone.

The publisher and the editorial board hope that this book will prove to be a valuable piece of knowledge for researchers, students, practitioners and scholars across the globe.

LIST OF CONTRIBUTORS

Stephen A. Adefegha, Ganiyu Oboh, Sunday I. Oyeleye and Kolawole Osunmo
Functional food and Nutraceutical Unit, Department of Biochemistry, Federal University of Technology, P.M.B. 704, Akure 340001, Nigeria

Anne-Mette S. Hansen, Henrik L. Frandsen and Arvid Fromberg
National Food Institute, Technical University of Denmark Mørkhøj Bygade 19, Søborg DK-2860, Denmark

Felipe Jiménez-Aspee, Samanta Thomas-Valdés, Ayla Schulz and Guillermo Schmeda-Hirschmann
Laboratorio de Química de Productos Naturales, Instituto de Química de Recursos Naturales, Universidad de Talca, Talca, Chile

Ana Ladio
Laboratorio Ecotono, INIBIOMA (CONICET)-Universidad Nacional del Comahue, Bariloche, Río Negro, Argentina

Cristina Theoduloz
Laboratorio de Cultivo Celular, Facultad de Ciencias de la Salud, Universidad de Talca, Talca, Región del Maule, Chile

Kamran Kheiralipour and Farshid Marzbani
Mechanical Engineering of Biosystems Department, Ilam University, Ilam, Iran

DeAnn J. Liska and Chad M. Cook
Biofortis Research, 211 E. Lake St., Addison, Illinois 60101

Ding Ding Wang
D&V Systematic Consulting, 1945 Eastchester Rd., Apt 26D, Bronx, New York 10461

John Szpylka
Silliker, a Mérieux NutriSciences Company, Chicago, Illinois 60601

Lembe Samukelo Magwaza
Department of Crop Science, School of Agricultural, Earth and Environmental Sciences, University of KwaZulu-Natal, Private Bag X01, Scottsville 3209, Pietermaritzburg, South Africa

Umezuruike Linus Opara
Postharvest Technology Research Laboratory, Department of Horticultural Science, Stellenbosch University, Stellenbosch 7602, South Africa
Postharvest Technology Research Laboratory, Department of Food Science, South African Research Chair in Postharvest Technology, Stellenbosch University, Stellenbosch 7602, South Africa

Paul J. R. Cronje
Citrus Research International, Department of Horticultural Science, Stellenbosch University, Stellenbosch 7602, South Africa

Sandra Landahl, Jose Ordaz Ortiz and Leon A. Terry
Plant Science Laboratory, Cranfield University, Bedfordshire, MK43 0AL, UK

Kambiz Mashayekhi, Siamak Mohammadi Chiane and Seyyed Javad Mousavizadeh
Department of Horticultural Science, Gorgan University of Agricultural Sciences and Natural Resources, Gorgan, Iran

Manizheh Mianabadi
Department of Biology, Faculty of Sciences, University of Golestan, Gorgan, Iran

Farshid Ghaderifar
Department of Agronomy, Gorgan University of Agricultural Sciences and Natural Resources, Gorgan, Iran

Samira Naderinezhad, Nasrin Etesami, Arefe Poormalek Najafabady and Majid Ghasemi Falavarjani
Department of Chemical Engineering, Isfahan University of Technology, Isfahan, 84156-8311, Iran

Sheilla Natukunda, John H. Muyonga and Ivan M. Mukisa
School of Food Technology, Nutrition and Bioengineering, Makerere University, Kampala, Uganda

Christina A. Nti
Department of Family and Consumer Sciences, University of Ghana, Legon, Ghana

Wisdom A. Plahar and Nana T. Annan
CSIR-Food Research Institute, Accra, Ghana

Ehigbai I. Oikeh and Ehimwenma S. Omoregie
Department of Biochemistry, Faculty of Life Sciences, University of Benin, PMB 1154 Benin City, Nigeria

Faith E. Oviasogie
Department of Microbiology, Faculty of Life Sciences, University of Benin, PMB 1154 Benin City, Nigeria

Kelly Oriakhi
Department of Medical Biochemistry, Faculty of Basic Medical Sciences, University of Benin, PMB 1154 Benin City, Nigeria

Ricard Rico
International Nut and Dried Fruit Council, Reus, Spain

Mònica Bulló and Jordi Salas-Salvadó
Department of Biochemistry and Biotechnology, IISPV, School of Medicine, Rovira i Virgili University, CIBERobn Physiopathology of Obesity and Nutrition, Instituto de Salud Carlos III, Madrid, Spain

Francisco Rodríguez-Gómez, Verónica Romero-Gil, Pedro García-García, Francisco Noé Arroyo-López and Antonio Garrido-Fernández
Food Biotechnology Department, Instituto de la Grasa (Agencia Estatal Consejo Superior de Investigaciones Científicas, CSIC) Campus Pablo de Olavide, Building 46. Ctra. Utrera, km 1., 41013 Seville, Spain

Xuan T. Tran and Paul D. Roach
School of Environmental and Life Sciences, University of Newcastle, Ourimbah, NSW 2258, Australia

Sophie E. Parks and John B. Golding
School of Environmental and Life Sciences, University of Newcastle, Ourimbah, NSW 2258, Australia
NSW Department Primary Industries, Central Coast Primary Industries Centre, Ourimbah, NSW 2258, Australia

Minh H. Nguyen
School of Environmental and Life Sciences, University of Newcastle, Ourimbah, NSW 2258, Australia
School of Science and Health, University of Western Sydney, Penrith, NSW 2751, Australia

Yousef Tavakolpour
Department of Food Science and Technology, College of Agriculture, Shiraz University, Shiraz, Iran

Marzieh Moosavi-Nasab
Department of Food Science and Technology, College of Agriculture, Shiraz University, Shiraz, Iran
Seafood Processing Research Group, College of Agriculture, Shiraz University, Shiraz, Iran

Mehrdad Niakousari
Department of Food Science and Technology, College of Agriculture, Shiraz University, Shiraz, Iran
Nanotechnology Institute, Shiraz University, Shiraz, Iran

Soroush Haghighi-Manesh
Department of Food Science and Technology, School of Agriculture, Tarbiat Modares University, Tehran, Iran

Yixiang Xu, Chyer Kim and Edward Sismour
Agricultural Research Station, Virginia State University, Petersburg, Virginia 23806

Sheanell Burton
Agricultural Research Station, Virginia State University, Petersburg, Virginia 23806
Department of Biology, Virginia State University, Petersburg, Virginia 23806

Aijun Yang and Andrew James
CSIRO Agriculture, 306 Carmody Road, St Lucia, Queensland 4067, Australia

Heather Smyth
Queensland Alliance for Agriculture and Food Innovation, The University of Queensland, St Lucia, Queensland 4072, Australia

Mridusmita Chaliha
Department of Agriculture, Fisheries and Forestry, Coopers Plains, Queensland 4108, Australia

Habtamu Fekadu Gemede
Department of Food Technology and Process Engineering, Wollega University, Nekemte, Ethiopia

Center for Food Science and Nutrition Program, Addis Ababa University, Addis Ababa, Ethiopia

Gulelat Desse Haki
Department of Food Science and Technology, Botswana Collage of Agriculture, Botswana University, Gaborone, Botswana

Fekadu Beyene
Department of Food Technology and Process Engineering, Wollega University, Nekemte, Ethiopia

Ashagrie Z. Woldegiorgis
Center for Food Science and Nutrition Program, Addis Ababa University, Addis Ababa, Ethiopia

Sudip Kumar Rakshit
Department of Chemical Engineering, Canada Research Chair (Tier 1), Lakehead University, Thunder Bay, ON, Canada P7B 5E1

Adegoke H. Bakare
Department of Hospitality and Tourism, Federal University of Agriculture, Abeokuta, Nigeria

Oluwatooyin F. Osundahunsi
Department of Food Science and Technology, Federal University of Technology, Akure, Nigeria

Joseph O. Olusanya
Department of Home Economics and Hotel Management, Tai Solarin University of Education, Ijebu Ode, Nigeria

Mohammadreza Asghari and Ali Rashid Hasanlooe
Department of Horticulture, Faculty of Agriculture, Urmia University, Urmia, Iran

Faith Agbozo
Department of Family and community Health, School of Public Health, University of Health and Allied Sciences, Ho (Hohoe campus), Ghana

Esi Colecraft
Department of Nutrition and Food Science, University of Ghana, Legon, Ghana

Basma Ellahi
Faculty of Health and Social Care, University of Chester, Chester, CH1 4BJ, United Kingdom

Index

A

Abelmoschus Esculentus, 169-170, 176-178

Agushie, 93-99

Air Temperature, 70-71, 75, 77

Alleviate Malnutrition, 169, 176

Allium Sativum, 63, 68-69

Ambient Temperature, 4, 72, 117, 145

Anacardium Occidentale, 107-108, 115-116

Anthocyanin, 20, 25, 29-31, 34, 61, 63-65, 67-68, 115, 143, 151-152, 196

Antimiocrobial, 100

Antinutrient, 169, 171, 176

Antioxidant, 3, 6, 8-11, 20, 22-25, 30, 32-34, 41, 47, 53, 56, 62, 80, 92, 100-103, 105-107, 109, 116, 142-147, 149-155, 157-159, 174, 178, 193, 195-201

Artocarpus Communis, 180-181, 191-192

B

Bioavailability, 43-44, 46, 53-54, 169-170, 174-178

Browning Reaction, 10, 40

C

Carbohydrate, 1, 6, 41, 46, 52, 63, 66, 68-70, 112, 169-175, 191

Caregiving, 202, 210

Cashew Nut, 107-108, 115-116

Catalase, 24, 195, 197, 199-200

Childhood Malnutrition, 202

Chiral-gc-ms, 12

Chlorophyll, 63-68

Citrus Limon, 100

Clove Bud, 1-2, 4-9

Composite Blends (CB), 180

Composite Flour Technology, 180

Condensed Tannin, 79, 84

Coronary Heart Disease, 1, 116, 172

Cyanidin Hexoside, 19, 25, 28

D

Diabetes Mellitus, 1, 47, 54

Drying, 70-72, 74-78, 88, 95, 99, 108, 136, 149, 170

E

Enantiomeric Composition, 12-13, 17

Enantioselective Gc, 12

Enzyme, 1, 10-11, 31, 57, 61, 63, 65, 68-69, 95, 109, 119, 197-198, 200

Ethanol Production, 151, 158

Extraction Method, 21, 56-58, 61, 82, 136, 144, 147

F

Fatty Acids, 31, 40, 49, 65, 107, 111, 134, 147, 149, 161, 165, 167, 177

Fermented Confectionery, 180

Flavanone Glycosides (FGS), 56

Flavonoid, 4, 6-10, 19-20, 22, 24, 28, 32, 57, 79, 82-88, 91, 151-157, 159, 201

Food Insecurity, 169, 177

G

Gac Fruit, 134-143

Grape Pomace, 88-89, 91, 151, 154, 156, 158-159

H

Hesperidin, 56-57, 59-61

High-performance, 56-57

Hydraulic Handling, 35

Hydrodistillation (HD), 144-145

Hydroxycinnamic Acids (HCA), 19, 30

L

Lactic Acid Bacteria, 117, 119, 121-122, 124, 132, 177

Lactobacillus, 109, 117-118, 131-133

Lipoxygenase, 160-162, 166-168

Liquid Chromatography (HPLC), 33, 56, 136

Lox Isomers, 161

Lycopene, 134-136, 140-141, 143

M

Maturation, 32, 134, 140-142, 158

Methyl Jasmonate, 195-196, 200-201

Mineral Bioavailability, 169

Momordica Cochinchinensis, 134, 142-143